The Eye in Contact Lens Wear

The Eye in Contact Lens Wear

Second Edition

J. R. Larke BSc PhD FBOA
Department of Optometry, University of Wales, Cardiff

BUTTERWORTH
HEINEMANN

Butterworth-Heinemann
Linacre House, Jordan Hill, Oxford OX2 8DP
225 Wildwood Avenue, Woburn, MA O1801-2041
A division of Reed Educational and Professional Publishing Ltd

A member of the Reed Elsevier plc group

OXFORD AUCKLAND BOSTON
JOHANNESBURG MELBOURNE NEW DELHI

First published 1985
Second edition 1997
Paperback edition 1999

British Library Cataloguing in Publication Data
A catalogue record for this book is available from the British Library

Library of Congress Cataloguing in Publication Data
A catalogue record for this book is available from the Library of Congress

ISBN 0 7506 4438 9

Typeset by Bath Typesetting Ltd
Printed in Great Britain at the University Press, Cambridge

Contents

Preface

I first became interested in the eye's response to contact lens wear thirty years ago. Following a suggestion by Otto Wichterle I designed the first soft lens to give satisfactory vision, and it rapidly became clear that this new type of lens interacts with the eye in subtle and complex ways. Today we know of twenty nine adverse reactions to contact lens wear and, to an extent, we know why these reactions occur. This knowledge has made successful contact lens management possible.

Contact lens knowledge has changed the way in which lenses are used. The daily disposable high water contact lens is unlikely to be surpassed and soft lenses are reaching their optimum usage as social wear lenses. Daily contact lens wear remains the realm of gas permeable lenses which have improved hugely in recent years. The blind pursuit of ever increasing 'DK' values is now over and finding an optimum balance of lens material properties has already borne fruit. Inexplicably no one appears to have asked 'why are gas permeable lenses uncomfortable?' which is, after all, the single major drawback to wide-scale acceptance. Extended wear remains the philosopher's stone of contact lens practice, forever enticing those who continue to fund research. No future extended wear lens can be considered safe until a satisfactorily low infection rate has been demonstrated in a clinical study whose size and cost would represent the single largest investment ever made by the contact lens industry.

John Larke

Acknowledgements

Three chapters of this book have been contributed by experts in their field:

My friend and former colleague Brian Tighe, Pro Vice Chancellor of Aston University, was kind enough to write Chapter 4 in conjunction with Valerie Franklin. Brian not only knows more about lens deposits than anyone else; he has developed the novel techniques which have made the acquisition of this information possible.

My friend Stuart Hodson had not previously written a review of the cornea in some thirty years of work on this topic. Not only has he now written the most authoritative description of the cornea, he has made it accessible; no one could ask for more.

John Dart and Fiona Stapleton persevered with my poor and incomplete communication to produce a definitive chapter on the risks and types of infection provoked by contact lens wear. I thank them for their effort, and also their patience in dealing with me.

Finally, I would like to pay tribute to many of the postgraduate students with whom I have worked over the years. To Pete, Dave, Nizar, Chris, Clair, Nabil, Chris B. Darsh, Stella and Bee Ling. Their research forms the largest single contribution to this book. I don't know what they learned from me, but I learned an awful lot from them.

Chapter 1

Anatomy of the eyelids

Introduction

The structure and action of the eyelids are important in contact lens wear.

Meibomian glands within the upper and lower lids secrete the lipid phase of the tear film which reduces tear evaporation rates. Contact lens wear may result in partial or complete obstruction of these glands. The resulting reduction in meibomian fluid causes adverse symptoms which, in severe cases, may prevent further wear. Although the mechanism of this reaction is now understood, no satisfactory treatment currently exists and management involves treating the symptoms rather than the underlying condition.

The act of blinking strongly influences lens wear. The movement of the upper lid over the edge of a hard lens gives rise to discomfort. Consequently, patients may modify blinking patterns, and a reduced blink excursion may lead to a portion of the cornea being almost continuously exposed, with resulting disturbance to the epithelium. Modifying lens specifications and restoring normal blinking habits, in affected patients, is often a necessary part of patient care. Long-term persistence of epithelial exposure has unpleasant sequelae which may eventually prevent lens wear.

Contact lenses may also, but rarely, affect the eyelids. Very occasionally, excessive manipulation of the lids during lens insertion and removal results in disinsertion of the aponeurosis of the levator palpebrae which gives rise to ptosis. Contact lenses may also, on very rare occasions, become embedded in the upper eyelid.

Anatomy of the eyelids

The eyelids are moveable structures overlying the anterior portion of the eye. Their role is essentially protective, and closely associated with the production, and subsequent distribution, of tears. In man, the upper eyelid extends downwards from approximately the line of the eyebrow, while the lower lid is continuous with the structures of the cheek. Temporally, the lids join at the lateral canthus, while nasally a medial canthus is formed, which encompasses the caruncle – a small protrusion of skin containing sweat and sebaceous glands. In many animals a third eyelid, the

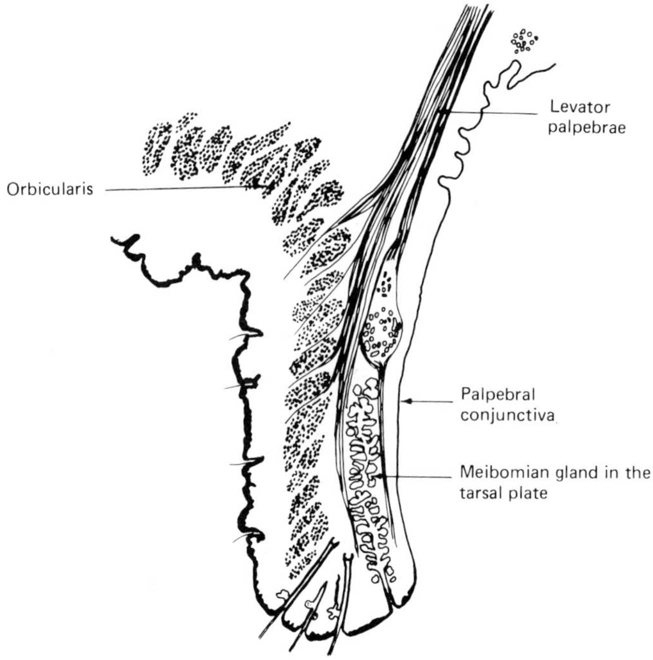

Figure 1.1 Diagram of the upper eyelid (redrawn from Wolff, 1933[34])

nictitating membrane, is present below the medial canthus. No such structure exists in man, although a possible vestigial remnant, the plical semilunaris, may be noted as a reddish fold on the lateral side of the caruncle.

The opening of the eyelids, the palpebral fissure, is approximately 30 mm long and 15 mm high. The palpebral fissure is not symmetrical, the lateral canthus being approximately 2 mm above an imaginary horizontal line drawn through the medial canthus, when the eyes are open. The situation is reversed, however, when the eyes are closed – the lateral canthus being slightly below the medial canthus.

The margin of each lid is approximately 2 mm broad. Anteriorly, two or three rows of hairs, the eyelashes, are found on a rounded surface, while posteriorly a much sharper junction is formed against the surface of the eye. Immediately in front of this margin, the openings of a line of tarsal glands may be noted. On the extreme nasal aspect of the lids, the opening to the lacrimal ducts, the lacrimal puncta, may be observed. It is via these ducts that excess tears drain from the eye.

The lids are bounded posteriorly by a mucous membrane, the palpebral portion of the conjunctiva. The conjunctiva is an envelope overlying not only the posterior surface of the lids, but also the anterior surface of the eye, where it becomes continuous with the epithelium of the cornea.

The eyelids are bounded anteriorly by the skin and posteriorly by the palpebral conjunctiva. Within these boundaries are found layers of striped muscle, layers of areolar tissue, and a fibrous layer containing the tarsal plates. The structure of the eyelid is illustrated in Figure 1.1.

The skin of the eyelids is probably the thinnest to be found on the body surface. It is highly elastic and much folded, only being fully extended when the eyes are closed. Its ultrastructure is similar to that of skin in other body sites.

Two layers of areolar tissue are found in the lids, one immediately beneath the skin and a second layer between the orbicularis and the tarsal plates. Both layers consist of loose connective tissue with little or no fat.

The orbicularis oculi surrounds the palpebral fissure, its overlying fibres being arranged symmetrically around the opening. It is innervated by the VIIth nerve and is responsible for lid closure. The muscle is divided into two portions: the palpebral and the orbital. The palpebral portion is confined to the lids and is responsible for involuntary blinking. The orbital portion extends beyond the lids, superiorly to the line of the eyebrow, and interiorly to the cheek; it is responsible for the voluntary closure of the lids.

The fibrous layers of the lids form semirigid structures which give form to both lids. The tarsal plates arise in medial and lateral ligaments and consist of dense fibrous and elastic tissue. The upper plate is larger than the lower, being approximately 30 mm long, 1 mm thick, and 11 mm high at the centre of the lid. The lower plate is similar in configuration, being a curved 'half-moon' structure, but it is less substantial, being only 5 mm high at its central point. The tarsal plates are of practical use in contact lens practice, as the rigidity of the upper plate allows the lid to be averted for inspection of the palpebral conjunctiva.

Immediately adjacent to the tarsal plates, and possibly continuous with them, is the orbital septum, a floating membrane which extends to the orbital margin.

The tendons of the levator palpebrae arise from this muscle and pass forwards to the upper lid where they become almost vertical. They are attached to:

1 The skin of the lid, which is reached via the fibres of the orbicularis
2 The tarsal plate by way of the superior palpebral muscle
3 The fornix of the conjunctiva.

The function of the tendon of the levator is to act as a site of attachment, thus enabling the lid to be raised.

The arteries of the lids are derived from the lacrimal and ophthalmic arteries. Branches of these vessels anastomose to form arterial arcades; a single arcade in the lower lid, and two arcades in the upper.

The veins of the lids are more numerous and larger than the arteries. They lie on either side of the tarsal plates and form plexus in the region of the upper and lower fornices.

Lymphatic fluid drains from the lid via two principal vessels. A superior lateral vessel drains lymph from the major portion of the upper lid and the lateral part of the lower lid, while an inferior medial vessel drains lymph from the extreme medial end of the upper lid and most of the lower lid.

Glands of the eyelid

The lacrimal gland

The lacrimal gland is by far the largest gland to be found in the anterior eye. It consists of two portions a large orbital or superior portion, and a smaller palpebral portion. This large lobulated gland is found in the lateral superior portion of the upper lid (Figure 1.2). The orbital portion lies under the fossa of the frontal bone and is separated from the palpebral portion by the tendons of the levator palpebrae. The palpebral portion is about one-third of the size of the orbital and lies above the lateral aspect of the upper fornix.

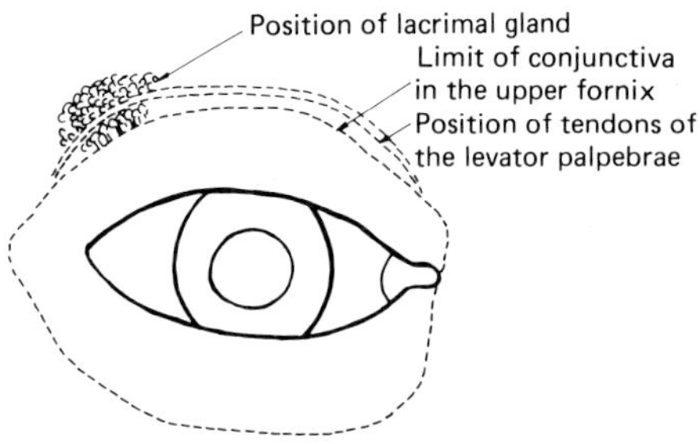

Figure 1.2 Diagram of the location of the lacrimal gland

The gland consists of numerous lobules, usually surrounded by fat. Each lobule contains a large number of secretory elements, which in turn consist of a layer of fat and a layer of cylindrical myoepithelial cells surrounding a central canal. The canals drain into interlobular ducts which, in turn, open into a series of larger ducts. The duct from the orbital portion passes through the palpebral portion.

Ciliary glands (the glands of Moll)
Ciliary glands are modified sweat glands associated with the eyelashes. The secretory portion is lined with secretory fatty granulations. Ducts from the ciliary glands may terminate near the base of an eyelash, or lead to the duct of a gland of Zeis.

The glands of Zeis
The glands of Zeis are rudimentary sebaceous glands associated directly with an eyelash. They perform the same function as other sebaceous glands, producing oily fluid for the hair follicle.

The meibomian (tarsal) gland
The meibomian glands are found in the upper and lower lids in the dermis of the tarsal plates. They are modified sebaceous glands of holocrine origin approximately 0.5–1 cm long. The glands are tree-like structures joined to the lid surface by a central duct which may become blocked. The glands terminate in a well-defined zone on the lid margin at the junction of the skin and the palpebral conjunctiva (see Plate 1). There are thirty to forty glands in the upper lid and twenty to thirty in the lower.

Meibomian fluid Meibomian fluid is, under normal circumstances, a clear, colourless oil. The oil is almost wholly composed of a complex mixture of lipids whose composition is now well established and described in Chapter 3 (Tear film composition – lipid phase). Although the melting point of the individual lipids in meibomian fluid is typically in the region of 100–160°C, the fluid as a whole begins to melt at 32°C and has completed melting by 36°C. The cause of this dramatic reduction in melting point is the ability of each constituent lipid to act as a solvent for all other lipids resulting in a complex and, possibly, somewhat structured fluid. Such structure may be important for the proper functioning of meibomian oil whose role is to spread over the surface of the tear film and reduce tear evaporation. Small changes in the structuring of meibomian oil invariably result in a rise in melting point. Such increases result in a material which at normal body temperature initially resembles clear oil then an opalescent grease and then, as melting point rises further, a semisolid wax. The appearance of such material is indicative of a clinical condition known as meibomian gland dysfunction.

Meibomian gland dysfunction

Meibomian gland dysfunction, as a contact lens related phenomenon, was probably first reported by Korb and Henriquez in 1980[20]. Meibomian gland dysfunction may be regarded as a change in the physical appearance of material expressed from meibomian glands without accompanying signs of infection.

Diagnostic criteria

Signs

The signs of meibomian gland dysfunction are:

1 Changes in the appearance of the clear oil expressed from meibomian glands
2 In severe cases, an absence of gland secretion
3 Inspissation of secretions in the glands
4 Irregularity of the eyelid margins
5 Dilation or enlargement of the glands
6 Accompanying tear foam in approximately half of affected patients (see Plate 2).

Symptoms

1 Dry eye problems in severely affected patients
2 Poor 'smeary' vision among contact lens wearers.

Pathogenesis

The mechanism of meibomian gland dysfunction is an increase in the level of keratin protein in meibomian oil. In affected patients the increased levels of keratin protein are the result of increased levels of keratinization in the ductal epithelia. In severe cases this increase in keratinization extends to both the epithelial and the subepithelial layers. Increased levels of keratinization were first proposed in an animal model by Jester *et al.*[17], while increased levels of keratin protein in human subjects suffering from meibomian gland dysfunction were first demonstrated by the author and Ong[27]. A photograph of antibody reactions to purified material obtained from the meibomian glands of normal and dysfunctional subjectives is shown in Figure 1.3.

Incidence

Altered meibomian gland oil appearance is a not uncommon observation among young non-contact lens wearing patients. Approximately 20% of subjects who are not wearing contact lenses have meibomian oil whose appearance is not wholly clear upon expression. However, very few – approximately 6% – have wholly opaque or waxy material expelled from their glands. Among contact lens wearers, these figures rise to 30% and 11% respectively. More strikingly, few, if any, young non contact lens wearers report the symptoms of dryness and reduced vision which are apparent among contact lens wearers. In contact lens wear about 10% of patients present with symptoms of 'smeary vision' or 'dryness' which can be attributed to changes in the appearance of material expelled from their meibomian glands. The reasons for this is readily apparent. One of the principal functions of meibomian oil is to spread

: Comparison of staining intensity with cytokeratin antibodies.

Anti-cyto keratin	Keratin standard	Normal meibomian fluids	Abnormal meibomian fluids
CK 8, 18, 19	+	+	++
CK 7	+	+/–	++
CK 8	++	+/–	+
CK 14	+++	+/–	++
CK 19	+/–	+/–	++
AE1/AE3	+++	+/–	++

Intensity of staining:

+/– : equivocal
+ : weak/poor
++ : moderate
+++ : high intensity

(a)

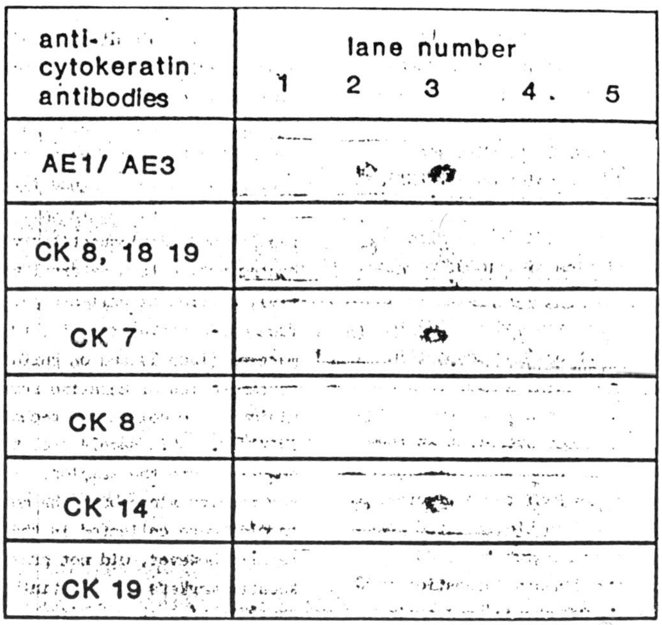

Developed blot of meibomian fluids using all 6 anti-cytokeratins. Lane 1: conjunctiva; lane 2: eyelid skin; lane 3: keratin standard; lane 4: normal meibomian fluids; lane 5: abnormal meibomian fluids

(b)

Figure 1.3 The response of meibomian fluid from normal and abnormal glands to 6 anti-cytokeratins. A keratin standard together with conjunctiva and eyelid skin is given for reference

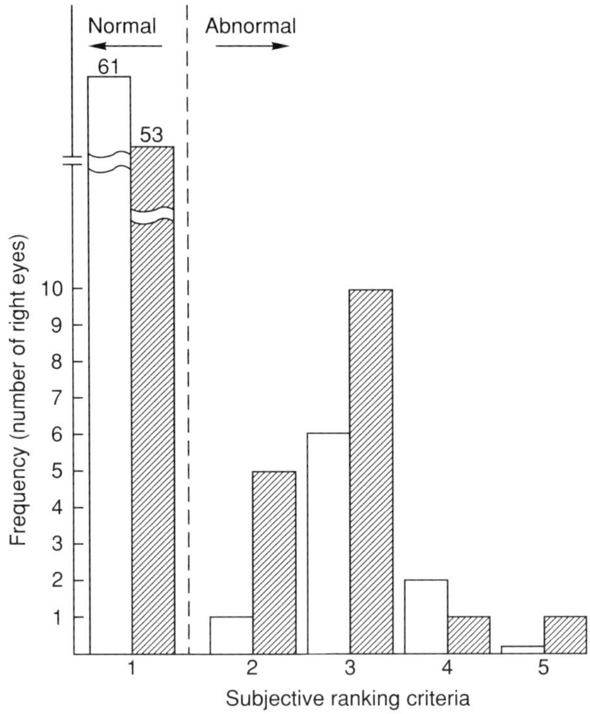

Figure 1.4 Distribution in the appearance of material expelled from the meibomian glands of contact ▨ and non-contact □ lens wearers in an age and gender matched group of young people

uniformly over the tear film and reduce tear evaporation. In non contact lens wearers even rather opaque material can apparently perform this function satisfactorily. In contact lens wear the grease and wax from dysfunctional glands adheres to the contact lens and reduces the patient's vision producing the symptoms of 'smeariness'. In addition, the continuity of the lipid tear layer is somewhat disrupted by the presence of the contact lens and this is further compromised by the semisolid material from a dysfunctional gland which leads to increased tear evaporation rates and the subjective impression of 'dryness'. The distribution in the appearance of material expelled from the meibomian glands of contact and non-contact lens wearers is illustrated in Figure 1.4.

Among elderly people, the incidence of meibomian gland dysfunction is very high. Among volunteers aged 64–86 years, the author and Ong could only find 12% of subjects with normal meibomian oil appearance. Of the remaining 88%, of the examined group approximately half had 'greasy' material expelled from their glands while the remaining half had 'waxy' material in the expelate. About one-quarter of all the elderly people we examined complained of 'dry or gritty' eyes and these subjects had clearly dysfunctional meibomian glands. The reasons for this increase in older people would seem readily apparent. Ageing is associated with increasing levels of skin keratinization and it would seem that this increased level of keratinization extends not only to the skin but to the epithelia of the ductal lining of the meibomian glands as well. The incidence of meibomian gland dysfunction in a group of elderly subjects compared with a younger group of patients is illustrated in Figure 1.5.

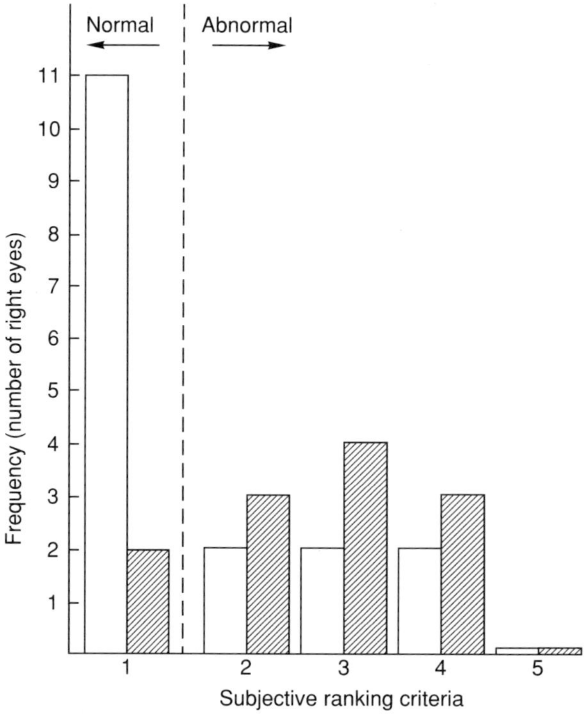

Figure 1.5 A comparison of the appearance of human meibum in an 18–24 year old □ and 64–86 year old ▨ age group

Ranking the appearance of meibomian gland function

A ranking system, devised by the author and Ong which is used in the contact lens clinic of the University of Wales, Cardiff, utilizes the appearance of material expelled upon mild digital pressure from the orifices of meibomian glands. Material may be gently expelled from the gland orifice by pressing upward along the line of the glands with a finger or more usually a thumb. Greater pressure may be required in patients with dysfunctional glands where a fold of lower eyelid may be gently squeezed between thumb and first finger. Some practice is required with this technique as material from normal glands spreads rapidly over the lower eyelid where it is lost to observation, while very dysfunctional glands may fail to expel any material due to gland blockage with insipiated waxy 'plugs' of material. However, practice by the practitioner will help to familiarize the differences between patients and the ranking system provides a quick and useful recording system:

Rank 1 'Normal'. Clear fluid expelled upon mild digital pressure from all gland orifices.

Rank 2 'Mild dysfunction'. Greasy fluid expelled upon mild digital pressure from all gland orifices.

Rank 3 'Moderate dysfunction'. Opaque fluid expressed upon moderate digital pressure, one or two glands may fail to expel material.

Rank 4 'Severe dysfunction'. Waxy material expressed upon forceful digital pressure. Up to half the observed glands may fail to expel any material.
Rank 5 'Very severe dysfunction'. Fine filamentary wax expelled upon forceful digital pressure. More than half the observed glands may fail to expel any material.

Treatment

Treating meibomian gland dysfunction presents considerable difficulties. At present, no treatment for raised levels of ductal epithelial keratinization exists, and treatment is concerned with attempting to alleviate symptoms rather than resolving the underlying cause. Perhaps the most successful palliative measure is hot compresses. This remedy which has apparently been known to medicine since ancient times consists of warming the eyelids in an attempt to melt material which may be causing gland obstruction. Hot spooning, a variant of the hot compress technique, has been used to some effect by the author. A 2 cm strip of lint is wrapped around the head of a domestic teaspoon. The lint and spoon are immersed in warm water and then held against the closed eyelids. The purpose of the spoon is to retain the heat of the warm water; even so, repeated application is invariably necessary. The eyelids are warmed in this manner for about 5 minutes each morning and evening for a period of 4–6 weeks. This procedure seems to give relief to some patients, although it may require to be repeated every few months.

Blinking

Blinking occurs as a spontaneous partial or complete closure of the palpebral fissure. The action involves the orbital portion of the orbicularis and is an involuntary autonomic response to a wide variety of stimuli. In man, blinking occurs 5–15 times per minute, while in other animals it is far less frequent. In rabbits for example, blinking occurs only 4 or 5 times an hour. This marked difference in blink rate between species is not wholly understood. It is possible that the known differences in tear fluid composition between species may affect blink rates, as may differences in the stimuli for blinking. In man, a range of stimuli may evoke a blink reflex. Auditory, perceptual and emotional stimuli have been demonstrated to have a marked effect on blink rate, and theories of blinking include the evaporation of tears, and the repeated action of the lids in spreading the film of tears over the eye to improve the optical resolution of the cornea.

Lid pressure during blinking

During blinking the upper lid moves rapidly downwards to meet the lower. The forces exerted on the eye during this activity are surprisingly high[6], and may be accompanied by transient rises in intraocular pressure. However, due to the configuration of the obicularis these forces are not applied uniformly to the eye but show a displacement towards the lacrimal duct (Figure 1.6). The effect in contact lens wear is to produce a rotational effect on the lens. This may be readily observed with the aid of a slit lamp biomicroscope. By observing a mark on the lens periphery, and asking the patient to blink, a rotation of the lens will occur, which will reverse as the upper eyelid withdraws. This effect has little significance in spherical lens wear, although it may contribute to epithelial trauma, but it is of great importance in the fitting of toric lenses.

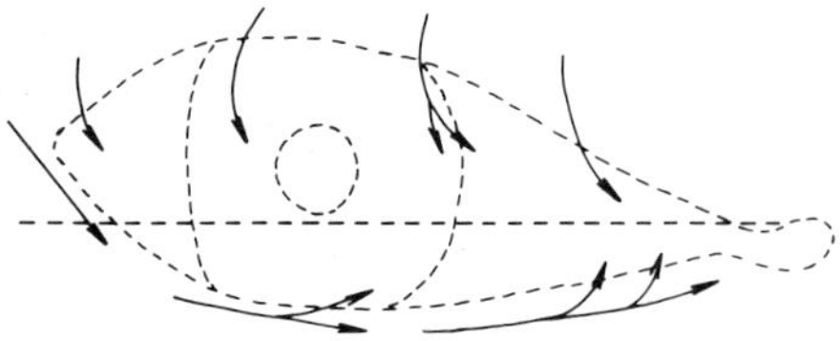

Figure 1.6 An illustration of the direction of forces applied to the eye during blinking (reproduced by permission of Haberich, *Contacto*, 1968[14])

Blink characteristics and contact lens wear

It is a common clinical observation that blink rate alters in the early stages of contact lens wear. Blink rate rises from a mean of seven blinks per minute to approximately 18 blinks per minute over the first 6 hours of hard lens wear[35], and both blink amplitude and duration are affected[4]. The initial and dramatic changes in blink characteristics will be familiar to contact lens practitioners, as will the longer term changes. Much of the discomfort of hard lens wear arises from the passage of the back of the upper lid over the edge of the lens. Patients soon acquire the habit of blinking less completely than prior to lens wear, as this improves comfort levels. However, this may give rise to difficulties, as the portions of the cornea not covered by either the contact lens or the lid can suffer from exposure keratitis.

Clinical problems associated with blinking

Characteristic superficial corneal disturbance has been associated with incomplete or inefficient blinking in contact lens wear[7,18,21,23,31]. The disturbance may take the form of 'severe punctate staining of the epithelium at the nasal temporal, and less frequently inferior margins of the cornea and is often accompanied by hyperaemia of the adjacent scleral vessels and/or some degree of corneal clouding'[31]. The corneal disturbance usually stains with both 2% sodium fluorescein and 1% rose bengal, and is frequently referred to as 'three and nine o'clock stain'[23] (Figure 1.7). The aetiology of this form of disturbance has not been experimentally established, although the reported work gives good circumstantial evidence for an association between corneal exposure and incomplete or disturbed blinking.

Attempts to alleviate 'three and nine o'clock stain' may take two forms. Fitting thinner and smaller lenses may result in less obstruction to the passage of the lids over the lens, and voluntary exercises to correct incomplete blinking may result in a more even distribution of tear fluid. In practice both approaches may be worthy of consideration. The practical limits to making lenses smaller and thinner are usually

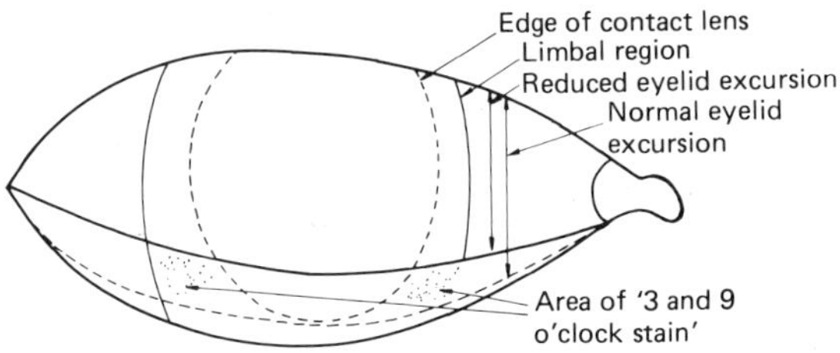

Figure 1.7 An illustration of limbal exposure keratitis (based on a drawing by Lester, 1978[21])

determined by visual considerations and, although the writer was sceptical upon first hearing of the suggestion of 'blinking exercises', there have been numerous instances when this approach has proved successful[30]. It is frequently important that the condition is alleviated at an early stage; persistent long-term 'three and nine o'clock stain' may lead to conjunctival involvement with the possibility of corneal infiltrates, and delan formation. In long-standing cases treatment is frequently unsuccessful, and it is important to deal with the situation in its initial stages.

Exposure keratitis is by no means uncommon, being occasionally present in non-lens wearers[5] and present in as many as one in ten hard lens wearers[30]. However, it has not been reported in soft lens wearers, where incomplete closure results in 'inferior closure stain'.

Inferior closure stain

In soft lens wearers inferior closure stain is an occasional complication which can arise from poor blinking, among other factors. The symptoms are inferior limbal redness and mild discomfort, while the signs are inferior corneal or interpalpebral conjunctival punctate stain, associated with inferior limbal hyperaemia. The aetiology of the condition has been examined by a number of workers and it is known that the pre-lens tear film is significantly less stable than the pre-corneal tear film in hydrogel lens users[11] and the majority of hydrogel lenses dehydrate during wear[1,3,8]. This may cause lens parameter changes, altered oxygen transmissibility and may cause epithelial desiccation[16]. The amount of dehydration varies with lens type; greater dehydration has been shown for high water content compared with low water content, and for ionic compared with non-ionic materials[9].

Inferior arcuate staining has been reported in asymptomatic hydrogel lens wearers[19,36]. This may be attributable to localized drying within the interpalpebral region, combined with a metabolic mechanism, due to insufficient tear exchange causing trapped debris in this region. Similar findings have been reported with thin high water content hydrogel lenses in some individuals[16] where epithelial desiccation is thought to have occurred due to pervaporation through the lens. Andrasko[1] reported a more rapid reduction in the water content of thin hydrogel lenses during wear, compared with thick lenses. However, Guillon *et al.*[13] showed similar levels of desiccation staining for a range of lens thicknesses under adverse environmental conditions. Desiccation staining was shown to be associated with a rapidly destabilizing pre-lens tear film and a thinning lipid layer[13]. These studies support a desiccation mechanism whereby excessive evaporation from the lens front surface within the interpalpebral region causes dehydration of the underlying cornea.

Management can present some problems as there appears to be a large intersubject variability in the presence and severity of such staining[8,16]. However, management aims to improve the stability of the pre-lens tear film. Strategies include use of polymers with a reduced free-to-bound water ratio, which show reduced *in vivo* dehydration. Increasing lens thickness, improved lens hygiene, management of lid disease and topical lubricants may reduce staining. Refitting with lid attached gas permeable hard contact lenses (GP-HCLs) may be helpful as these lenses rewet the inferior conjunctiva even when the blink amplitude is decreased.

Blinking and corneal oxygen

Hard lenses, which are essentially impermeable to the passage of oxygen, are fitted to

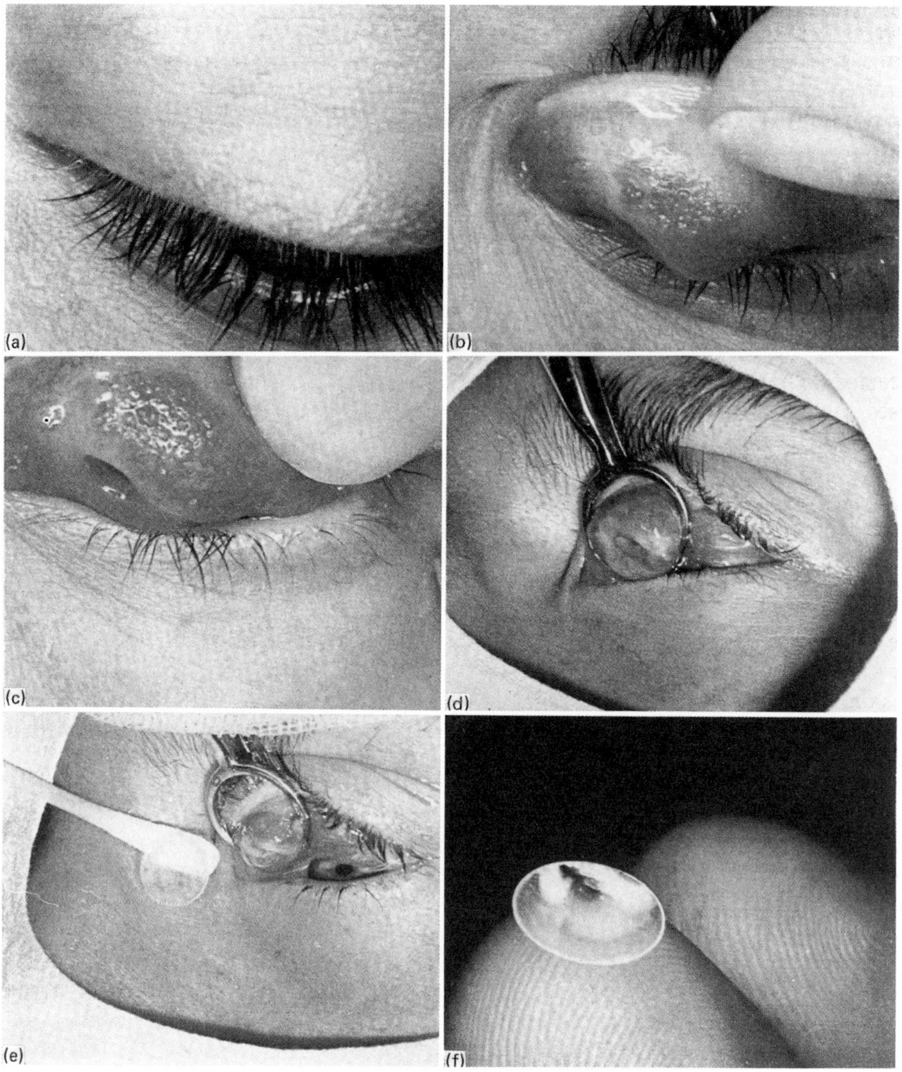

Figure 1.8 A 'lost' contact lens. (*a*) A moderate ptosis of the left upper lid in association with a small firm swelling near the medial canthus; (*b*) eversion revealing a papillary conjunctivitis; (*c*) double eversion revealing a small draining sinus; (*d*) lacrimal probe detects the presence of a hard object with a definite 'click'; (*e*) and (*f*) contact lens easily removed at operation accompanied by a considerable amount of mucopurulent material (reproduced by kind permission of Ellis Shenken and the *Canadian Medical Association Journal*, 1969[32])

allow the interchange of tear fluid, containing dissolved oxygen, beneath the lens during wear. Blink frequency is one of three variables which influence corneal oxygen tensions in hard lens wear. This question is considered in Chapter 7.

Ptosis secondary to contact lens wear

Acquired ptosis is a common ophthalmological disorder which may arise from many causes[2]. However, among contact lens wearers it is a rare condition which may arise from excessive manipulation of the upper eyelid during lens insertion and removal[10]. Acquired ptosis is a condition that is readily recognized, although it may occasionally be confused with severe cases of giant papillary conjunctivitis (see Chapter 2), where a considerably thickened conjunctiva can cause a not dissimilar appearance. Examination of affected patients has shown the aponeurosis of the levator palpebrae to be disinserted and treatment is effected by surgical reattachment to the superior tarsal border.

Contact lenses 'lost' in the eyelid

Occasional instances have been reported in which patients have 'lost' contact lenses, which have subsequently been found to have become embedded in the upper lid[12,22,24,25,26,28,29,32,33].

Probably the best-illustrated case was that reported in Canada by Ellis Shenken in 1969. Photographs taken at the time by Mr Frederick Sanger and Mr Gunter Golt of Scarborough General Hospital, Toronto, are reproduced with Ellis Shenken's permission in Figure 1.8. The patient presented with moderate ptosis of the left upper lid, and a slight intermittent mucous discharge. There was a history of contact lens wear, and a contact lens had been 'lost' in a fracas some 40 months previously. The patient had suffered some swelling and ecchymosis of the lid following the dispute and had visited a general medical practitioner who had been unable to detect the contact lens.

Upon everting the lid 'a papillary conjunctivitis, with a firm ulcerated edge above the tarsal ridge' was noted. Double eversion revealed a 'small drawing sinus in the left upper palpebral conjunctiva near the inner canthus and extending into the fornix over the indurated mass'[5]. A hard object was detected with a lacrimal probe and a contact lens was removed at surgery.

The features reported by Ellis Shenken are similar to those of other reported cases. Ptosis of the lid is invariably present together with a mucous discharge, which may cause the lids to adhere together.

A wise precaution before issuing a replacement hard lens to a patient who reports a lost lens, is a careful examination of the upper fornix with double lid eversion.

References

1 Andrasko, G. J. (1983). *International Contact Lens Clinic*, **10**, 22–28
2 Beard, C. (1976). In *Ptosis*. St Louis, USA: C. Mosby
3 Brennan, N. A., Efron, N., Bruce, A. S., Duldig, D. I. and Russo, N. (1988). *American Journal of Optometry and Physiological Optics*, **65**, 277
4 Brown, M., Chinn, S., Fatt, I. and Harris, M. G. (1973). *Journal of the American Optometric Association*, **44**, 254
5 Callender, M. (1980). Personal communication
6 Conway, H. D. and Richmond, M. (1982). *Journal of the American Optometric Association*, **59**, 13
7 Dickinson, F. (1971). *British Journal of Physiological Optics*, **26**, 22
8 Efron, N., Brennan, N. A., Bruce, A. S., Duldig, D. L. and Russo, N. J. (1987). *CLAO Journal*, **13**, 152–156

9 Efron, N. and Young, G. (1988). *Ophthalmology and Physiological Optics*, **8**, 253–256
10 Epstein, G. and Putterman, A. M. (1981). *American Journal of Ophthalmology*, **91**, 634
11 Faber, E., Golding, T. R., Lowe, R. and Brennan, N. A. (1991). *Optometry and Vision Science*, **68**, 380–384
12 Green, W. R. (1963). *Archives of Ophthalmology*, **69**, 23
13 Guillon, J.-P., Guillon, M. and Malgouyres, S. (1990). *Ophthalmology and Physiological Optics*, **10**, 343–350
14 Haberich, F. J. (1968). *Contacto*, **12**, 24
15 Henriquez, A. S. and Korb, D. R. (1981). *British Journal of Ophthalmology*, **65**, 108
16 Holden, B. A., Sweeney, D. F. and Seger, R. (1986). *Clinical Experiments in Optometry*, **69**, 103–107
17 Jester, J. V., Nicolaides, N., Kiss-Palvovolgyi, I. and Smith, R. E. (1989). *Investigative Ophthalmology and Vision Science*, **30**, 936
18 Kersely, H. J. (1977). *Journal of the British Contact Lens Association*, **1**, 15
19 Kline, L. N., DeLuca, T. J. and Fishjburg, G. M. (1979). *Journal of the American Optometric Association*, **50**, 353–357
20 Korb, D. R. and Henriquez, A. S. (1980). *Journal of the American Optometric Association*, **51**, 243
21 Lester, R. W. (1978). *International Contact Lens Clinic*, **15**, 61
22 Long, J. C. (1962). *American Journal of Ophthalmology*, **56**, 309
23 Mackie, I. A. (1972). *Transactions of the Ophthalmological Society of the United Kingdom*, **91**, 129
24 Michaels, D. D. and Zugsmith, G. S. (1963). *American Journal of Ophthalmology*, **55**, 1057
25 Nicolitz, E. and Flanagan, J. C. (1978). *Archives of Ophthalmology*, **96**, 2238
26 Older, J. J. (1979). *Annals of Ophthalmology*, **11**, 1393
27 Ong, B. L., Hodson, S. A., Wigham, T., Miller, F. and Larke, J. R. (1991). *Current Eye Research*, **10**, 1113
28 Oshima, T. (1966). *Folia Ophthalmologica Japonica*, **17**, 103
29 Richter, S., Sherman, J., Horn, D. and Zelaznick, S. (1979). *Journal of the American Optometric Association*, **50**, 372
30 Sabell, A. G. (1980). Personal communication
31 Sarver, M. D., Nelson, L. and Polse, K. A. (1969). *Journal of the American Optometric Association*, **40**, 310
32 Shenken, E. (1969). *Canadian Medical Association Journal*, **101**, 295
33 Smalling, O. H. (1971). *Journal of the American Optometric Association*, **42**, 755
34 Wolff, E. (1933). *Anatomy of the Eye and Orbit*. London: H.K. Lewis
35 York, M., Ong, J. and Robbins, J. C. (1971). *American Journal of Optometry*, **48**, 461
36 Zadnick, K. and Mutti, D. (1985). *International Contact Lens Clinic*, **12**, 110

Chapter 2

Conjunctiva

Introduction

The conjunctiva covers the posterior surface of the lids and the anterior surface of the eye, excluding the cornea. For many years it was a tissue disregarded by contact lens practice which was almost wholly concerned with the effects of contact lens wear on the cornea. However, in 1974 the ophthalmologist, Thomas Spring from Victoria in Australia, described an allergy-like condition on the conjunctiva covering the upper tarsal plate, which was similar in appearance to 'spring catarrh'[17]. Within a short period of time the aetiology of the condition was being exhaustively examined by Mathea Allansmith and her colleagues at the Retina Institute in Boston. Practical measures to alleviate the problem were being examined by a number of commercial laboratories, in particular Allergan Pharmaceuticals of Irvine, California.

The conjunctiva was not to be disregarded again. In the years since 1974 the allergic condition now known as contact lens association papillary conjunctivitis (CLAPC) has become one of the most carefully examined and documented reactions to contact lens wear.

CLAPC closely resembles vernal conjunctivitis. The signs are characterized by the presence of changes in the conjunctiva of the upper lid, while the symptoms are itchy eyelids and mucous discharge. The condition occurs in hard, soft and gas permeable lens wear.

The patient suffering from CLAPC is difficult to treat. In hard lens wear, modifying the lens edge form is the most satisfactory approach. Reducing the thickness of the lens, working a front edge bevel and asking the laboratory for a reworked well polished edge is often productive. However, the patient may have to discontinue lens wear to allow the condition to subside, and recurrence is always possible.

In soft lens wear, the problem is common with uncleaned lenses but it can also arise where apparently satisfactory cleaning regimens have been followed. Where no attempt has previously been made to remove lens surface contaminants, frequent cleaning with a proteolytic enzyme is the first step in treatment. As with hard lenses, a period of discontinued lens wear is often necessary. Where lens cleaning has been satisfactory, or where very heavily contaminated lenses are involved, replacement lenses are necessary. A radical change in lens materials may be indicated where the reaction has been provoked by apparently clean lenses. However, recurrence is

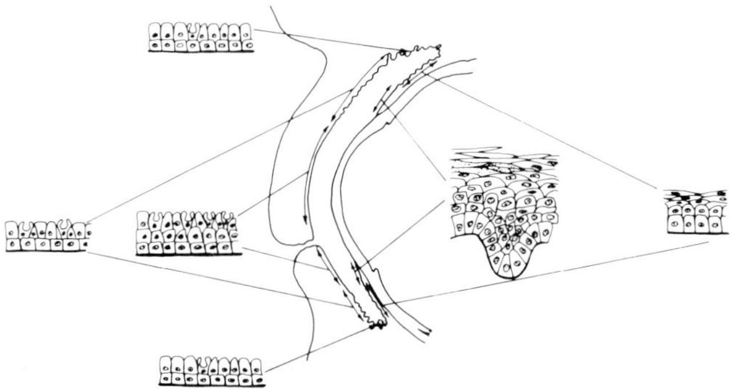

Figure 2.1 Regional variations in the conjunctival epithelium

always a difficulty with CLAPC and a realistic assessment of clinical prospects is important. As with some other adverse reactions to contact lens wear, CLAPC is easier to prevent than it is to cure.

Anatomy of the conjunctiva

The conjunctiva is a thin mucous membrane lining the posterior portion of the lids, and the anterior portion of the eye. It is continuous with the skin of the lid margins where a discernible interface is formed in the epithelium between the keratinized outer layers of the skin, and the non-keratinized cells of the conjunctiva.

The number of cells in the differing conjunctival zones varies. In the palpebral conjunctiva the number of cell layers becomes reduced and the squamous cells give way to columnar or cuboidal cells. In the fornices, a third layer of polyhedral epithelial cells, which are not present in the immediately adjacent areas, is found. The bulbar conjunctiva is the thinnest of the three regions and is essentially transparent. In this zone, only two layers of cells may be found. Regional variations in the conjunctival epithelium are shown in Figure 2.1.

A surprisingly high number of inflammatory cells is found in the normal conjunctiva. In the epithelium and substantia propria of the conjunctiva, some 70% of all cells are either lymphocytes or neutrophils, while in the substantia propria mast cells and plasma cells are found. However, eosinophils and basophils are not present in the epithelium or substantia propria[3]. This finding has a particular relevance to contact lens practice, as these cells are present in the conjunctiva of patients suffering from CLAPC[4].

Goblet cells of the conjunctiva

Goblet cells are found in most regions of the conjunctiva. They are large oval glands, principally producing mucus, which is discharged over the surface of the conjunctiva. The cells are produced continuously in the basal layer of the epithelium and migrate forwards. After discharging their contents they desquamate into the tear film. Goblet cells are found in the fornices, but decrease in number in the bulbar and palpebral conjunctiva, being entirely absent at the limbus and lid margins.

The distribution of goblet cells in man has been carefully examined[13] using novel techniques of whole conjunctival mounts obtained at post mortem, and conjunctival

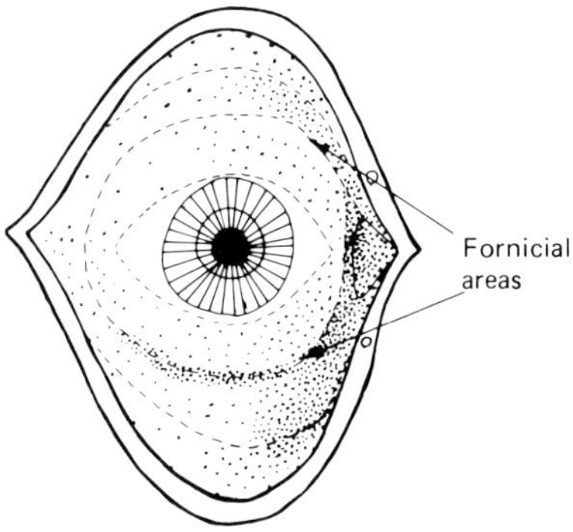

Figure 2.2 The distribution of goblet cells in man (reproduced by permission of Kessing, *Acta Ophthalmologica*, 1966[13])

biopsies obtained *in vivo* (Figure 2.2). The incidence of goblet cells has been quantified and well defined mucous crypts not previously thought to occur in man[9] have been demonstrated. The crypts fall into three categories:

1 A net-like system, which includes the structures first described by Henle in 1866
2 Saccular and branched crypts
3 Intraepithelial crypts.

The distribution of crypts is illustrated in Figure 2.3

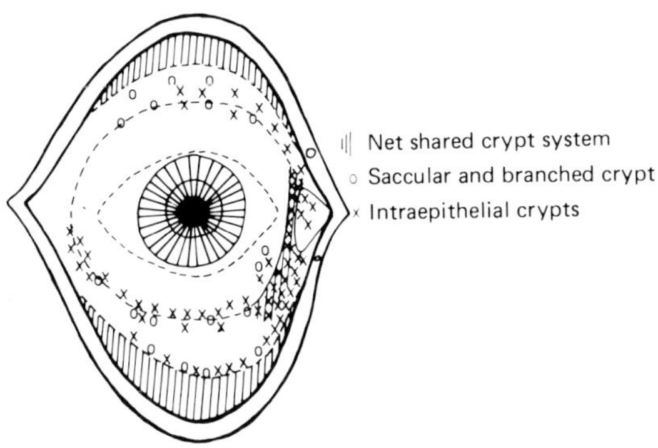

Figure 2.3 The distribution of conjunctival crypts (reproduced by permission of Kessing, *Acta Ophthalmologica*, 1966[13])

Conjunctival papillae

The conjunctiva shows evidence of regular small protrusions on the nasal and temporal aspects – the conjunctival papillae. The papillae are extensions of the underlying substantia propria and consist of connective tissue infiltrated with lymphocytes. It is important in contact lens practice to distinguish between these papillae, which are a normal feature of the conjunctiva, and papillae in the tarsal area which are indicative of CLAPC. The distribution of normal conjunctival papillae and those found in giant papillary conjunctivitis is shown in Figure 2.4.

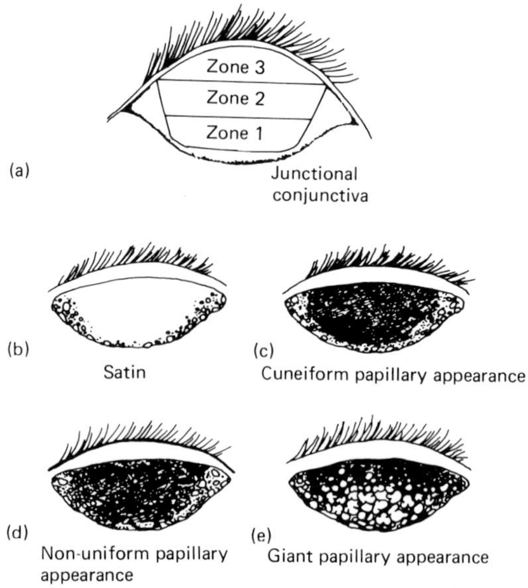

Figure 2.4 An illustration of the location and appearance of conjunctival papillae. (*a*) Normal papillae are found in the junctional conjunctiva, while those associated with contact lens associated papillary conjunctivitis are found in zones 1, 2 and to a lesser extent, 3; (*b*) 'satin smooth' appearances of a normal conjunctiva devoid of papillae in zones 1, 2 and 3; (*c*) uniform small papillae (4–8 mm) often found in normal eyes and also contact lens wearers; (*d*) non-uniform papillae with some papillae 0.4–0.8 mm in diameter. Occasionally found in normal eyes but more often seen in contact lens wearers; (*e*) giant papillae greater than 1 mm in diameter present in zones 1 and 2. This appearance is only seen in contact lens wearers suffering from CLAPC (reproduced by permission of Allansmith *et al.*, *American Journal of Ophthalmology*, 1977[5])

Blood vessels

The conjunctiva is well supplied with arteries and veins, the palpebral conjunctiva particularly so. The arteries of the conjunctiva are derived from the peripheral arcades, the marginal arterial arcades and the anterior ciliary arteries. The conjunctival veins follow the distribution of the arteries, although they are more numerous. For the most part they drain into the palpebral veins. The vessels of the conjunctiva are mobile, particularly those of the bulbar portion, and move with the conjunctiva when it is displaced. The vessels of the conjunctiva have a particular interest for contact lens practice. The fine meshwork of vessels of the palpebral conjunctiva provides the majority of available oxygen to the cornea in sleep. It is this supply of oxygen which is affected in extended contact lens wear.

In addition, the limbal arcades act as the origin for new-vascularization into the cornea, which occurs in certain forms of contact lens wear.

Lymphatics

Lymphatic fluid from the conjunctiva drains via a superficial plexus of vessels beneath the blood capillaries to deeper and larger vessels in the tarsal plates. Drainage from the fibrous layer follows a similar route to that from the lids.

Innervation

The nerve supply of the conjunctiva is derived from the short ciliaries, the lacrimal, the infratrochlear, the supratrochlear and the supraorbital nerves. The nerves may terminate in either:

1 Free endings (the nerves having lost their myelin sheaths)
2 The end bulbs of Krause, which are round bodies surrounded by connective tissue.

It is interesting to note that the area of the palpebral conjunctiva adjacent to the lid margins, is as sensitive to touch as the corneal surface and displays a similar loss of sensitivity in contact lens wear[14].

Conjunctival glands

Glands of Krause

The glands of Krause are located in subconjunctival connective tissue above the upper fornix. The glands are supplementary lacrimal glands and have the same structure as the main lacrimal gland. There are 42 glands in the upper lid and 6 to 8 in the lower, situated mainly on the lateral aspect of the lid. The ducts from each gland unite to form a single principal duct which opens directly into the fornix.

Glands of Wolfring

The glands of Wolfring are also accessory lacrimal glands, although they are somewhat larger than the glands of Krause. They are situated in the tarsal plate between the ends of the tarsal glands. There are 2 to 5 glands in the upper lid of each eye and a further 2 glands at the inferior edge of the lower tarsal plate.

Glands of Henle

Evaginations of the palpebral conjunctiva occur between the fornices and the tarsal area. Formerly thought to have little significance, they have now been identified as mucous crypts. The glands of the conjunctiva are illustrated in Figure 2.5.

Contact lens associated giant papillary conjunctivitis

Papillary changes in the upper tarsal conjunctiva as a result of soft lens wear were first reported in 1974[17]. Subsequent reports described similar reactions to hard contact lenses[5], ocular prostheses[18] and incompletely covered nylon sutures following cataract surgery[8]. The clinical signs and symptoms are very similar to those of vernal conjunctivitis.

Contact lens associated papillary conjunctivitis has been defined as 'a papillary reaction of the tarsal conjunctiva of the upper lid in which the papillae reach a diameter of one millimetre or more, are elevated, and are associated with symptoms of mucus or itching or both'[16].

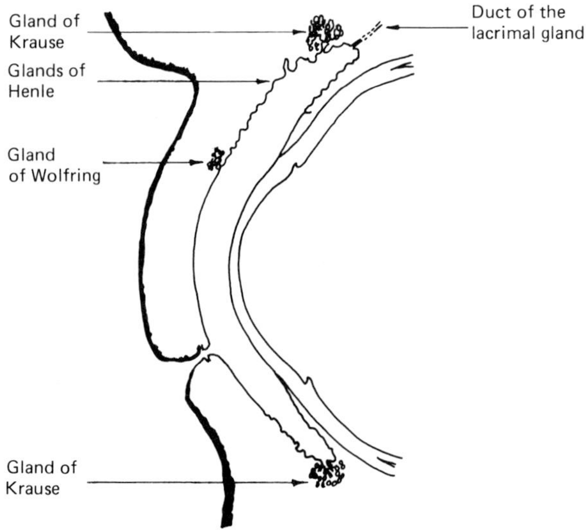

Figure 2.5 The glands of the conjunctiva

Although this early definition of CLAPC proved useful, it rapidly became apparent that cases of conjunctival disturbance were occurring without the presence of *large* papillae. Nowadays, a more satisfactory definition would include changes in the transparency of vascular 'trees' in papillae which may be much less than 1 mm in diameter. Reduced lens wearing times are associated with mild grades of CLAPC, while in its most advanced form, lenses cannot be worn for more than a few minutes without intense itching and mucous discharge.

The signs and symptoms of CLAPC have been summarized and descriptions of the four stages of CLAPC are given in Tables 2.1 and 2.2.

Although provoked by hard, soft and gas permeable lens wear, there are differences in the timescale and appearance of the conditions. Among soft lens wearers, the most likely time of onset is from 3 to 18 months of lens wear. In hard lens wear many years may elapse before the condition becomes manifest. CLAPC is probably the most usual cause of acquired intolerance to hard lens wear. In gas permeable lens wear the condition may be provoked at almost any stage of lens wear. The earliest onset of CLAPC seen by the author occurred after 4.5 weeks of gas permeable lens wear; a quite exceptionally early occurrence.

The appearance of the papillae provoked by hard and soft lens wear is also different. Papillae in soft lens wearers have a generally rounded appearance with smooth elevated contours. The papillae may be found over the entire conjunctival surface or may be limited to the tarsal zone with little progression towards the lid margin. In hard lens wear, the papillae are generally less raised and their tops have small depressions. Papillae in hard lens wear are generally fewer in number and isolated to part of the tarsal zone. Very occasionally, single large papillae are seen as the result of hard lens wear. Photographs of papillae provoked by hard and soft lens are shown in Figure 2.6.

The aetiology of CLAPC is associated with changes in the cells of the conjunctiva[10,11]. A fine examination of the surface of the conjunctival cells in successful lens wearers shows changes in the appearance and distribution of

Table 2.1 The signs of giant papillary conjunctivitis (reproduced by permission of Allansmith *et al.*, *American Journal of Ophthalmology*, 1977[5])

Stage	*Lens condition*	*Size and elevation of papillae*	*Morphology*	*Staining of tops of giant papillae with 2% fluoroscein*	*Hypuraemia and oedema*	*Method of diagnosis*	*Mucus on conjunctiva*	*Corneal condition*
1 Pre-clinical	***	Baseline	Baseline	***	***	Symptoms only	***	***
2 Early clinical	Light coating	Elevation of normal papillae and initial formation of giant papillae	Clover-like formations	Occasional staining of papillae	None or mild erythoma	u.v. light 2% fluoroscain high power on slit lamp	Usually mild, in sheets over papillae	Rare mild puncuate staining supariorly
3 Moderate	Moderate to heavy coating	Increased number, size and elevation	Occasional mushroom forms	Staining during exacorbution	Variable erythoma and oedema	Slit lamp, sometimes naked eye	Heavy sheets strands, globe	Like Stage 2 but less rare
4 Severe or terminal	Heavy coating	Flattening of apex of elevation and progression of Stage 3	More of Stage 3	More papillae staining	Erythoma more common, oedema variable	Naked eye	Severely increased	Occasional white arcuate infiltrate in superior cornea

Table 2.2 The symptoms of giant papillary conjunctivitis (reproduced by permission of Allansmith *et al.*, *American Journal of Ophthalmology*, 1977[5])

Stage	*Mucus or discharge in morning*	*Itching on removal of lens*	*Awareness of lens during wear*	*Vision with lens*	*Development of mucus while lens is worn*	*Lens wearing time*	*Itching while lens is worn*	*Lens movement*
1 Pre-clinical	Minimal increase over normal	Mild	***	***	***	***	***	***
2 Early clinical	Moderate increase over normal	Increased	Lens awareness late in day	Slight blurring late in day	***	***	Mild by end of day, variable	***
3 Moderate	Moderate to heavy	Moderate to severe, but variable	Increased awareness throughout day	Moderate blurring; increased blinking required to see	Mucus accumulates on lens or eye; patient may pick mucus out of inner canthus	Begins to decrease, but often little	Mild to moderate, variable	Small increase
4 Severe or terminal	Heavy; eye lids stick together, must be prised apart	Same as Stage 3	Distress or pain while wearing lenses	Depends on mucus secretions deposits on lens	Marked mucus secretion	Total loss of tolerance; pain on insertion of lens, depending on condition	Mild to severe, variable	Lens moves so much it may be pulled off cornea

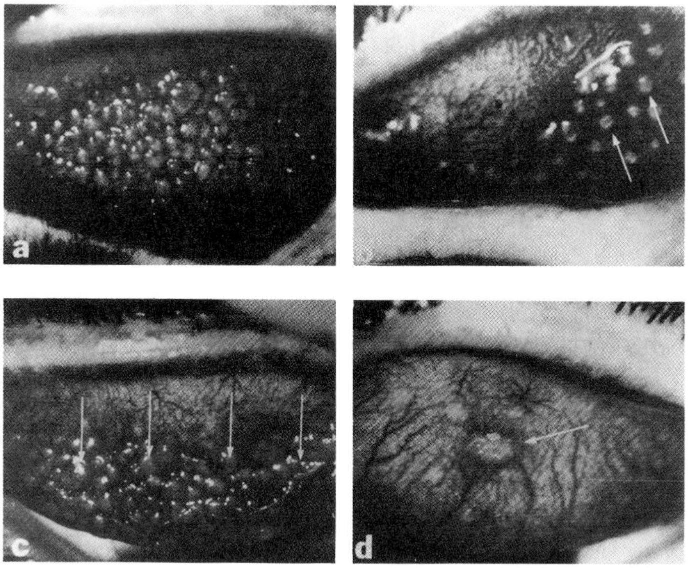

Figure 2.6 Different clinical types of giant papillary conjunctivitis. (*a*) Diffuse type with papillae over entire conjunctiva (soft lens wearer); (*b*) isolated papillae (hard lens wearer); (*c*) zonal type with papillae in tarsal area (soft lens wearer); (*d*) single papillae (hard lens wearer) (reproduced by permission of Richmond and Allansmith, *International Ophthalmology Clinic*, 1981[16])

microvilli. In the patient suffering from CLAPC the microvilli become white and tufted and there are gross cell changes. Cell shape becomes disturbed as the papillae push forward from the deeper layers of the conjunctiva. The conjunctiva thickens and, as the papillae are formed, the surface area of the conjunctiva increases by a factor of two[16].

The mechanical trauma that is a feature of hard lens wear may be present for many years and may provoke no more than changes in the microvilli of the surface cells of the conjunctiva. In CLAPC, whether it be provoked by hard, soft, or gas permeable lens wear, some further process takes place which leads to a dramatic increase in the total number of cells in the conjunctiva[2]. However, this increase in cell numbers is not accompanied by a change in cell density. As the number of cells increases, the conjunctiva simply becomes thicker, and it may well be that the convoluted nature of the papillae is the response by the conjunctiva to accommodate the increased number of cells.

As the number of cells increases, the type of cells also varies. In CLAPC, mast cells, eosinophils, and basophils, which are normally absent, are found in the epithelium. Both eosinophils and basophils, which are similarly absent from the substantia propria, are now found in this layer. However, there is no change in the density of lymphocytes and plasma cells which are found in similar concentrations in both the normal and CLAPC affected conjunctivae.

As the conjunctiva becomes grossly affected by the CLAPC, the conjunctival production of mucus increases dramatically. To the normal production of mucus by the goblet cells, is added mucus produced by secretory vesicles formed in the non-goblet epithelial cells[12]. Clinically, the observation of increased mucus levels forms one of the most important signs in the diagnosis of CLAPC.

Early detection and diagnosis

Early recognition of CLAPC is of some importance. Appropriate treatment is more successful in the early stages of this adverse reaction to contact lens wear. Since the size of the papillae is no longer considered a reliable diagnostic criterion, how then is the distinction made between a conjunctiva whose appearance has been changed by contact lens wear but which still remains clinically quiet and a conjunctiva which is active and in the early stages of the progression of the reaction? In the author's experience, there are two signs which are of importance: the transparency of the conjunctiva; and the presence of fine mucus strands in the tear film. As the conjunctival response to contact lenses passes from a clinically quiet to a clinically active state, the transparency of the conjunctiva is adversely affected by the increase in the number of inflammatory cells and the increase in the number of goblet cells. A conjunctiva which was initially clear will first become opalescent and later opaque. In this respect the appearance of the underlying vessels is of some help. Blood vessels viewed through a clear conjunctiva will appear red, while those viewed through an opalescent conjunctiva will appear pink and those viewed through an opaque conjunctiva will disappear. The appearance of 'pink' blood vessels which, prior to contact lens wear were red, coupled with the appearance of fine mucus strands in the tear film is probably the earliest diagnostic criterion of CLAPC.

Prevention and treatment

Prevention

Preventing CLAPC is dependent upon effective measures being taken to avoid stimulating the essential mechanism responsible for provoking this condition[1]. Unfortunately, the precise nature of this mechanism is unknown at the time of writing. The close similarity of CLAPC to vernal conjunctivitis, which is a complex immunological condition, suggests that CLAPC is also an atopic condition. The presence of mast cells, basophils and eosinophils gives strong support for the contention that CLAPC is a hypersensitivity reaction[4]. However, if this is the case the antigen has not been unequivocally established[16].

The presence of individual characteristics, and antigens on contact lenses, has been postulated in a hypothetical model which includes CLAPC (GPC) and vernal conjunctivitis (Figure 2.7).

Should this hypothetical model be validated, contact lens practitioners can take a number of practical steps to at least reduce the possibilities of provoking CLAPC:

1 In prospective soft lens wearers:
   (a) Pay particular attention to any evidence of an atopic case history
   (b) Take all reasonable measures to remove potential antigens from the lens surface. Daily lens cleaning with a suitable surfactant to remove lipids and some mucus should augment the weekly use of proteolytic enzymes to remove protein residues
2 In prospective hard lens wearers:
   (a) Pay particular attention to lens edge characteristics. Controlling the lens

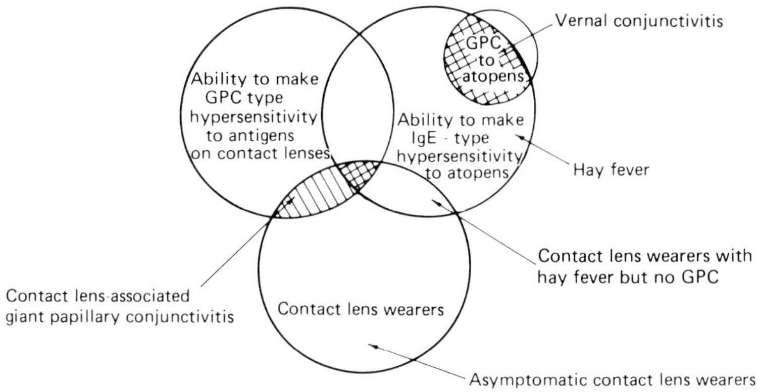

Figure 2.7 A hypothetical model of the relationship between contact lens wear, giant papillary conjunctivitis (GPC), vernal conjunctivitis and hypersensitivity (reproduced by permission of Richmond and Allansmith, *International Ophthalmology Clinic*, 1981[16])

centre thickness will also control the peripheral thickness. Lenses of even comparatively low minus power (−2 to −3 dioptres) can be lenticulated and the extent of lenticulation can be increased as power is increased

(b) Arrange for regular polishing of the lenses paying particular attention to polishing lens edges

3 In prospective gas permeable lens wearers:

(a) Combine the measures in (1) and (2). The growing evidence of protein accumulation on gas permeable contact lenses suggests the need to use proteolytic enzymes regularly, although perhaps not with the same frequency as in soft lens wearers

(b) Lens centre thickness can also be reduced to very low levels. Lenses of centre thickness 0.06 to 0.08 mm are not widely available, although not all have the same edge form.

Treating CLAPC if the patient wishes to continue lens wear is by no means easy. The simplest and most effective measure is for the patient to abandon lens wear. Should they do so, the signs and symptoms are invariably resolved and there is no current evidence of recurrence. However, many practitioners, the author included, feel that it is appropriate to respect the patient's wishes and make the best possible efforts for a return to satisfactory lens wear if the patient desires this. The measures that can be taken include those already described in preventing the condition and frequently involve the temporary cessation of lens wear. If a soft lens is old or cannot be cleaned satisfactorily, a replacement can be obtained. In soft lens wear, a radical change in lens material from a HEMA to a non-HEMA containing polymer and vice versa, may be beneficial. Similarly, in hard lens wear, replacement with a thin gas permeable lens may be appropriate, although it is wise to institute weekly cleaning with a proteolytic enzyme if this is contemplated. In affected gas permeable lens wearers, hard lenses may be supplied with appropriately formed edges. Whatever course of action is taken, it is wise to inform the patient of the trial and error nature of the exercise, and also of the possibility of recurrence when the signs and symptoms have subsided and lens wear is resumed.

Treatment

Once diagnosed, CLAPC may be treated with compounds which act by mast cell stabilization, since it is the degranulation of basal cells which underlies the condition. One topical ocular preparation is currently available – sodium cromoglycate (Opticrom). In addition, one further preparation, lobaxamaide, has been examined for efficiency in controlling CLAPC.

Opticrom (sodium cromoglycate) Sodium cromoglycate was first synthesized in 1965. It acts as a mast cell stabilizer by inhibiting the release of preformed chemical mediators such as histamine, serotonin, heparin, platelet-activating factor, eosinophil chemotactic factor, neutrophilic chemotactic factors and others. Initially, it was thought that sodium cromoglycate acted by inhibiting cell wall transport, thus in turn inhibiting mast cell degranulation. More recently, it has been shown that Opticrom may selectively and rapidly phosphorylase a 78 000 Dalton protein in the mast cell membrane responsible for terminating secretion and restabilizing the mast cell after degranulation[6].

Sodium cromoglycate has been found to be effective in the treatment of ocular signs and symptoms that have no apparent underlying allergic diathesis. Thus, sodium cromoglycate has a role in the treatment of CLAPC which goes beyond its ability to act as a mast cell stabilizer.

The effectiveness of Opticrom as a treatment for CLAPC. A number of studies on the efficacy of sodium cromoglycate have been carried out. Buckley 1987[7], studied the effect of sodium cromoglycate and placebo in a group of patients with CLAPC. During the treatment, lens wear was continued and no attempt was made to improve lens hygiene. In the patient sample, 41% did not adhere to an adequate lens care regimen. None of the 19 hard lens wearers used protein removal tablets and 8 used no cleaning solution. Of the soft lens wearers, 6 used no cleaning solution, 4 stored their lenses in unpreserved saline without heating them and 11 used no protein removal tablets. The patients were asked if they felt their treatment had been effective: 78% of the patients treated with cromolyn sodium and 50% of those given placebo, felt that the treatment had been either moderately or very successful. After 6 weeks of treatment the patients were assessed by clinicians and they found that the treatment had been moderately or very successful in 72% of the patients treated with sodium cromoglycate and in 22% of the patients treated with placebo. Independent assessment based on examination of photographs revealed moderate improvement in 68% of the sodium cromoglycate treated patients and 6% of the placebo treated patients. The results showed that sodium cromoglycate was significantly more effective than placebo in treating CLAPC.

Treatment of CLAPC with lodoxamide The lodoxamides are a new class of inhibitors of mediator release, which are biologues of sodium cromoglycate, but have greater intrinsic activity. Studies show that lodoxamide compounds are bifunctional. Low doses of the drugs inhibit histamine release by binding the calcium which normally triggers release; however, at high concentrations, calcium is forced into the cell and histamine release increases. A single dose of lodoxamide will stimulate guanylate cyclase and inhibit guanylate phosphodiesterase which breaks down the cyclic GMP. The enzymes that increase cyclic GMP located on the cell membrane mediate the enhancement through cholinergic stimulation of guanylate cyclase which, in turn, stimulates synthesis of cyclic GMP. Lodoxamide compounds stimulate guanylate cyclase resulting in the formation of more cyclic GMP. Lodoxamide inhibits guanylate phosphodiesterase which breaks down cyclic GMP, as the cyclic GMP increases, histamine comes out of the cell.

Comparative studies of lodoxamide versus sodium cromoglycate as a treatment for CLAPC have indicated that lodoxamide is at least as effective as cromoglycate and may result in fewer side effects. However, although potentially useful in the treatment of allergic conditions, lodoxamides have not at the time of writing been approved for clinical use.

Clinical management

As with so many clinical conditions, prevention is better than cure. The measures referred to in Prevention and treatment will reduce the incidence of CLAPC from approximately 40% to about 7%, provided the patients comply with the advice given by the contact lens practitioner. Among those patients who still present with signs and symptoms after daily and weekly cleaning to remove potential antigens from the lens surface, treatment is best effected by 3 months' supply of Opticrom after lens wear has been discontinued. This invariably leads to a rapid resolution of symptoms, although papillae are often still found in the conjunctiva covering the tarsal plate area of the upper eyelid. Once resolved, many patients wish to return to contact lens wear and this presents problems for the practitioner, since the incidence of recurrence is high.

In general, most patients can only achieve limited lens wear without running an unacceptably high risk of recurrence. Perhaps social wear of a soft lens of a material different to that previously used for 4 or 5 hours, 2 or 3 times a week is the best that can be hoped for. As this needs to be accompanied by careful and frequent lens cleaning with surfactant and enzyme systems, attempts to return to all day wear are usually unsuccessful with recurrence taking 3–9 months. Although sodium cromoglycate can be used once to accelerate the recovery from symptoms, its repeated use is not justified and after recurrence contact lens wear should be abandoned.

References

1 Allansmith, M. R. (1963). *Journal of Allergy*, **34**, 535

2 Allansmith, M. R., Baird, R. S. and Greiner, J. V. (1979). *American Journal of Ophthalmology*, **87**, 171

3 Allansmith, M. R., Greiner, J. V. and Baird, R. S. (1978). *American Journal of Ophthalmology*, **86**, 250

4 Allansmith, M. R., Korb, D. R. and Greiner, J. V. (1978). *Ophthalmology*, **85**, 766

5 Allansmith, M. R., Korb, D. R., Greiner, J. V., Henriquez, A. S., Simon, M. A. and Finnemore, V. M. (1977). *American Journal of Ophthalmology*, **83**, 697

6 Allansmith, M. R. and Ross, R. N. (1986). *Survey of Ophthalmology*, **30**, 229

7 Buckley, R. J. (1987). *British Journal of Ophthalmology*, **71**, 239

8 Collin, H. B. (1980). *Australian Journal of Optometry*, **63**, 251

9 Duke-Elder, S. (1961). *System of Ophthalmology*, Vol. II. London: Kimpton

10 Greiner, J. V., Covington, H. I. and Allansmith, M. R. (1977). *American Journal of Ophthalmology*, **83**, 892

11 Greiner, J. V., Covington, H. I. and Allansmith, M. R. (1978). *American Journal of Ophthalmology*, **85**, 242

12 Greiner, J. V., Kenyon, K. R., Henriquez, A. S., Korb, D. R., Weidmann, T. A. and Allansmith, M. R. (1980). *Archives of Ophthalmology*, **98**, 1843

13 Kessing, S. V. (1966). *Acta Ophthalmologica*, Suppl. 95, 133

14 Lowther, G. E. and Hill, R. M. (1968). *American Journal of Optometry*, **45**, 587
15 Morgan, G. (1971). *Transactions of the Ophthalmological Society of the United Kingdom*, **91**, 457
16 Richmond, P. P. and Allansmith, M. R. (1981). *International Ophthalmology Clinic*, **21**, 65
17 Spring, T. F. (1974). *Medical Journal of Australia*, **1**, 449
18 Srinivasan, B. D., Jakobiec, F. A., Iwamoto, T. and De Voe, A. G. (1979). *Archives of Ophthalmology*, **97**, 892

Chapter 3

Tears

Introduction

The tear film is a complex layer of liquid covering the anterior surface of the eye. Derived from a number of sources, it fulfils a variety of roles. The presence of the film significantly increases the optical resolution of the eye by 'covering' the many fine irregularities of the corneal surface. Proteins present in the film act together to inhibit microbiological contamination. The film accepts the cellular debris desquamated from the epithelium, and due to the action of the lids, these are 'washed' from the surface of the eye. Dissolved oxygen present in the film is consumed by the cells which is invariably affected by contact lens wear. The ordered arrangement of the film reduces evaporation and prevents the anterior eye from 'drying out'.

The composition of the tear film is affected by contact lens wear. The lipid phase is disrupted in some forms of lens wear and tear evaporation rates may increase. Dissolved tear salt concentrations are affected and some changes may occur in the relative concentration of different proteins.

Components of the tear film can become associated with the contact lens in the form of surface deposits. These deposits comprise varying ratios of the differing substances to be found in tears. Some would appear to be loosely attached to the lens surface and may be removed by manual cleaning. Others are more firmly associated with the lens and cleaning with biochemically active systems is necessary for removal

Structure of the tear film

The structure of the tear film has been much discussed, with both three layer and single layer models proposed in conjunction with thicknesses ranging from 6–40 μm. There is strong evidence to support the view that the outer layer of the tear film consists of lipid, although not in a regularly arranged manner. Beneath the lipid layer is an aqueous layer containing dissolved salts, protein and glycoproteins at a concentration that may vary cross-sectionally. The tear film behaves as a non-newtonian fluid exhibiting low viscosity when mobile and high viscosity when stationary. However, it is almost certainly conceptually wrong to regard the tear film as a fluid; recent evidence strongly suggests that the tear film is a structured gel.

Recent claims that the tear film is as much as 40 μm thick have, in this author's view, arisen from a faulty technique. The 40 μm thick measurement was achieved using a laser interference technique, requiring two reflections, one from the tear film surface and the second from the tear/epithelial interface. In this author's opinion the second reflection came instead from the basement membrane of the epithelium which exhibits a marked difference in refractive index to its surrounding tissues rather than from the tear epithelium interface which does not. The reliable measurements made some years ago of 6–10 μm[32,52,89] remain the best estimates of the true thickness of the tear film.

The tear film attains its thickness 'from the moment after the blink'[62] and thereafter shows no evidence of drainage, although in the absence of further blinking, slight thinning of the film as a result of evaporation has been seen[69].

The superficial lipid layer is principally derived from the tarsal (meibomian) glands. The aqueous phase is wholly derived from the main and the accessory lacrimal glands and the conjunctival goblet cells.

The function of the lipid layer has long been held to be the reduction of evaporation from the aqueous phase[54,72]. However, it has also been suggested that the non-polar nature of the surface layer is an important factor in preventing surface contamination of the film with highly polar skin lipids, which would lead to rapid and dramatic 'break up' of the tear film[42].

The aqueous phase of the tears contains the wide variety of both organic and inorganic substances to be found in tears. In addition to the principal inorganic ions, as many as 60 proteins are present in the tears, together with a variety of biopolymers and glycoproteins, glucose and urea.

The tear volume and flow rate

Estimating tear volume and tear flow rates presents considerable technical difficulties. Reflex tear production may be provoked by a wide variety of stimuli under the mildest of conditions. Probably the most reliable estimate so far achieved is that obtained using the decay characteristics of sodium fluorescein instilled into the lower marginal tear strip. By plotting the apparent fluorescein concentration against time, an estimate of tear volume has been achieved. This method gives a value for the tear volume of 7.0 μl ($\pm$2.0 μl)[1]. By comparing the data for tear volume with that achieved from an objective fluorophorometer[62], an estimate of 1.2 μl/min has been made for tear production rates. A similar, but somewhat lower estimate, has also been made for tear production rates using a radioactive tracer[81].

Tear production rates reduce with age, declining from an average value of approximately 2 μl/min at 15 years of age, to less than 1 μl/min at 65 years of age[35,57].

Given values for tear volume and production rates, it is possible to determine the tear turnover rate of the human eye. The reported measured values[71,81] are in close agreement, 16% and 15% per minute, but are lower than the calculated values made from experiments in which Schirmer strips are introduced into the eye[59].

The distribution of the pre-corneal tear film

The tear film is not evenly distributed over the ocular surfaces, but forms a distinct meniscus at the lid margins; the marginal tear strips, or 'lakes'. The volume of tears in this area has been estimated to be approximately 3 μl[71]. The volume of tears covering the cornea is approximately 1 μl, while a further 3–4 μl are distributed in an even manner over the conjunctiva[1,62].

Tear film dynamics

Although it is possible to ascribe differing volumes to the tear film located in differing parts of the anterior surface of the eye, the tears are not static. The act of blinking has a substantial effect upon the film and the marginal strips. Frank Holly[42] described the effect on the tear film during blinking thus:

> As the upper lid moves downwards the superficial lipid layer is compressed. As it thickens, it begins to exhibit interference colours. The whole lipid layer together with the associated biopolymers is compressed between the lid edges and can be contained there even in the closed eye due to the small thickness of the lipid layer in the open eye. Lipid epiphora almost never occurs as the compressed lipid layer between closed eye lipids has a thickness only of the order of 0.1 μm.
>
> When the eye opens, at first the lipid spreads in the form of a monolayer against the upper eyelid. In this spreading process the limiting factor is the motion of the eyelid. The spreading of the excess lipid follows, and in about one second the duplex (multimolecular) lipid layer is formed. The spreading lipid drags some aqueous tears with it, thereby thickening the rear film. The magnitude of this effect is controlled by the size and shape of the tear meniscus adjacent to the lid edges. As soon as there are insufficient tears to form a saturated meniscus, a local thinning adjacent to the meniscus takes place, which effectively prevents further fluid flow from the meniscus to the tear film.

Although it is now generally accepted that the lipid layer of tears does not form a 'duplex multimolecular lipid layer', the general concept of tear dynamics described by Holly probably holds true.

The sequence of events described by Frank Holly is shown diagrammatically in Figure 3.1.

Further insight into the dynamic distribution of tears has been provided by experiments in which sodium fluorescein was instilled into the marginal tear strip via a fine polythene tube. A 'black line' was observed between the marginal tear strip and pre-corneal film and fluorescein was observed not to migrate across this boundary. The black line was ascribed to the superficial oily layer lying close to the epithelial cell surface, and it was further observed that 'freshly secreted tear fluid runs around the tear strip from above to below without passing over the corneal or conjunctival surface'[62].

Surface tension of the tear film

The surface tension of the tear film is of particular importance in contact lens wear. It is necessary, both for optical considerations and for the maintenance of epithelial and conjunctival integrity, that a contact lens is wetted by a uniform layer of tears[78].

The surface tension of tears has been assessed dynamically by measuring the force required to pull a fine ring out of an annular pool of tears contained within a circular depression on a scleral shell. As a result of this experiment, a figure of 46.24 dynes/cm has been proposed for the surface tension of tears. This value may be too high. In experiments utilizing contact angle goniometry the values of 40–42 dynes/cm have been reported[44].

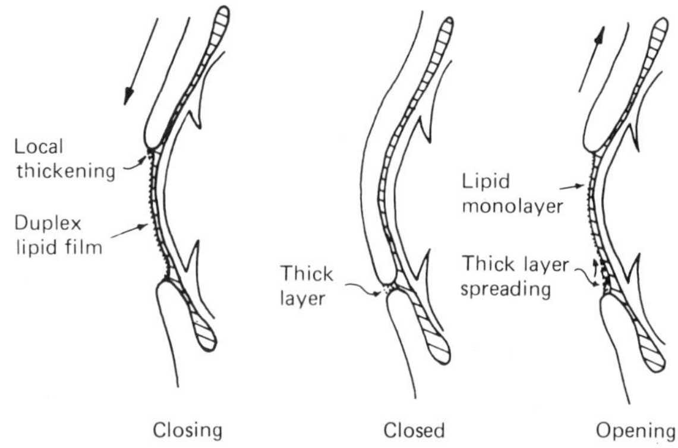

Figure 3.1 Dynamic events during blinking (reproduced by permission of Holly, *American Journal of Optometry*, 1980[42])

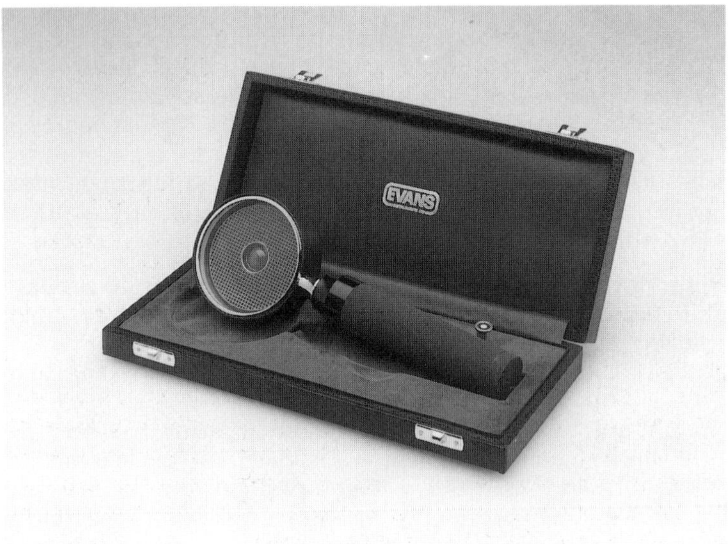

Figure 3.2 The Loveridge grid for the clinical measurement of non-invasive tear film break up time

Tear film break up time

Tear film break up time (often referred to as BUT) is a complex phenomenon which is often considered in relation to contact lens wear. If the tear film is considered solely as a thin film bounded by a layer of lipids and the epithelial interface then the surfaces should be able to approach one another to within a few nanometres before rupture occurs; a process which, in man, would take several minutes. Since tear film break up times of as little as 10 seconds are occasionally observed in prospective contact lens wearers other factors are clearly at play.

Tear film break up times have, in the past, been measured with the aid of sodium fluorescein. Unfortunately this technique is flawed. The action of sodium fluorescein instilled onto the eye is to solubilize the lipid layer of the tear film and the break up

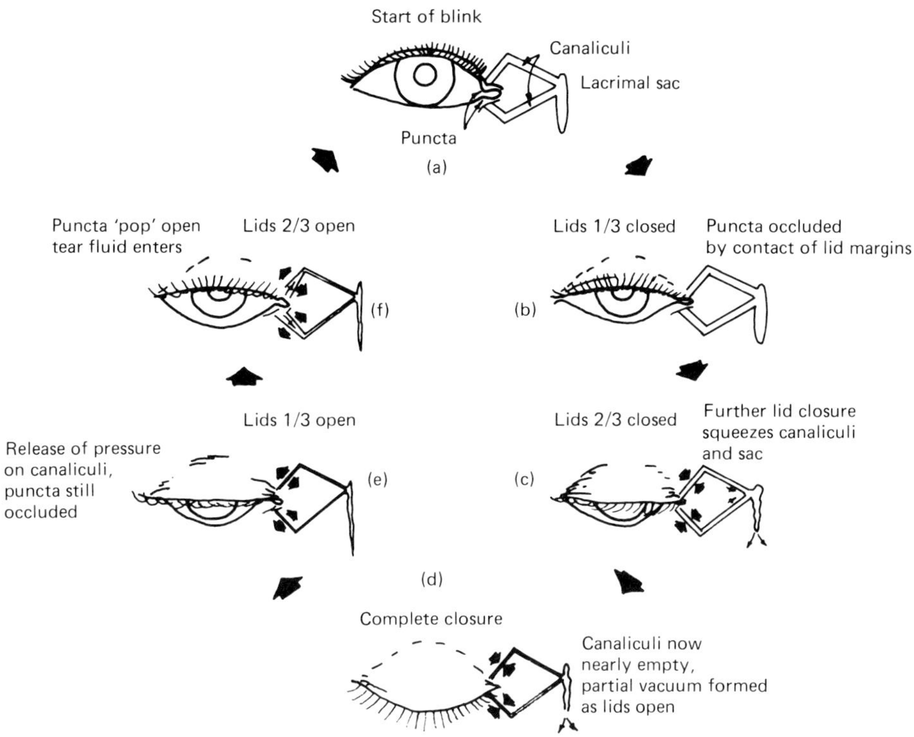

Figure 3.3 Mechanism of blinking (reproduced by permission of Doane, *Ophthalmology*, 1981[23])

time is the time taken for this event to occur. Since this time is dependent on the amount of fluorescein instilled onto the eye in the first place it can have no clinical value. Satisfactory non-invasive tear film break up times were first measured by Tiffany[97] who showed that mean tear film break up times were between 25 and 35 seconds and that they were reproducible (± 5 seconds). The original device for measuring break up time was a modified bowl perimeter with a grid pattern on the inner surface. More recently, Loveridge and the author have developed a clinically useful modification of the original instrument (Figure 3.2) which replaces the circular grid of a keratoscope with a squared grid for break up time. Although tear film break up times can now be reliably and practically measured the absolute value is of less clinical relevance than the detection of very short break up times which are indicative of tear film instability. Measurements of less than 10 seconds are associated with a variety of conditions among which 'dry eye' predominates. While not all preclude contact lens wear, the majority are contraindications to contact lens wear, particularly soft lens wear.

Tear film drainage

Tears drain from the eye via:

1 The lacrimal puncta due to the act of blinking
2 By osmotic flow across the conjunctiva.

Blinking and tear film drainage

High speed photography has revealed many of the subtle features of the drainage of tears during blinking. At the starting phase of the blink the openings of the puncta elevate and seal together during the downward movement of the upper lid. Muscular contraction compresses the elastic walls of the canaliculi and lacrimal sac[33,86], overcoming the slightly negative pressure within the sac, and tears are expelled into the nasal passages. Once in the nose the tears are wholly absorbed by the nasal mucosa and dyes added to the eye do not appear in a nasal discharge unless excess lacrimation has occurred. As the eyes open after a blink, the walls of the canaliculi expand forming a suction until the puncta come suddenly apart and draw in fresh tear fluid. The sequence of events during blinking is shown in Figure 3.3.

Osmotic flow across the conjunctiva

Measurement of the electrical potential of the conjunctiva shows it to be approximately 25 mV, negative with respect to blood[62]. A potential of this order suggests active sodium transport with an accompanying water flow across the conjunctiva. Although the extent of water flow will vary with the circumstances, the very thin film of relatively stagnant fluid over the conjunctiva may well be appropriate for a significant loss of water from the tears into the conjunctiva via this route.

Tear film composition

Lipid phase

The composition of human tear lipid was probably first described in 1897 as 'cholesterol, fatty acids and fat'[79]. A number of attempts have subsequently been made to analyse the lipids of the meibomian glands[3,9,21,25,62,76,77]. A principal difficulty in the analysis is the small amount of material that may be mechanically expelled and collected from the gland orifices. Larger amounts of material may be collected from excised bovine glands collected after partial dissection of the gland openings[76]. The improved amounts of material collected in this manner show a marked similarity to much smaller expelled samples collected post-mortem from both man and animals. A contaminate of lipid found in man but virtually absent in bovine samples is hydrocarbons. Hydrocarbons may arise from airborne petrochemicals or cosmetics and can account for approximately 7.5% of human samples. A comparative table of major lipid classes is given in Table 3.1. The large size and number of meibomian glands suggest that the eye has a considerable requirement for fatty material. Lipids are required to prevent wetting of the skin of the lids adjacent to the eye and to contain the tears. Some is spread over the tears forming the outermost layer of the film and reducing evaporation. This spreading action may be aided by the particular nature of the fatty acids found in lipids which form an unusual group of high molecular weight compounds[77]. It has been suggested that considerable variations in lipid composition exist between different individuals[97]. However, there are considerable technical difficulties in the analysis of the very small samples that can be obtained from live subjects and the close similarity between post-mortem samples of human and bovine fluid suggest that 'the requirement for lipids on the eyelids of man and animals is much the same and strictly defined'[26].

Table 3.1 Comparative lipid composition for bovine and human meibomian samples (prepared from data in Nicolaides *et al.*, *Investigative Ophthalmology*, 1981[76])

	Sterol esters	*WA esters*	*Material in the diester region*	*Triacyl glycerols*	*Material in the post triacyl glycerol region*	*Free sterols*	*Free fatty acids*	*Polar lipids*
Bovine samples	31.7	31.2	11.4	1.6	2.8	3.0	5.1	13.3
Samples from man	29.5	35.0	8.4	4.0	3.2	1.8	2.1	16.0

All values % by weight

Table 3.2 A summary of reported values for human tear and serum electrolyte concentrations (mmol/l) (reproduced by permission of Van Haeringen, *Survey of Ophthalmology*, 1981[101])

	Na^+	K^+	Ca^{2+}	Mg^{2+}	Cl^-	HCO_3^-	*Reference*
Tears	120–170	6–26	–	–	118–138	–	95
	80–161	6–36	–	–	106–130	–	64, 70, 90
	145	24	–	–	128	26	13
	134–170	26–42	0.5–1.1	0.3–0.6	120–135	–	94
	–	–	0.4–0.8	–	–	–	102
	–	–	0.4–1.0	0.5–1.1	–	–	5
	–	–	0.4–1.1	–	–	–	58
	–	–	0.3–2.0	–	–	–	110
Serum	140	4.5	2.5	0.9	100	30	Average of normal

Aqueous phase

The aqueous phase of the tears comprises the major component of the film, comprising some 98% of its total thickness. It is a complex dilute solution of both inorganic electrolytes and low and high molecular weight organic substances.

Electrolytes
The main cation found in the aqueous phase of the tear film is sodium. The concentration of sodium at 145 mmol/mm is similar to that reported for serum, although the concentration of potassium, the other principal cation found in tears, is three to six times higher than its concentration in serum. Other cations are also found in small amounts in tears, principally magnesium and calcium. Calcium is of interest to contact lens practice as it is often present in lens deposits. The concentration of calcium in tears is low; approximately 0.53±0.12 (s.d.) mmol/l[45,100].

The two principal anions found in tears are chloride and bicarbonate ions. Chloride and bicarbonate concentrations are very similar to those reported for serum[13]. The concentrations of tear electrolytes are shown in Table 3.2.

Electrolytes and osmotic pressures
The three main tear electrolytes, sodium, potassium, and chloride ions, contribute towards the osmotic pressure exerted by the tear fluid. Differences between individuals and between the eye being open or closed have been reported[94] (Table 3.3). Of particular interest to contact lens practice is the observation of an increase in osmotic pressure when the eyes are open. This has been held to be the reason for observed changes in corneal thickness first reported in rabbits[73] and later observed in man[66].

Table 3.3 Human tear osmotic pressure (mOsm/kg) (reproduced by permission of Terry and Hill, *Archives of Ophthalmology*, 1978[94])

Subject	*Waking hours*				*Prolonged lid closure*			
no./sex	*N*	$\bar{X}$	*s.d.*	*Range*	*N*	$\bar{X}$	*s.d.*	*Range*
1/M	70	314	6.1	302–329	6	285	2.2	283–289
2/M	70	318	4.8	306–326	6	284	2.3	282–287
3/M	70	305	4.7	295–317	6	288	3.6	285–293
4/F	70	315	4.7	308–326	6	283	2.5	280–287
5/F	70	308	7.7	292–323	6	284	1.4	282–286
6/F	70	297	6.2	289–319	*			
Men only	210	312	5.2	301–324	18	286	2.7	283–290
Women only	210	307	6.2	296–323	12	284	1.9	281–287
All subjects (averages)	420	310	5.7	299–323	30	285	2.4	282–288
Equivalent sodium chloride solution (%)	...	0.97	0.02	0.93–1.01	..	0.89	0.01	0.88–0.90

*Subject was not available for this phase of the study.

Bicarbonate concentrations, tear pH and buffering capacity
The presence of bicarbonate and carbonate ions in the tear film may contribute towards the maintenance of pH. Tear film pH has been reported to be very slightly acidic, approximately 6.8, following eyelid closure, and slightly alkaline, 7.3–7.6, when the eyes are open[18]. The acidic 'shift' observed in lid closure is probably

attributable to the obstruction of carbon dioxide effluxing through the cornea (approximately 20 μl/cm[30]) with the formation of an increased concentration of weakly dissociated carbonic acid when the lids are closed. The observed changes in tear film pH would probably be greater were it not for the presence of bicarbonate ions in the film. Using a challenge technique comprising 1 μl of 0.1 M sodium hydroxide solution, a shift of 2.5–3.0 pH units occurs when this solution is added to samples of human tears, while a shift of 3.5–4.0 pH units occurs when the solution is added to a similar volume of unbuffered saline.

Low molecular weight organic substances

Glucose Glucose is present in tears only in very low concentrations. Raised glucose levels may be seen in diabetes but these values are attributable to raised tissue fluid levels rather than raised tear levels.

Amino acids The free amino acids present in tears have not been identified at the time of writing, but may be present in a concentration that is three to four times the level reported for serum.

Urea The concentration of urea in tears is reported to be similar to that of plasma[95], suggesting unrestricted passage across the blood/tear barrier of the lacrimal gland[106].

Tear proteins The aqueous phase of tears contains a remarkably complex mixture of both locally produced and serum derived proteins. Using a novel technique of crossed immunoelectrophoresis, Gachon and co-workers[36] have identified at least 60 protein components, some of which were immunologically indistinguishable from serum homologues, while others were clearly distinguishable and of specific tear origin. Although tear proteins have been considered to consist of a mixture of albumin, globulin and lysozyme, it is apparent that this classification is overly simple for this complex biological fluid. A list of some currently identified tear proteins is given in Table 3.4.

The immunoglobulins The immunoglobulins comprise one of the five major groups of tear protein. In common with secretions covering other exposed mucosal surfaces, the major immunoglobulin has been shown to be 'secretory' IgA[46,63,65,88,98,107].

Secretory IgA is a dimer formed from two IgA units and a secretory component. Individual IgA polymers are synthesized in plasma cells from where they may migrate into the intercellular spaces of the acinar of the gland. Upon entering an adjacent cell, the IgA becomes associated with a secretory component formed from within the cell, and the newly arranged dimer migrates to the lumen of the gland and hence becomes incorporated in the tears[53]. A diagram which illustrates the formation of secretory IgA is shown in Figure 3.4.

The concentration of secretory IgA in tears has been variously estimated as: 21.2 mg/100 μl (standard deviation 2.6 mg/100 μl)[63], 9–50 mg/100 μl[14], 17 mg/100 μl[65], 30 mg/100 μl[19] and 10.7 mg/g of total protein.

The role of secretory IgA in tears is almost certainly part of the defence mechanisms of the external eye. Locally produced secretory IgA is thought to be far more effective in combating the invasion of microorganisms through mucosal surfaces than serum IgA, and also to be effective in neutralizing certain viruses and responding to certain specific antigens[65]. In addition to secretory IgA, single IgA chains have been reported to be present in tears[49,62,63].

Table 3.4 Some proteins identified in tears

1 *Principal tear proteins**	
Secretory immunoglobulin A	
Lysozyme	
Lactoferrin	
Albumin	
Specific tear albumin	
2 *Further proteins*	
Immunoglobulin G	Beta lysin (?)
Immunoglobulin M	Transferrin
Immunoglobulin D	Antichymotrypsin
Immunoglobulin E	Antitrypsin
Complement component C3	Prostaglandins
Complement component C4	Zinc alpha II glycoprotein
Histamine	Ceruloplasmin (?)
3 *Enzymes from the lacrimal gland*	
(In addition to lysozyme)	
Alpha galactosidase	Amalysase
Beta hexosaminidase	Hexokinase
Beta glucuronidase	Glutamate pyruvate
Acid phosphatase	Transaminase
Alkaline phosphatase	
4 *Enzymes from the corneal and conjunctival epithelium*	
Lactate dehydrogenase	Glucose-6-phosphase
Malate dehydrogenase	Dehydrogenase
Pyruvate kinase	Sorbitol dehydrogenase
Isocitrate dehydrogenase	Glutamate dehydrogenase
Aldolase	Glutamate oxalacetate

* A necessarily arbitrary classification based mainly on the electrophoretic separation of Gachon *et al.*, (1979)[36]. See text.

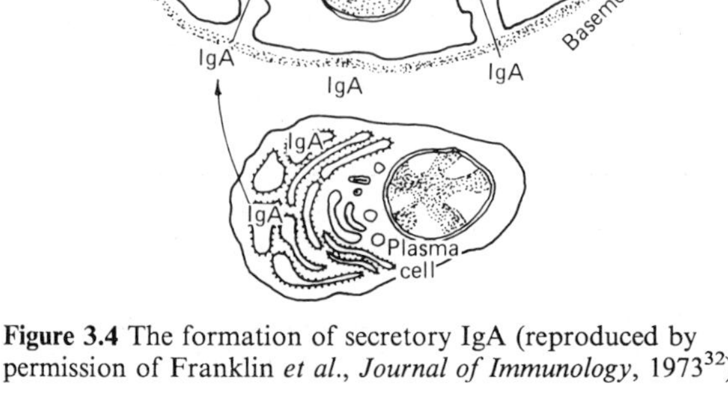

Figure 3.4 The formation of secretory IgA (reproduced by permission of Franklin *et al.*, *Journal of Immunology*, 1973[32])

Although IgG is the main immunoglobulin in serum, it is present in tears in a lower concentration than IgA[19,63]. A comparison of immunoglobulin concentration in tears and serum is given in Table 3.5. The concentration of immunoglobulins in tears changes in response to infection, and it has been suggested that a transduction of serum proteins into tears occurs in 'inflammation from whatever cause'[65].

Of the remaining immunoglobulins, low concentrations of IgM, IgD and IgE have occasionally been observed in tears[14,63].

Table 3.5 Comparison of amount of total protein and immunoglobulin in tears and serum by ratio (from McClellen *et al.*, 1973 and reproduced by permission of McClellan *et al.*, *American Journal of Ophthalmology*, 1973[65])

	Average amount (g/l)		*Ratio*
Substance	*Tears*	*Serum*	*Tears/serum*
Total protein	80	650	1:8
IgG	1.4	100	1:70
IgA	1.7	17	1:10
IgM	0.5	10	1:18
IgD	0.1	1.1	1:11
IgE	25*	200*	1:8

*in ng/ml

Complement Although individual proteins of the complement system have been known for some time[10,19], it was not until the work of Yamamoto and Allansmith[110] that the presence of all nine of the components of the complement system were detected in tears. Following the Yamamoto study, Kijistra and Veerhuis[56], when seeking to detect the complement system in tears, found instead an anti-complementary factor. This factor appears to be associated with the protein binding properties of lactoferrin, which would prevent complement activation on the ocular surface following serum leakage under inflammatory conditions.

The albumins Although early electrophoretic studies of the tear proteins revealed the presence of a substance having a similar mobility to serum albumin, it was observed that the majority of this protein would not complex as an antisera with human serum albumin[28,49]. Hence the majority of albumin in tears may be considered to be immunologically distinct from serum albumin, and has come to be known as 'tear albumin'[49] or 'human tear pre albumin'[50]. Using the SDS-page technique a molecular weight of approximately 21 000 Daltons has been determined and this protein is not found in serum, spinal fluid, saliva or urine[51]. The nature of tear pre albumin has been examined in a number of species[12] and the presence of specific tear pre albumin has been demonstrated in the tears of man, rabbit, guinea-pig, chicken and monkey. It has been shown that it is synthesized by the lacrimal gland rather than derived as a modified serum homologue, as is the case with IgA. Although tear pre albumin has been demonstrated to produce a single line on conventional gel column electrophoresis[49], improved techniques[36] using a novel form of crossed immunoelectrophoresis have demonstrated the presence of more than one component and genetic polymorphism with five discernible types of tear albumin has been observed[6].

The role of tear pre albumin may be similar to that of a number of other tear proteins in that it is part of the defence mechanism of the eye. The lysis of

Micrococcus lysodeikticus is reported to be enhanced by the activity of an 'anodal tear protein'[56], almost certainly specific tear pre albumin. A clearer identification of tear albumin as a bactericide together with lysozyme and a glycoprotein has recently been provided, although individual bactericidal assays have yet to be undertaken.

Lysozyme (mucopeptide N-acetyl muramyldehydrolase) Lysozyme forms one of the major protein constituents of tears, and was the first tear protein whose antimicrobial properties were identified and described[83]. The name 'lysozyme' was suggested from the ability of this protein enzyme to cleave a mucopeptide found in the cell wall of *M. lysodeikticus*[31]. The ability of lysozyme to cause cell wall lysis is limited to a relatively small number of Gram-positive bacteria, and its role in the defence mechanisms of the external eye is not wholly clear.

Lysozyme may be separated from the other proteins present in tears by conventional gel column electrophoresis and has the lowest isoelectric point of the major tear proteins. However, it is positively charged at physiological pH and is therefore considered to be an anodal tear protein. Two isoenzymes of lysozyme exist and these may be electrophoretically resolved under appropriate conditions[38,89]. The origin of tear lysozyme is thought to be synthesis in the lacrimal gland. Structurally, tear lysozyme closely resembles serum lysozyme, but there is little or no correlation between serum and tear lysozyme concentrations and both may become independently altered in a number of systemic and ocular conditions[80].

The concentration of lysozyme in tears has been estimated at between 0.83 and 2.06 g/ml[38,74], although this value and that of the other principal tear proteins is somewhat affected by the method of collection[8]. Lysozyme levels appear largely unaffected by circadian patterns but a marked reduction in concentration has been observed in polluted environments[88] and some disease states[5,29]. The electrophoretic mobility of tear lysozyme from 50 subjects has been examined[2], but no significant difference has been observed in mobility, suggesting that lysozyme cannot be used as a genetic marker in a manner similar to that employed for some haemoglobulins.

The activity of human tear lysozyme is greater than that of lysozyme obtained from hens' eggs, although they both act as catalysts for the same biochemical reaction[11].

Lactoferrin Lactoferrin, which forms approximately 25% by weight of the total tear protein[55], is common to a number of external secretions. This protein has both bacteriostatic and complexing properties[15] and can reversibly bind two atoms of iron. The source of lactoferrin is the acinar epithelium of the main and accessory lacrimal glands[32].

Lactoferrin, which is present in a number of forms[37], plays an important role in the eyes' defence against microbiological contamination. Although at one time thought to be principally concerned with iron binding activities, more recent work has shown that lactoferrin has a direct effect on certain strains of bacteria[4]. In addition, lactoferrin plays a role in the rate of production of macrophage-derived colony stimulating factors[7,16].

Lactoferrin may also a play a role in inflammatory ocular conditions where serum leaks into the tear film. The tear protein has been shown to inhibit the formation of C3 convertase of the classical complement system, thus preventing the formation of the biologically active fragments, C3A and C5A[106]. However, the physiological role of lactoferrin in the tear film is by no means wholly understood at the time of writing.

Non-lysozymal antibacterial factor Claims for the presence in tears of a low molecular weight potent non-lysozymal antibacterial factor (NLAF) have been made[34,96].

The possible identification of NLAF as beta lysin, an antibacterial substance known to be present in other body fluids, has been proposed. However, there are a number of inconsistencies in the published literature and platelets, which are a major source of beta lysin, are not known to be present in tears. The difficulties of satisfactory assay procedures for lysozyme in tears has been emphasized by a number of writers[27,85], and it is possible that NLAF in tears is a spurious observation arising from a faulty technique.

Transferrin, the serum counterpart of lactoferrin, can be found in tears[11,36,49,51], but only in the presence of inflammation or if there is mild trauma provoked by tear collection.

Ceruloplasmin Ceruloplasmin, a copper carrying protein, has been reported to be present in tears[49,88], at a concentration which varies from its serum counterpart. However, ceruloplasmin was not detected by Gachon *et al.* in 1979[36], who concluded 'attempts to establish the presence of ceruloplasmin have never been successful'. The analytical procedure described by Gachon and his co-workers is a careful and thorough separation and identification of human tear proteins. The absence of ceruloplasmin in their analysis must raise doubts about the presence of this protein in tears.

Proteinase inhibitors The presence of proteinase inhibitors, alpha I antichymotrypsin and alpha I antitrypsin, has been demonstrated[82] and confirmed in tears[36]. Both substances are present in low concentrations and their role is thought to be associated with inhibiting the action of certain proteolytic enzymes, both from ocular tissues and bacteria. Support for the inhibition of bacterial enzymes has been provided from the observation of an increased concentration of alpha I antitrypsin during bacterial infections of the conjunctiva and cornea, and it has been suggested that the assay of alpha I antitrypsin could be used as an aid in diagnosis of ocular infections[112]. A further antiproteinase, alpha II macroglobulin, has also been detected in tears[36].

Prostaglandins The presence of prostaglandin E in tear fluid has been demonstrated[22]. Using radioimmunoassay techniques, with specific antisera, low concentrations (25–137.5 pg/ml) of this protein have been found to be present in tear samples collected with Schirmer strips from 'normal' eyes, while substantially raised concentrations have been observed in patients suffering from vernal conjunctivitis and chronic trachoma. The role of prostaglandins is that of one of the mediators of the inflammatory process and intraocular injection of prostaglandins has been found to provoke a response characteristic of ocular inflammation[109].

Histamine Histamine concentrations in tears from 'normal' subjects and those suffering from vernal conjunctivitis have been reported[1]. The mean values for normal subjects were 10.3 ng/ml (±9.43 s.d.) while the values for samples collected from subjects suffering from vernal conjunctivitis were 38.2 ng/ml (±40.83 s.d.).

Acid hydrolases derived from the lacrimal gland (Alpha galactosidase, beta hexosaminidase, beta glucuronidase, acid phosphatase and alkaline phosphatase.) The presence of six acid hydrolases in tear fluid has been reported[91,105]. The source of five of the six acid hydrolases is thought to be the lysozomes of the secretory cells in the lacrimal gland's acini, which have been shown to be particularly well endowed with secretory granules[87]. The lysozomal enzymes may form particular hydrolytic functions within the cell during tear secretion. The sixth acid hydrolase, alkaline phosphatase, is thought to be derived from the epithelial cells of the lacrimal glands which have been demonstrated to have a high level of activity of this enzyme.

Amylase The origin of tear amylases is thought to be the lacrimal gland and studies of its isoenzyme pattern suggest that it is synthesized by the gland rather than derived from blood[102]. The concentration of amylase in tears is low, its concentration being 625–4000 μg/l and this value is markedly affected by lacrimation rates[102].

Hexokinase and glutamate-pyruvate transaminase Both hexokinase and glutamate-pyruvate transaminase have been identified in tears[104]. The presence of these two enzymes, when lactate dehydrogenase is absent, suggests that their origin is to be found in the lacrimal gland rather than in the cells of the corneal epithelium.

Enzymes derived from the corneal epithelium and conjunctiva The enzymes lactate dehydrogenase, malate dehydrogenase, pyruvate kinase, isocitrate dehydrogenase, aldolase glucose-6-phosphate dehydrogenase, sorbitol dehydrogenase, glutamate dehydrogenase and glutamate oxalacetate transaminase have been identified in tears[104]. These enzymes are derived from the energy producing metabolism of the epithelial cells[53,104] and not the lacrimal gland as had been previously suggested. The concentration of these enzymes in tears is low and markedly affected by the method of collection[104]. During collection with Schirmer strips, mild trauma is caused to the epithelial cells of the conjunctiva and detectable quantities of enzymes may be obtained. However, if glass 'capillary' tubes are used, very little disturbance is caused to the eye and few, if any, of the enzymes are detected. Whichever method of collection is used, the main enzyme detected is lactate dehydrogenase, with the remainder of the enzymes being present in very low concentrations.

The isoenzyme pattern of lactate dehydrogenase in tears of man shows a typical M (muscle) type configuration[53]. This finding indicates that this enzyme is derived from the energy producing metabolism of the corneal epithelium. Changes in isoenzyme pattern can occur in some forms of ocular disease[52]. In herpes simplex or conjunctivitis an unusual isoenzyme pattern consisting of six rather than five bands is sometimes found. This may represent the binding of lactate dehydrogenase to immunoglobulins; a phenomenon known to occur in blood[101].

Zinc alpha II glycoprotein The presence of glycoproteins in the aqueous phase of the tear film has been reported[97]. The glycoprotein has been characterized as zinc alpha II glycoprotein[40]. Glycoproteins make up the 'mucous' content of the ocular secretions.

The 'mucous' phase

At one time it was considered that the mucous phase of the tear film formed an interface between the tears and epithelium which rendered the epithelial surface wettable by tears[43]. This is now known not to be the case. The fine surface of the superficial cells is highly interdigitated with numerous microplicate and microvilli and the surface is readily wetted by tears.

The major source of tear glycoprotein is undoubtedly the conjunctival goblet cells. However, mucus secreting cells have also been found in the acini of the human lacrimal gland[24]. The presence of glycoproteins in lacrimal fluid uncontaminated by fluid from other glands would suggest a further source for tear glycoproteins, in addition to the conjunctival cells[58]. Although the term 'mucus' has been widely used to describe tear glycoprotein there is no clear agreement as to the constituents of this component of the tear film. A largely insoluble mucoid gel has been observed with a high carbohydrate to protein ratio[75]. It is considered that this material consists of polymers, containing about 70% carbohydrate, which are cross-linked. However, the glycoprotein complexes are likely to be bound to lipids in the high molecular weight fraction region of greater than 10^5 Daltons[20]. Some plasma proteins present in mucus may also complex with lipids although to a much lesser extent than the high molecular weight fractions. It is also possible that these complexes are transiently attached to the epithelial surface although the nature of this association is unknown at the time of writing.

The function of tear glycoprotein is also not wholly clear. Despite some recent extravagant claims for tear mucus, it is likely that tear glycoprotein has at least two primary roles. First, tear glycoprotein renders the tear film 'non-newtonian', that is to say that when stationary it exhibits a high viscosity, while in motion during blinking it has a low viscosity approaching that of water. This non-newtonian attribute undoubtedly aids tear film spreading during the blink and it may add to tear stability thereafter. The second role of tear mucus is to adhere to the many fine contaminants which the tear film continuously encounters. The carbohydrate component of tear glycoprotein forms fine spiral sugar arms to which many of the smaller contaminants of the tear film readily adhere, and are lost to the eye surface during the normal process of tear film drainage. These two roles are the traditional role of mucus in the body as a whole.

Contact lens induced changes in the tear film

The most obvious change in the tear film induced by contact lens wear is the dramatic increase in tear production rate on lens insertion. Not only do production rates alter but tear tonicity levels also decline to equivalent plasma levels, as evaporation has a negligible effect on the large volume of continuously produced tear. However, the effect on tear production, as indicated by chloride ion levels, is relatively short-lived[96] and within a week or so lacrimation is apparently back to normal.

The volume and composition of tears in the adapted contact lens wearer may be affected by contact lens wear. Reduced tear flow as the result of a 'fatigue block' in the efferent nerves to conjunctival sensory impulses has been postulated as a mechanism for promoting deposit formation in soft lens wearers. An examination of tear flow rates in soft lens wearers has shown an absence of this type of response[92]. However, among contact lens wearers there is evidence for raised tear osmolarity levels as compared to normal[60] (Figure 3.5). A possible reason for these raised levels is increased tear evaporation rates as a result of contact lens induced disruption to the lipid phase of the tear film[99].

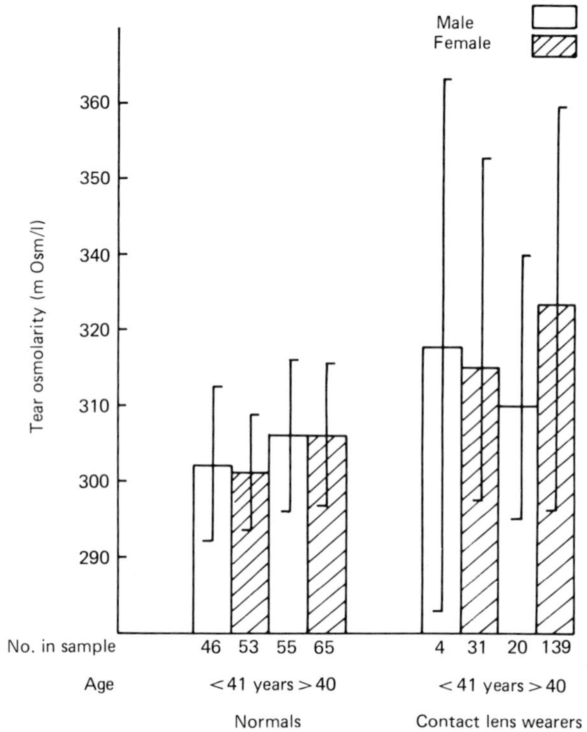

Figure 3.5 A comparison of tear osmolarity levels in normals and contact lens wearers (all types) of at least three months' duration (reproduced by permission of Linsey Farris, Stuchell and Mandell, *Ophthalmology*, 1981[60])

The surface appearance of the lipid phase may be photographed by a novel technique developed by Jean-Pierre Guillon[37] which utilizes crossed polaroids and the specularly reflected image of the slit lamp light source. Since the thickness of the lipid phase is of the same order of magnitude as light, colours produced by interference within the film may be used for measurement purposes. Generally it is found that the normal eye, which has a lipid phase thickness of about 100 nm, has greyish appearance, while as thickness increases fringes of red, orange, yellow, green and eventually blue may be seen.

In addition to measurement, the general appearance of the film gives a qualitative impression of lipid phase continuity. This technique can be utilized clinically by observing the appearance of the lipid phase between blinks.

In soft lens wear, with a new or clean lens, the lipid phase is similar in appearance and behaviour to the non-lens wearing eye. However, when surface deposits or defects are present the film becomes unstable.

In hard corneal lens wear, the lipid phase is absent over the anterior lens surface. However, interference colours may be observed arising from the thicker aqueous phase drying on the surface. The coloured fringes appear in a narrow zone along the drying border. In the area surrounding a corneal lens a lipid layer may be observed and it would appear that the edge of a hard lens forms a barrier to the spreading of

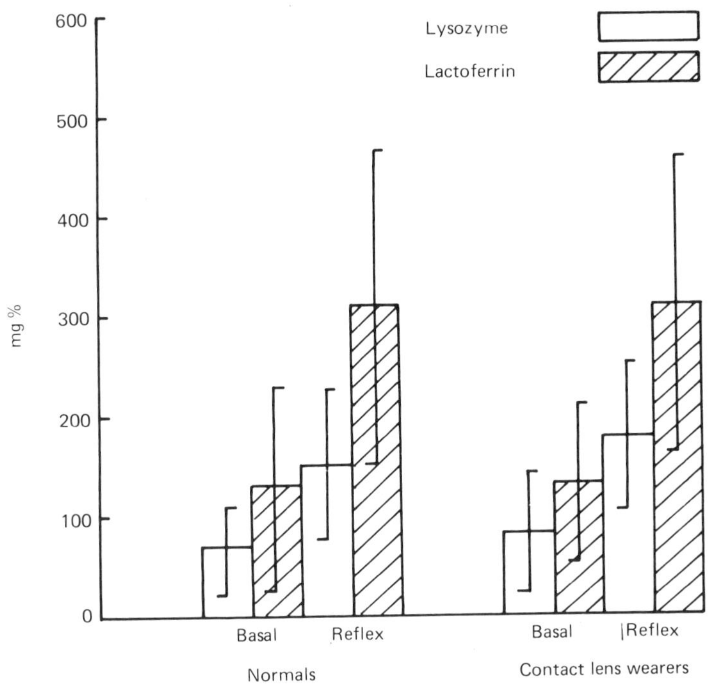

Figure 3.6 Lysozyme and lactoferrin concentrations in basal and reflex tears in normals and contact lens wearers (Reproduced by permission of Stuchell, Linsey Farris and Mandell, *Ophthalmology*, 1981[93])

lipid over the surface of the lens. Examples of lipid phase appearance in the normal and contact lens wearing eye are shown in Plate 3.

A disturbance to lipid phase continuity suggests the possibility of increased evaporation rates in contact lens wearers. Devices to measure tear evaporation rates have been described[39,84] and increased evaporation rates have been observed in various forms of contact lens wear[39,99]. The extent of the increase in evaporation rates so far observed is consistent with the reported changes observed in tear osmolarity levels. The practical effect of these changes may be to reduce corneal swelling in adapted wearers. However, the author is not aware of experimental work causally relating these events.

In addition to disturbed tear lipid levels, markedly raised levels of cholesterol have been suggested as a cause of intolerance to contact lens wear[111]. The elevated levels were observed in obesity, the middle 3 months of pregnancy, and the use of diuretics. Lenses worn by patients subject to these conditions had recurrent oily deposits which gave rise to reduced vision and discomfort. The tear cholesterol levels measured in these patients were extremely high and in excess of equivalent plasma levles. A comparison of tear and plasma cholesterol levels has shown tear cholesterol levels to be much lower than plasma[103]. This finding is consistent with differences in protein levels which may be a relevant observation as α- and β-lipoproteins are involved in cholesterol transport in other body fluids. The very marked discrepancy in the reported cholesterol levels found in the different studies[103,111] must cast some doubt on the observation of tear cholesterol levels as a cause of contact lens intolerance.

In addition to the lipid phase of the tear film, some of the proteins in the aqueous region have also been examined[38]. The mean concentration of lysozyme and lactoferrin, in a general group of differing types of contact lens wearers, has been observed to be similar to non-lens wearers (Figure 3.6). However, some individuals within the group had markedly raised levels of both these tear proteins.

Among a carefully monitored group of differing types of soft lens wearers, total protein and major protein fractions were initially observed to decrease due to hypersecretion and then to return to a level below the pre-wear value. In addition, some changes were noted in lysozyme concentrations suggesting some absorption of lysozyme into high water content hydrogels with large (400–600 nm) interchain spaces[38].

Little further information appears to be available on the composition of tear proteins in contact lens wear. In recent years some insight has been gained into the way in which the tear proteins act together to keep the surface of the eye free of disease. It is very likely that contact lens wear affects this process and this area is worthy of further research.

References

1 Abelson, M. B., Soter, N. A. and Simon, M. A. (1977). *American Journal of Ophthalmology*, **83**, 417

2 Allansmith, M. R., Drell, D., Anderson, R. P. and Newman, L. (1971). *American Journal of Ophthalmology*, **71**, 525

3 Andres, J. S. (1970). *Experimental Eye Research*, **10**, 223

4 Arnold, R. R., Russell, J. E., Champion, W. J., Brewer, M. and Fauthier, J. J. (1982). *Infection and Immunology*, **35**, 792

5 Avisar, R., Menache, R. and Shaked, P. (1977). *American Journal of Ophthalmology*, **87**, 148

6 Azen, E. A. (1976). *Biochemical Genetics*, **14**, 225

7 Badgy, G. C., Rigas, U. D., Bennet, R. M., Vandenbank, A. A. and Garewal, H. S. (1981). *Journal of Clinical Investigation*, **68**, 56

8 Barnett, E. V. (1968). *Journal of Immunology*, **100**, 1093

9 Baron, C. and Blough, H. A. (1976). *Journal of Lipid Research*, **17**, 373

10 Bluestone, R., Easty, D. L., Goldberg, L. S., Jones, B. R. and Pettit, T. H. (1975). *British Journal of Ophthalmology*, **59**, 279

11 Bonavida, B. and Sapse, A. T. (1968). *American Journal of Ophthalmology*, **66**, 70

12 Bonavida, B., Sapse, A. T. and Sercarz, E. E. (1969). *Nature*, **221**, 375

13 Bothelho, S. Y. (1964). *Scientific American*, **211**, 78

14 Brauninger, G. E. and Centifanto, Y. M. (1971). *American Journal of Ophthalmology*, **72**, 558

15 Broekhuyse, R. M. (1974). *Investigative Ophthalmology*, **13**, 550

16 Broxmeyer, H. E., Smithyman, A., Eger, R. R., Meyer, P. A. and de Sousa, M. (1978). *Journal of Experimental Medicine*, **148**, 1052

17 Callender, M. (1981). Personal Communication

18 Carney, L. G. and Hill, R. M. (1976). *Archives of Ophthalmology*, **94**, 821

19 Chandler, J. W., Leader, R., Kaufman, H. E. and Caldwell, J. R. (1974). *Investigative Ophthalmology*, **13**, 151

20 Chao, C.-C. W., Vergnes, J. P. and Brown, S. I. (1983). *Experimental Eye Research*, **36**, 139

21 Cory, C. G., Hinks, W., Burton, J. L. and Shuster, S. (1973). *British Journal of Dermatology*, **89**, 25

22 Dhir, S. P., Garg, S. K., Sharma, Y. R. and Lath, N. K. (1979). *American Journal of Ophthalmology*, **87**, 403

23 Doane, M. G. (1981). *Ophthalmology*, **88**, 403

24 Dohlman, C. H., Friend, J. and Kalevar, V. (1976). *Experimental Eye Research*, **22**, 359

25 Ehlers, N. (1961). *Acta Ophthalmologica*, **45**, 718

26 Ehlers, N. (1965). *Acta Ophthalmologica*, Suppl. 81, 136

27 Ensink, F. T. E. and Van Haeringen, N. J. (1977). *Ophthalmology Research*, **9**, 366

28 Erickson, O. F., Feeney, L. and McEwen, W. K. (1956). *Archives of Ophthalmology*, **55**, 800

29 Eylan, E., Ronen, D., Romano, S. and Smetana, O. (1977). *Investigative Ophthalmology*, **16**, 850

30 Fatt, I. (1968). *Experimental Eye Research*, **7**, 413

31 Fleming, A. (1922). *Proceedings of the Royal Society*, **93**, 306

32 Franklin, R. M., Kenyon, K. R. and Tomasi, T. B. (1973). *Journal of Immunology*, **110**, 984

33 Frieberg, T. (1918). *Zeitschrift für Augenheilkunde*, **39**, 266

34 Friendland, B. R., Anderson, D. R. and Forster, R. K. (1972). *American Journal of Ophthalmology*, **74**, 52

35 Furukama, R. E. and Polse, K. A. (1978). *American Journal of Optometry*, **55**, 69

36 Gachon, A. M., Verrelle, P., Betail, G. and Dastugue, B. (1979). *Experimental Eye Research*, **29**, 539

37 Guillon, J.-P. (1982). *Journal of the British Contact Lens Association*, **5**, 84

38 Haggerty, C. (1979). Doctoral Thesis, University of Aston in Birmingham

39 Hamano, H., Hori, M. and Mitsunaga, S. (1980). *Japanese Journal of Ophthalmology*, **22**, 101

40 Hedin, C. A. (1977). *Archives of Dermatology*, **113**, 1533

41 Holly, F. J. (1973). *International Ophthalmology Clinic*, **13**, 73

42 Holly, F. J. (1980). *American Journal of Optometry*, **57**, 252

43 Holly, F. J. and Lemp, M. A. (1971). *Experimental Eye Research*, **11**, 239

44 Holly, F. J., Patter, J. T. and Dohlman, C. H. (1976). *Experimental Eye Research*, **24**, 479

45 Huth, S. W., Hirano, P. and Leopold, I. H. (1980). *Experimental Archives of Ophthalmology*, **98**, 122

46 Iwata, S. (1973). *International Ophthalmology Clinic*, **13**, 29

47 Iwata, S., Lemp, M. A., Holly, F. J. and Dohlman, C. H. (1969). *Investigative Ophthalmology*, **8**, 613

48 Jones, L. T. (1966). *American Journal of Ophthalmology*, **62**, 47

49 Josephson, A. A. and Lockwood, D. W. (1964). *Journal of Immunology*, **93**, 532

50 Josephson, A. A. and Wald, A. (1969). *Proceedings of the Society for Experimental and Biological Medicine*, **131**, 677

51 Josephson, A. A. and Winer, R. S. (1968). *Journal of Immunology*, **100**, 1080

52 Kahan, I. L. and Ottovay, E. (1975). *Albrecht Von Graefes Archiv für Ophthalmologie*, **194**, 267

53 Kahan, I. L. and Ottovay, E. (1975). *Experimental Eye Research*, **20**, 129

54 Keith, C. G. (1967). *Transactions of the Ophthalmological Society of the United Kingdom*, **87**, 85

55 Kijlstra, A., Jeurissen, S. H. M. and Konig, K. M. (1983). *British Journal of Ophthalmology*, **67**, 199

56 Kijlstra, A. and Veerhuis, R. (1981). *American Journal of Ophthalmology*, **92**, 24

57 Kirchner, C. (1964). *Klinische Monatsblätter für Augenheilkunde*, **144**, 412

58 Kreuger, J., Sokoloff, N. and Bothelho, S. Y. (1976). *Investigative Ophthalmology*, **15**, 479

59 Lambert, D. W., Foster, C. S. and Perry, H. D. (1979). *Archives of Ophthalmology*, **97**, 1082

60 Linsey Farris, R., Stuchell, R. N. and Mandell, I. D. (1981). *Ophthalmology*, **88**, 852

61 Linton, R. G., Curnow, D. A. and Riley, W. J. (1961). *British Journal of Ophthalmology*, **45**, 718

62 Liotet, S. (1979) *Nouvelle Presse Medicale*, **8**, 3893

63 Little, J. M., Centifanto, Y. M. and Kaufman, H. E. (1969). *American Journal of Ophthalmology*, **68**, 898

64 Lowther, G. E., Miller, R. B. and Hill, R. M. (1970). *American Journal of Ophthalmology*, **47**, 266

65 McClellan, B. H., Whitney, C. R., Newman, P. L. P. and Allansmith, M. R. (1973). *American Journal of Ophthalmology*, **76**, 89

66 Mandell, R. B. and Fatt, I. (1965). *Nature*, **208**, 292

67 Masson, P. L., Heremans, J. F. and Dive, C. (1976). *Clinica et Chimica Acta*, **14**, 735

68 Maurice, D. M. (1973). *International Ophthalmology Clinic*, **13**, 103

69 Maurice, D. M. and Mishima, S. (1969). *Experimental Eye Research*, **9**, 43

70 Miller, R. B. (1970). *American Journal of Ophthalmology*, **47**, 773

71 Mishima, S., Gasset, A., Klyce, S. D. and Baum, J. L. (1966). *Ophthalmology*, **5**, 264

72 Mishima, S. and Maurice, D. M. (1961). *Experimental Eye Research*, **1**, 39

73 Mishima, S. and Maurice, D. M. (1961). *Experimental Eye Research*, **1**, 46

74 Mizukawa, T. (1971). *Acta Societatis Ophthalmologicae Japonicae*, **75**, 1953

75 Moor, T. X. and Tiffany, J. M. (1979). *Experimental Eye Research*, **29**, 291

76 Nicolaides, N., Kaitaranta, J. K., Rawdah, T. N., Macey, J. I., Boswell, F. M. and Smith, R. E. (1981). *Investigative Ophthalmology*, **20**, 522

77 Nicolaides, N. and Ruth, E. C. (1982/83). *Current Eye Research*, **2**, 93
78 Norn, M. S. (1969). *Acta Ophthalmologica*, **47**, 880
79 Pes, O. (1897). *Archivo di Ottalmologia*, **5**, 82
80 Pietsch, R. L. and Perlman, M. E. (1973). *Archives of Ophthalmology*, **90**, 94
81 Puffer, M. J., Neault, R. W. and Brubaker, R. F. (1980). *American Journal of Ophthalmology*, **89**, 369
82 Rennert, O. M., Kaiser, D., Sollberger, H. and Jollier-Jemelka, S. (1974). *Human Genetics*, **23**, 73
83 Ridley, F. (1928). *Proceedings of the Royal Society of Medicine*, **21**, 1495
84 Rolando, M. and Refojo, M. J. (1983). *Experimental Eye Research*, **36**, 25
85 Ronen, D., Eylan, E. and Romano, A. (1975). *Investigative Ophthalmology*, **14**, 479
86 Rosengreen, B. (1972). *Ophthalmologica*, **164**, 409
87 Ruskell, G. L. (1975). *Cell Tissue Research*, **158**, 121
88 Sapse, A., Bonavida, B., Stone, W. and Sercarz, E. E. (1968). *American Journal of Ophthalmology*, **66**, 76
89 Sapse, A. T., Bonavida, B., Stone, W. and Sercarz, F. E. (1969). *Archives of Ophthalmology*, **81**, 815
90 Schmidt, P. P., Schoessler, P. and Hill, R. M. (1974). *American Journal of Optometry*, **51**, 84
91 Singer, J. D., Cotlier, E. and Krimmer, R. (1973). *Lancet*, **ii**, 1116
92 Sorensen, T., Taagehoj, F. and Christensen, U. (1980). *Acta Ophthalmologica*, **58**, 182
93 Stuchell, R. N., Linsey Farris, R. and Mandell, I. D. (1981). *Ophthalmology*, **88**, 858
94 Terry, J. E. and Hill, R. M. (1978). *Archives of Ophthalmology*, **96**, 120
95 Thaysen, J. H. and Thorn, N. A. (1954). *American Journal of Physiology*, **178**, 160
96 Thompson, R. and Gallardo, E. (1941). *American Journal of Ophthalmology*, **24**, 635
97 Tiffany, J. M. (1978). *Experimental Eye Research*, **27**, 289
98 Tomasi, T. B. and Bienenstock, J. (1968). *Advances in Immunology*, **9**, 1
99 Tomlinson, A. and Cedarstaff, T. H. (1983). *American Journal of Optometry*, **60**, 167
100 Uotila, M. H., Soble, R. E. and Savory, J. (1972) *Investigative Ophthalmology*, **11**, 258
101 Van Haeringen, N. J. (1981). *Survey of Ophthalmology*, **26**, 84
102 Van Haeringen, N. J., Ensink, F. and Glasius, E. (1975). *Experimental Eye Research*, **21**, 395
103 Van Haeringen, N. J. and Glasius, E. (1975). *Experimental Eye Research*, **20**, 271
104 Van Haeringen, N. J. and Glasius, E. (1976). *Experimental Eye Research*, **22**, 267
105 Van Haeringen, N. J. and Glasius, E. (1976). *Ophthalmic Research*, **8**, 367
106 Van Haeringen, N. J. and Glasius, E. (1977). *Albrecht von Graefes Archiv für Ophthalmologie*, **202**, 1
107 Vannas, A. and Ruusuvaara, P. (1977). *Klinische Monatsblätter für Augenheilkunde*, **170**, 873
108 Veerhuis, R. and Kijlstra (1982). *Experimental Eye Research*, **24**, 257
109 Whitelocke, R. A., Eakins, K. E. and Bennett, A. (1974). *Proceedings of the Royal Society of Medicine*, **66**, 429
110 Yamamoto, G. K. and Allansmith, M. R. (1979). *Ophthalmology*, **88**, 758
111 Young, W. H. and Hill, R. M. (1973). *American Journal of Optometry*, **50**, 12
112 Zirm, M. and Ritzinger, I. (1978). *Klinische Monatsblätter für Augenheilkunde*, **173**, 221

Chapter 4

Lens deposition and spoilation

B. Tighe and V. Franklin

Introduction

It is perhaps not immediately obvious that the use of polymers for contact lenses represents an example of the biomedical application of synthetic materials. The use of quite similar materials in joint replacement, heart valves, membrane oxygenators and haemodialysis membranes presents specific problems associated with, for example, their biocompatibility, strength and permeability that might seem to be absent in contact lenses. This is certainly not the case, however, and the general biomedical principle of designing the material to give a balance of properties appropriate to the particular environment is of prime importance.

Although polymethyl methacrylate was used for many years as the standard 'hard' contact lens material, its properties are far from ideal. It was not, however, until hydrogel polymers (water-swollen networks based on hydrophilic monomers) appeared on the scene that any serious competitor emerged. Because hydrogels were soft and much more comfortable, thought was given for the first time to the question of overnight wear. This requires a careful balance of properties to accommodate the requirements of the three essential features of the ocular environment, namely the cornea, the eyelid and the tears.

An appropriate demonstration of the way in which soft contact lenses have influenced the development of hydrogel chemistry is found in the patent literature[55]. Since the early work of Wichterle, principally on poly (2-hydroxyethyl methacrylate), more commonly known as polyHEMA, the contact lens field has provided the basis for the examination of many more such polymers and over one hundred patents appeared in the 1970s covering a wide range of molecular structures and compositions. Although only a small proportion of these have reached commercial status, the necessary toxicology and clinical work has produced a useful introductory evaluation of several hydrogels of widely differing chemistry. There are currently available many different hydrogel contact lens materials, containing between 30 and 80% by weight of water and based on lightly cross-linked (around 0.5–1.0%) combinations of various monomers including HEMA, vinyl pyrrolidone, glycidyl methacrylate, glyceryl methacrylate, methoxyethyl methacrylate, cyclohexyl methacrylate, methyl methacrylate, methacrylic acid and substituted acrylamides. Once a particular hydrogel has obtained the necessary regulatory (FDA) approval and a generic (USAN) name in the USA, it will often be sold by different manufacturers under different trade names. This is not unlike the situation with pharmaceutical products. Table 4.1 gives examples of compositions, trade names and generic (USAN) names of a range of hydrogel lens materials.

Table 4.1 Examples of soft contact lenses and lens materials

Name	*Manufacturer/ supplier*	*Principal components*	*Water content* (%)	*USAN nomenclature*
Accusoft	Ophthalmos Inc.	HEMA, PVP	47	Droxifilcon-A
Acuvue	Vistakon	HEMA, MA	58	Etafilcon-A
Aquaflex	UCO Optics	HEMA, VP, MMA	42.5	Tetrafilcon-A
Classic	Pilkington Barnes-Hind	HEMA, VP, MMA	42.5	Tetrafilcon-A
CSI	Pilkington Barnes-Hind	MMA, Glyceryl methacrylate	41	Crofilcon-A
Durasoft	Wessley-Jessen	HEMA, EEMA	30	Phemefilcon
Eurolens	Pilkington Barnes-Hind	HEMA	38	Polymacon
Flexlens	Flexlens Inc.	HEMA, VP	46	Hidilcon-A
Gelflex	Dow Corning	HEMA, MMA, TEGMA	36	Dimefilcon-A
Hydro-curve (1)	Soft Lenses Inc.	HEMA, VP	46	Hefilcon-A
Hydro-curve	Soft Lenses Inc.	HEMA, Diacetone acrylamide, MAA	55	Buficon-A
Hydron	Hydron Europe	HEMA	38	Polymacon
Menicon soft	Toyo Contact Lens	HEMA, VA, PMA	30	Mafilcon-A
Naturvue	Automated Optics	HEMA, VP	43	Hefilcon-A
Permalens	Pilkington Barnes-Hind	HEMA, VP, MA	71	Perfilcon-A
Permaflex	Pilkington Barnes-Hind	MMA, VP	74	Surfilcon-A
Sauflon-70	Contact Lens Mfg	VP, MMA	70	Lidofilcon-A
Sof-form	Salvatori	HEMA, BMA	43	Deltafilcon-A
Softcon	American Optical	HEMA, PVP	55	Vifilcon-A
Soflens	Bausch and Lomb	HEMA	38	Polymacon
Softmate II	Pilkington Barnes-Hind	HEMA, Diacetone acrylamide, MAA	55	Bufilcon-A
Weicon	Titmus Eurocon	HEMA	38	Polymacon

Abbreviations: AMA, alkyl methacrylate; BMA, butyl (probably isobutyl) methacrylate; EEMA, ethoxyethyl methacrylate; HEMA, 2-hydroxyethyl methacrylate; MA, methacrylic acid; MMA, methyl methacrylate; PMA, pentyl methacrylate; PVP, poly(vinyl pyrrolidone) (i.e. graft copolymer); TEGMA, triethylene glycol methacrylate; VA, vinyl acetate; VP, *N*-vinyl pyrrolidone.

Although several different monomer combinations are shown in Table 4.1, their behaviour is conveniently subsumed under the four USA classifications of generic soft lens materials ('low water content non-ionic' – group I, 'low water content ionic' – group II, 'high water content non-ionic' – group III, 'high water content ionic' – group IV). Of these, the high water content ionic materials are set apart by their relatively porous networks. They are the only group into which the low molecular weight (< 20 kDa) proteins can diffuse. The importance of this feature of group IV lens materials and spoilation will be discussed further at a later stage of this chapter. Of the remainder, the great similarity in behaviour stems from the fact that *N*-vinyl pyrrolidone and 2-hydroxyethyl methacrylate are almost invariably employed as the hydrophilic centres.

The three important aspects of the ocular environment, in terms of polymer design, are the cornea, the eyelid and the tears. The cornea is avascular and the need to ensure oxygen transport to the corneal surface governs the permeability requirement of the hydrogel. This is governed by the equilibrium water content of the gel. The eyelid dictates the range of acceptable mechanical properties, with comfort and retention of visual stability during the blink cycle dominating acceptable upper and lower limits of elasticity. The water content, although influential, is not the sole structural factor of importance here. The water structure within the gel, together with chain stiffness and interchain forces are capable of exerting a dominating influence. The interaction of the hydrogel with tears is an important example of interaction of a biomaterial with a complex biological environment. The behaviour has many similar features to that observed at other body sties and is a function of the surface properties of the hydrogel[45,55,56].

Although the design and successful use of contact lens materials requires attention to mechanical properties, which are controlled by polymer structure and cross-link density as well as water content, probably the most persistent problem of the last decade is biocompatibility. This topic is usually referred to as ocular compatibility, or spoilation, in the contact lens field. The problem of deposit formation on soft contact lenses may appear to be a unique phenomenon of fairly recent origin, however, this is not so. The underlying processes that govern this sort of interaction are common to many situations in which materials come into contact with biological solutions. Thus, the deposition of tear fluid debris, the clotting of blood on foreign surface, the formation of plaque, marine fouling and the fouling of membranes used in biochemical separations are all examples of the same fundamental phenomenon. The initiating processes in all these interactions are referred to as biological interface conversion processes and they can be readily studied in the eye, whereas they can only be studied with considerable difficulty in for example, blood contact devices. The reason for this is obvious. Whereas a contact lens may be removed and analysed after only a few minutes wear, it is exceedingly difficult to conceive of a surgical technique that would allow implantation and removal with equal rapidity in a blood contact situation. The eye, therefore, presents a unique opportunity for *in vivo* studies of biocompatibility provided that the detailed nature and composition of the tear film are sufficiently understood.

The nature and composition of the tear film (see Chapter 3)

The tear film covering the cornea was first suggested to have a three-layered structure by Wolff in 1954[62]. It is generally believed that this structure consists essentially of the superficial lipid layer, the aqueous below this, and an adsorbed mucin layer which adheres to the epithelium. The superficial lipid layer is believed to comprise

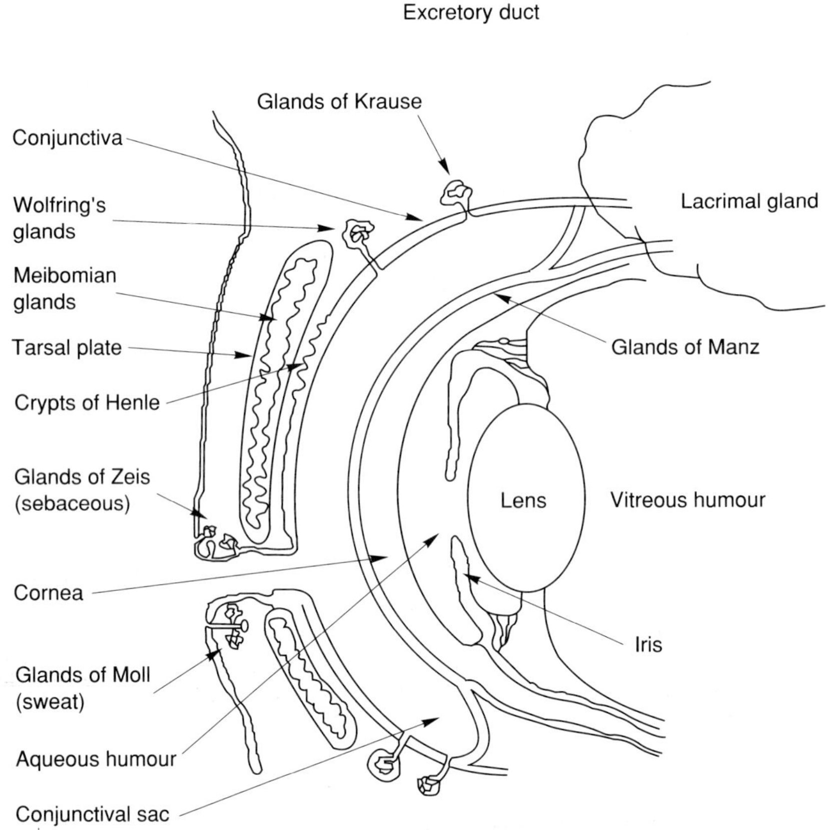

Figure 4.1 Cross-section though the anterior of the eye to show the location of the main tear-forming glands

about 1% of the total thickness (about 0.1 μm thick); the middle aqueous layer represents over 98% of the tear film and is 7 μm thick; and the inner mucoid layer is most commonly quoted as comprising under 0.5% of the film, being 0.02–0.05 μm thick. More recent observations have shown, however, that mucins become diluted towards the aqueous layer and interact with and mask the hydrophobicity of the lipids, making the delineation of different tear film layers somewhat arbitrary.

Human tears are formed by a group of glands collectively known as the lacrimal system. The secretory apparatus consists of the main and accessory lacrimal glands (source of the aqueous tear components), the meibomian glands (secrete lipids), and the conjunctival goblet cells (secrete mucous glycoproteins). The accessory lacrimal glands supply the minute-to-minute supply of tears, while the main lacrimal gland functions as a back-up reflex system by flooding the eye in response to injury, irritation of emotions (reflex tearing). Normal tear volume is between about 7.0–10.0 ml, and there is a continual secretion (non-reflex) rate of about 1 ml/min (the range of flow rates being 0.5–2.2 ml/min) from the accessory lacrimal glands. The various secretions contribute to a complex mixture which include proteins, enzymes, lipids, metabolites, electrolytes, hydrogen ions, and also drugs excreted in tears. The location and distribution of the glands responsible for tear formation are shown in Figure 4.1.

Protein components

These are found chiefly in the middle aqueous layer which originates from the main lacrimal gland located in the superior temporal aspect of the orbit, and from accessory lacrimal glands (glands of Krause and of Wolfring, the infraorbital gland, and the glands of the plica and the caruncle) lining the surface of the conjunctiva. The total concentration of proteinaceous substances in the tear fluid is variously estimated to be between 0.3–7.0% (800–2200 ml/100 ml). The concentration varies depending on whether the tears are unstimulated, emotion or irritant-induced. Using electrophoretic techniques, more than 60 protein components can be detected in normal tear fluid. Of these, more than 20 have been shown to be secreted by the lacrimal gland. The major tear proteins are albumin, tear specific pre albumin, lactoferrin, lysozyme and the immunoglobulins.

Lipid components

The superficial lipid oily layer is secreted by the meibomian glands and the glands of Moll and Zeis which are situated at the edge of the eyelids. The composition of meibomian lipids in humans has been found to vary considerably among individuals. The principal non-polar component of the tear film lipid has been identified as a mixture of waxes and sterol esters, with the sterol esters accounting for nearly one-third of the mixture. Chromatographic analysis has demonstrated the presence of all lipid classes in the meibomian secretion: hydrocarbons, wax esters, cholesterol esters, triglycerides and, in lesser amounts, diglycerides, monoglycerides, fatty acids, cholesterol and phospholipids

Mucus components

The inner mucoid layer is secreted by specialized conjunctival cells in the crypts of Henle and the glands of Manz. The composition of the mucus layer, which is the innermost layer of the tear film, has been analysed to be:

Salts	1.0%
Free protein	0.5–1.0%
Glycoprotein	0.5–1.0%
Water	>95%

The electrolyte content resembles that of serum or bile. Other constituents include immunoglobulins, salts, urea, glucose, leucocytes, tissue debris, and enzymes such as β-lysin, peroxidase and lysozyme. The glycoproteins, or mucins, are 50–80% carbohydrate, with the oligosaccharides attached to a protein backbone of molecular weight $2.0–15.0 \times 10^6$ Daltons, which is composed of about 800 amino acid residues. Serine and threonine comprise 40% of the total amino acid and form the O-glycosidic link with the side chains which cover approximately 63% of the backbone. The sugar side chains are composed of up to 12 sugar residues, which in human mucus secretions are made up of the same 5 monosaccharides; galactose, *N*-acetylgalactosamine, *N*-acetylglucosamine, fucose and *N*-acetylneuraminic acid (sialic acid). The link with the protein backbone is formed by galactose, and the terminal sugar group is either fucose or sialic acid. Other sugar residues may bear ester sulphate groups, and these, together with the sialic acid groups, provide mucin with its overall negative charge. The structure, which is illustrated in Figure 4.2,

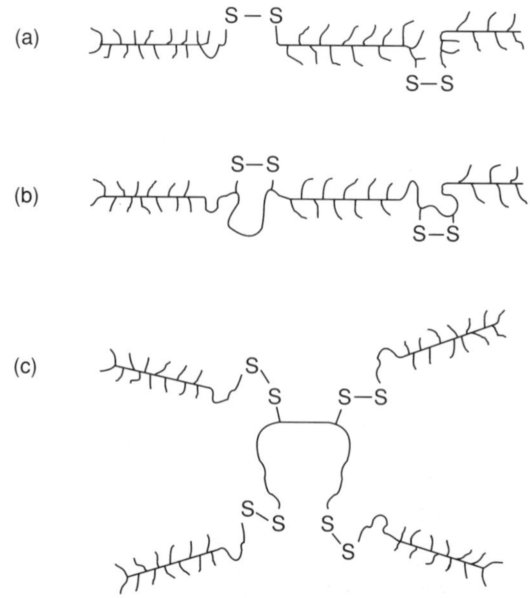

Figure 4.2 Proposed model of the mucus glycoprotein macromolecule: (*a*) subunits linked via disulphide bonds; (*b*) subunits linked via protein stabilized by disulphide bonds; (*c*) subunits joined as a tetramer

means that areas of both sugar and protein are exposed to the solution, although the former predominate. The presence of cysteine amino acids enables the formation of disulphide bridges between or within molecules, and proline residues allow the molecules to bend and assume random structures in solution. Cross-linking through disulphide bridges produces polymers of high molecular weight that bind to similar polymers by weak interactions of the carbohydrate chains to form a gel. Mucin has an important part to play in corneal wettability and tear stability, although the precise mechanisms of interaction with the corneal surface is a subject of current discussion. This chapter will deal with spoilation from two aspects. The first is the discrete analysis mechanisms used to study the ultimate spoilation phenomena as undoubtedly there is much to be learned about the biochemical species involved in the early stages of spoilation from these deposit forms. Second, because of the trend towards disposable and planned replacement lenses, the special aspects of these types of lenses will be considered.

Characterization of contact lens deposits and manifestations of lens spoilation

An important aspect of the role of hydrogels as contact lenses is the range and nature of these phenomena which are commonly collected together under the umbrella term 'spoilation'. Ironically, this only became a major materials problem with the advent of soft hydrogel lenses providing as they did greater comfort and allowing extended wear times. The term spoilation encompasses the physical and chemical changes in

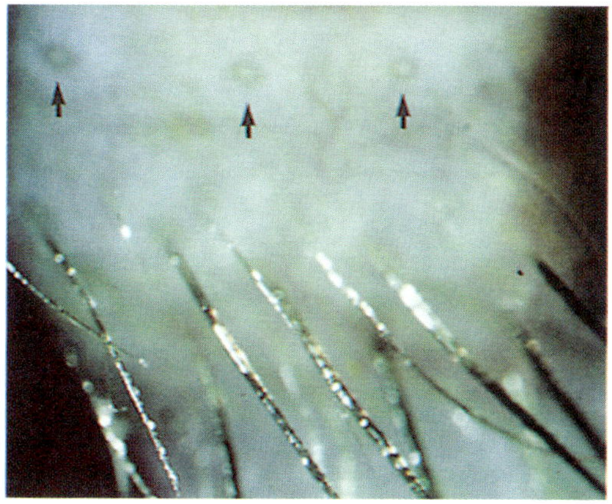

Plate 1 Openings of the meibomian glands

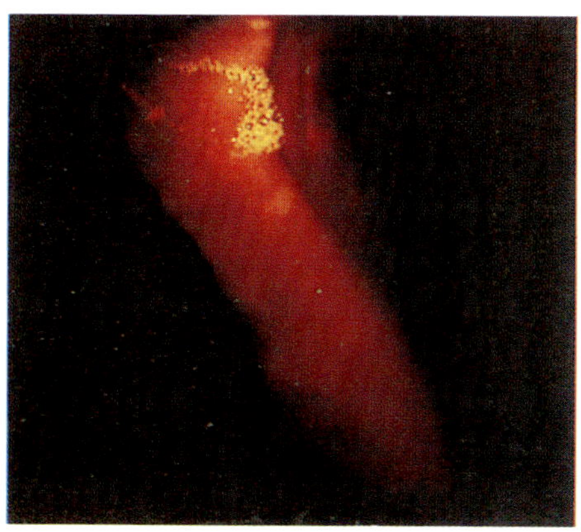

Plate 2 Foam in the tear film as a result of meibomian gland dysfunction (foam frequently flows in the opposite direction to tears and often accumulates at the temporal canthus)

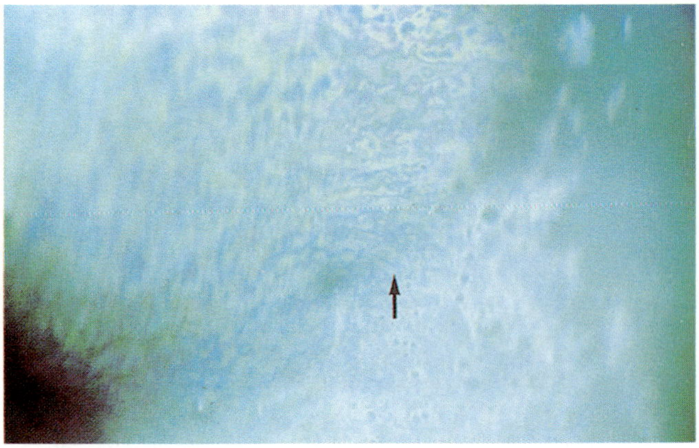

Plate 3 Tear lipid phase appearance. (*a*) Pre-corneal tear film: the lipid layer is continuous over the limbus where a local thinning is appearing (↑). Dust particles are trapped within this layer. The colours displayed denote a thicker than average layer. This is usually a favourable sign for contact lens wear. (*b*) Pre-contact lens tear film (PMMA lens). The localized interference colours are produced within the aqueous phase of the pre-lens tear film. Five visible fringes denote a thickness of approximately 1.5 μm. The lipid is absent from the front lens surface. The PMMA lens edge acts as a barrier to the spreading of the grey lipid layer visible outside the lens (0.01 μm thick). (*c*) Pre-contact lens tear film (low wetting angle material). The better wetting qualities of the lens are demonstrated by a thick pre-lens aqueous phase (20 fringes 4 μm) and the presence of a visible lipid phase ($=0.01$ μm) on the left of the picture (reproduced by permission of J. P. Guillon, 1983)

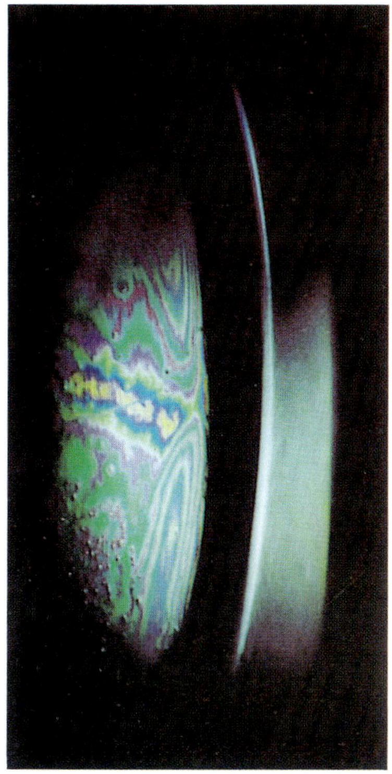

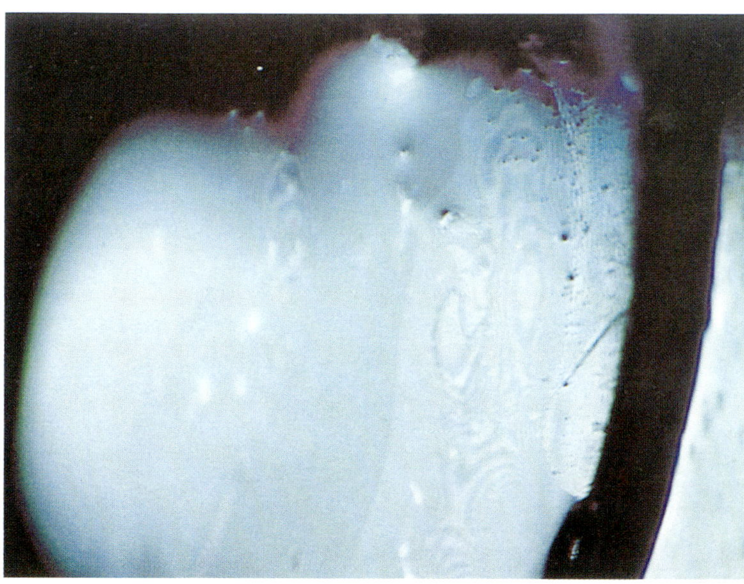

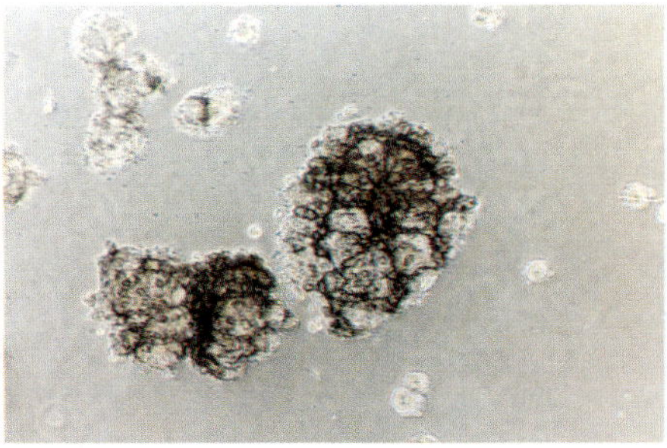

Plate 4 Discrete elevated deposit morphology. Phase contrast ×260

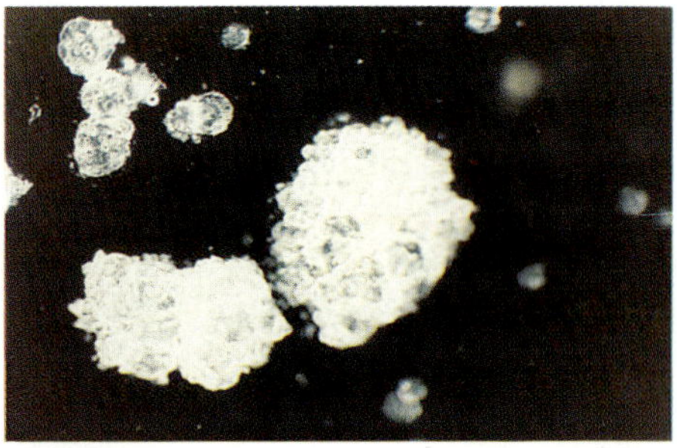

Plate 5 Discrete elevated deposit morphology. Darkfield ×260

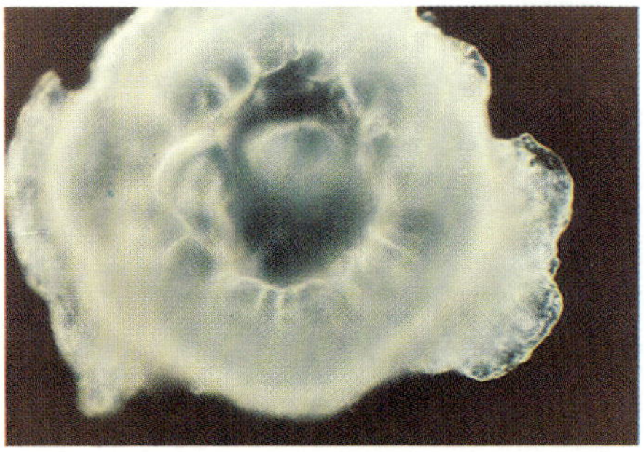

Plate 6 Discrete elevated deposit morphology, lobular component. Darkfield ×260

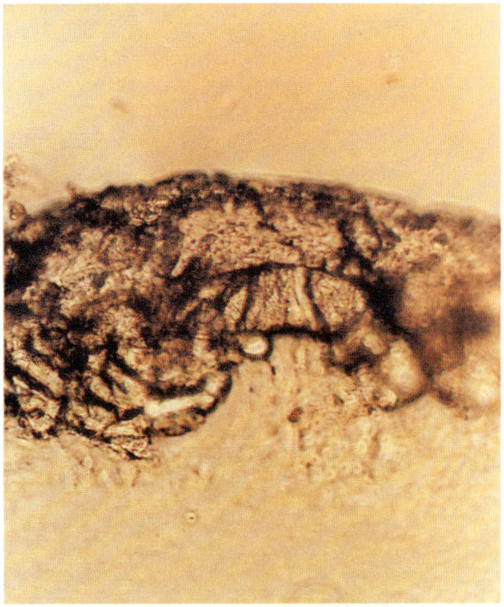

Plate 7 Longitudinal section (unstained) of a discrete elevated deposit. Phase contrast ×260

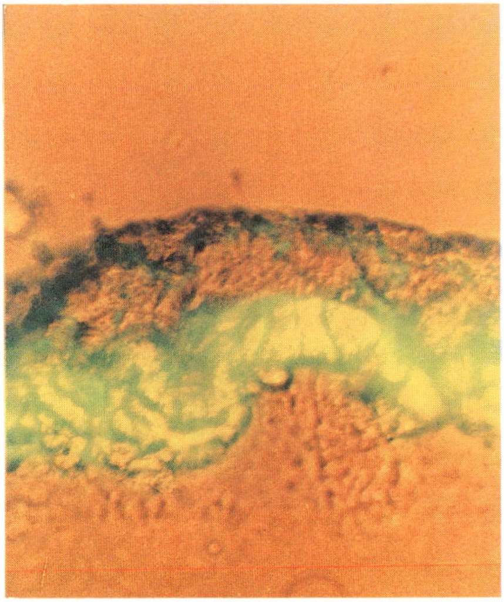

Plate 8 Autofluorescent profile of the longitudinal section shown in Plate 7. Phase contrast ×260

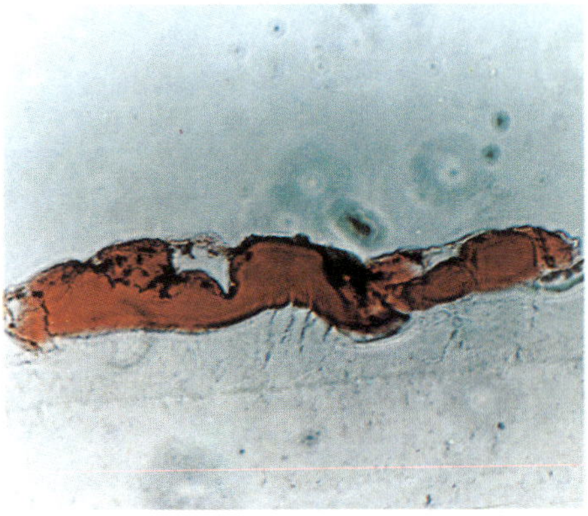

Plate 9 Longitudinal section (Oil Red O stained) of a discrete elevated deposit. Phase contrast ×260

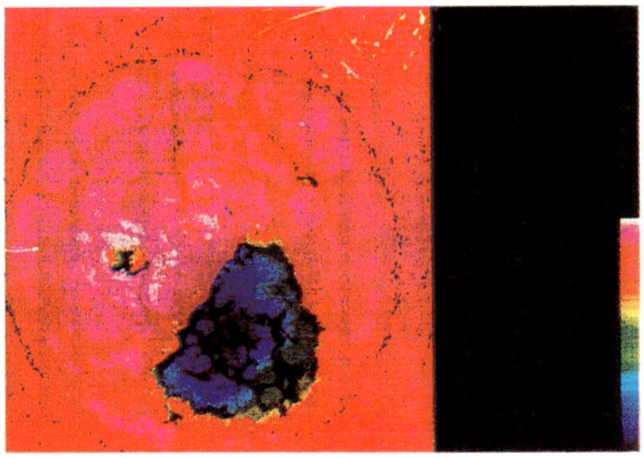

Plate 10 Pseudo-colour composite image of a discrete elevated deposit. Right-hand scale shows the distribution of colour from highest to lowest point in the deposit

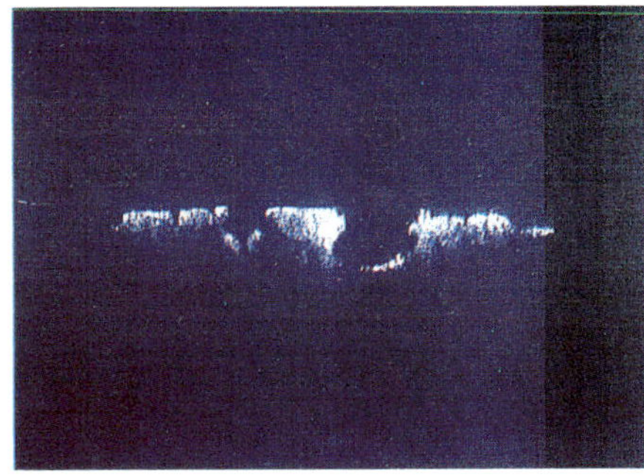

Plate 11 Section through discrete elevated white spot deposit. The images have been produced by reassembly of the individual layers collected in Plate 7

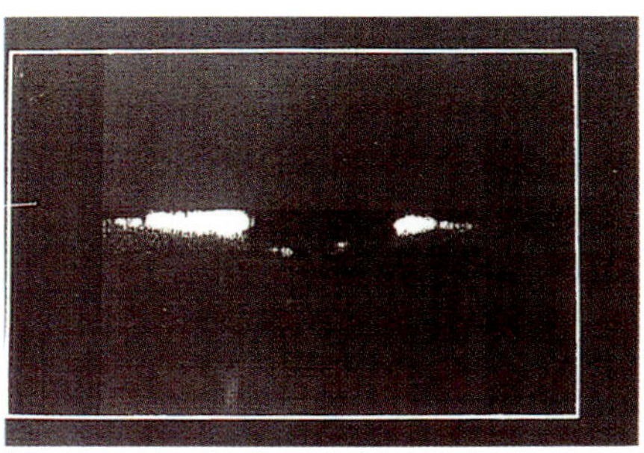

Plate 12 Section through discrete elevated white spot deposit. The images have been produced by reassembly of the individual layers collected in Plate 7

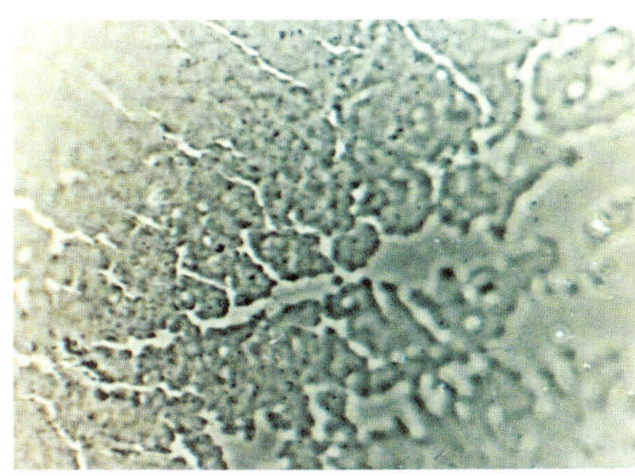

Plate 13 Optical photomicrograph of lens surface, typical white film coating. Phase contrast ×480

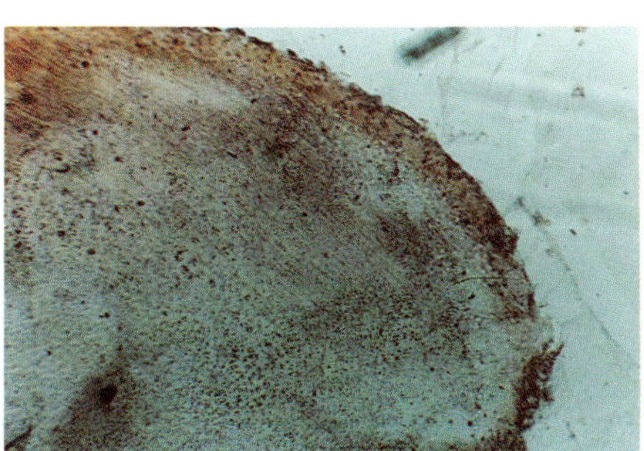

Plate 14 Stained section through lens with white film coating (perpendicular to optic zone, anterior to posterior surface). Von Kossa stain, phase contrast ×480

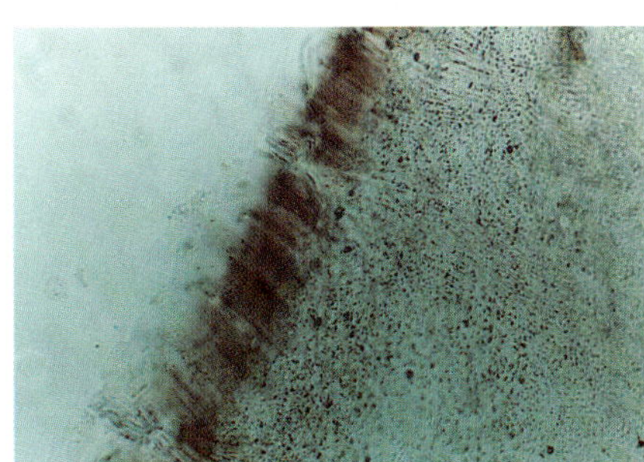

Plate 15 Stained section of lens with white film coating (parallel to and through optical zone of lens). Von Kossa stain, phase contrast ×480

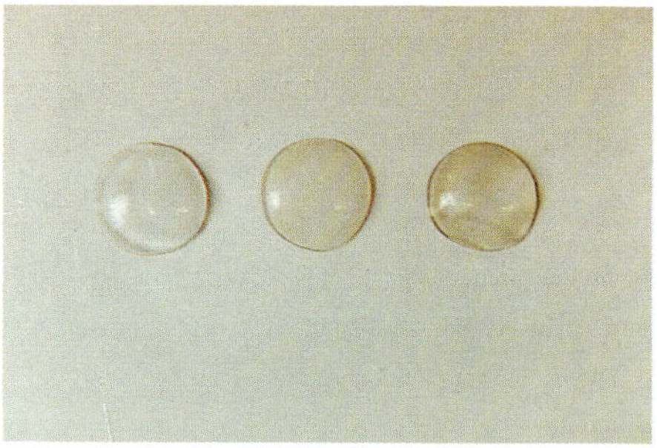

Plate 16 Three worn lenses illustrating various relatively early stages of the discoloration process

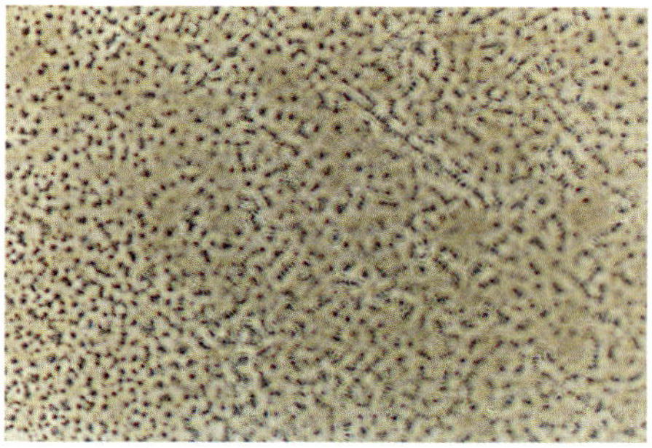

Plate 17 Optical micrograph of a typical yellow-brown lens viewed normal to the surface and showing clearly the individual pigment deposits

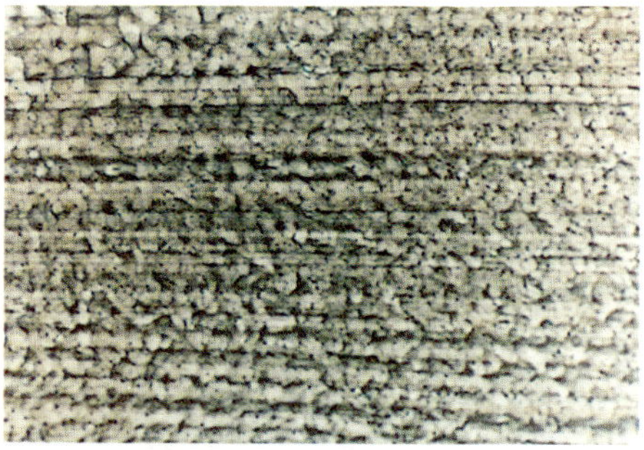

Plate 18 Optical micrograph of a section through the lens illustrating the even distribution of the pigment through the lens

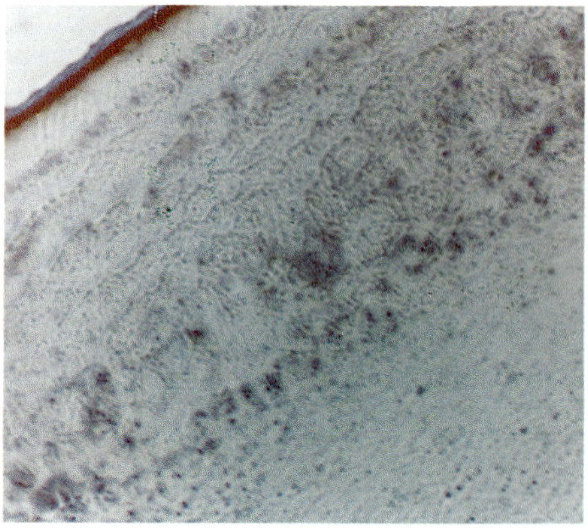

Plate 19 Optical micrograph of a phase contrast section of a yellow-brown lens. The lens surface is visible in the top left-hand corner

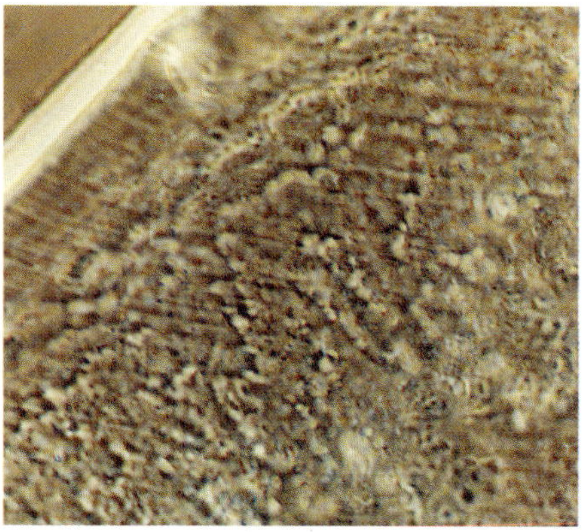

Plate 20 Optical micrograph of a section of a lens as Plate 19, but stained (blue) with Schmorl reagent

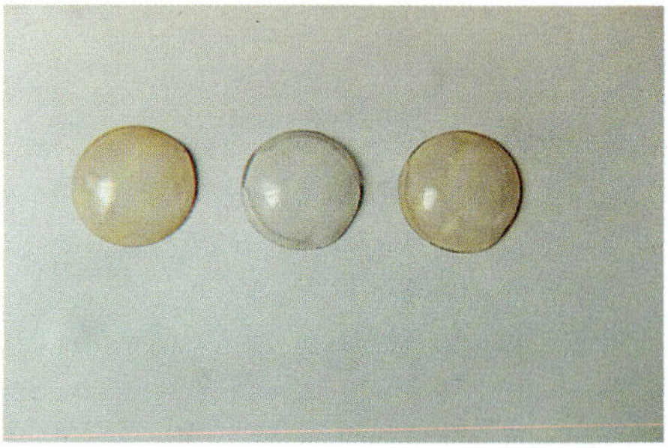

Plate 21 Examples of yellow-brown discoloured lenses produced by sorbic acid preserved saline in conjunction with thermal sterilization

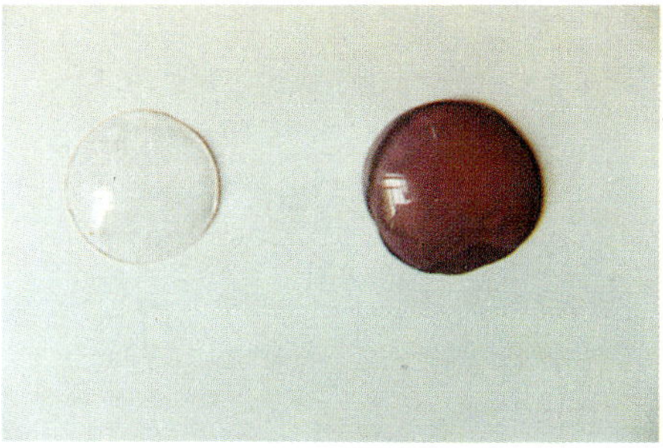

Plate 22 Retention of methyl orange dye by a 40% EWC HEMA lens (left) and a 70% EWC VP/MMA lens (right) after leaching in distilled water

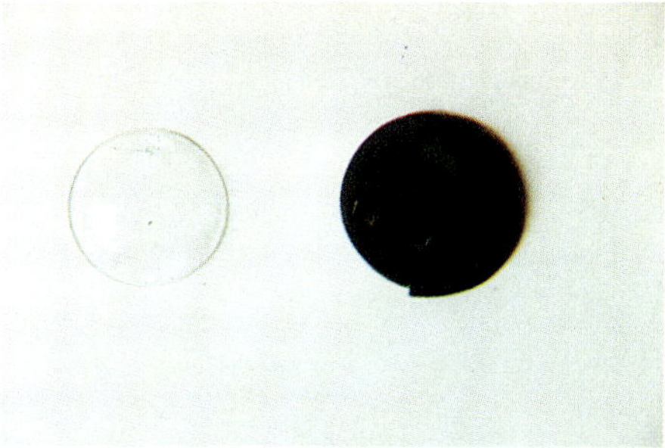

Plate 23 Retention of naphthol green dye by a 40% EWC HEMA lens (left) and a 70% EWC VP/MMA lens (right) after leaching in distilled water

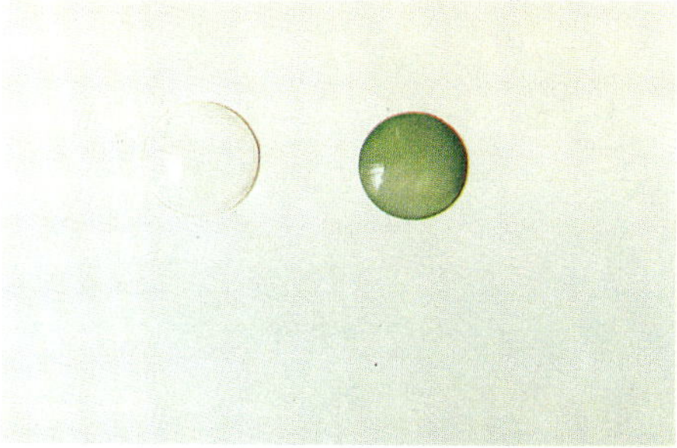

Plate 24 Retention of murexide dye by a 40% EWC HEMA lens (left) and a 70% EWC VP/MMA lens (right) after leaching in distilled water

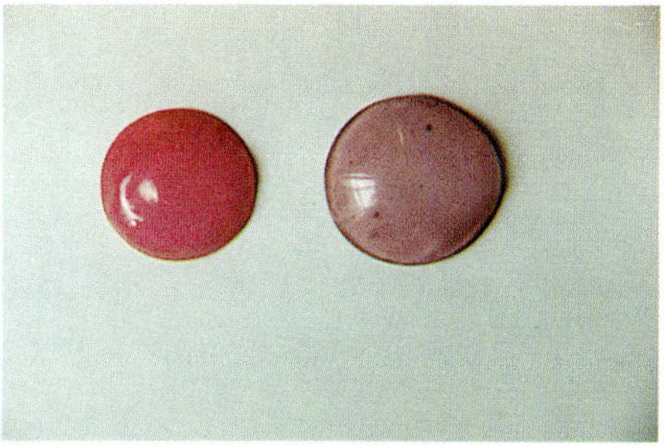

Plate 25 Retention of rhodamine B dye by a 40% EWC HEMA lens (left) and a 70% EWC VP/MMA lens (right) after leaching in distilled water

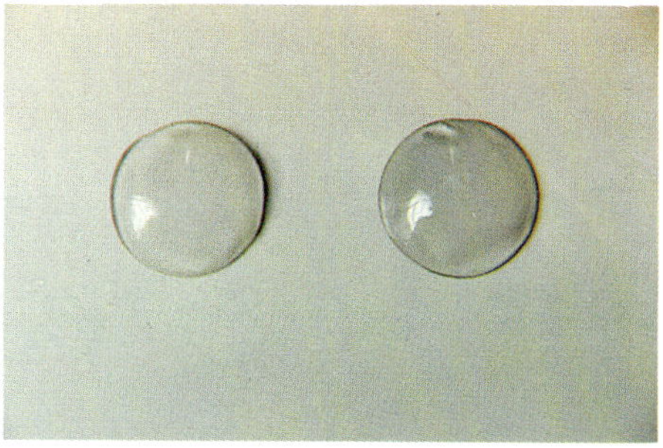

Plate 26 Two discoloured high water content vinyl pyrrolidone-containing lenses (Lunelle)

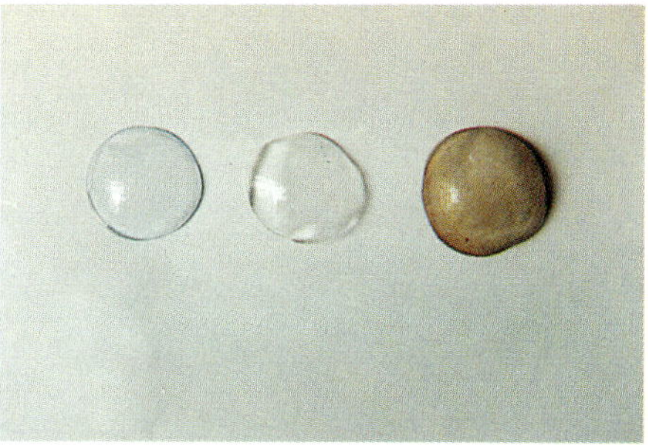

Plate 27 Three lenses discoloured with low levels of manganese

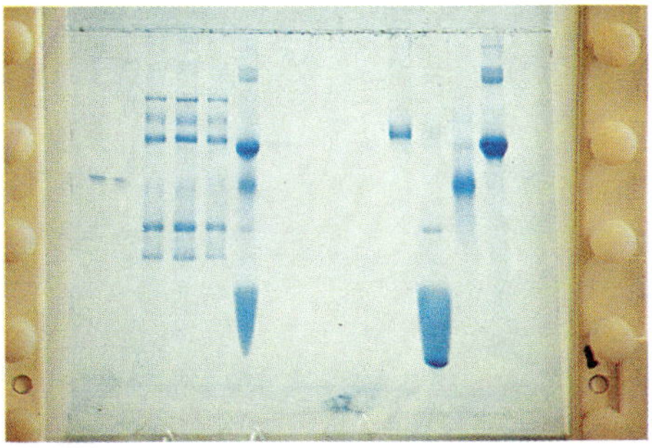

Plate 28 Electrophoresis gel stained with a conventional Coomassie blue stain

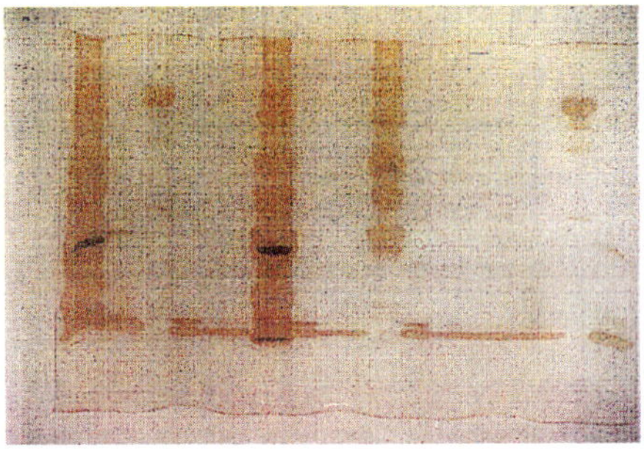

Plate 29 Polyacrylamide electrophoresis gel stained with silver stain

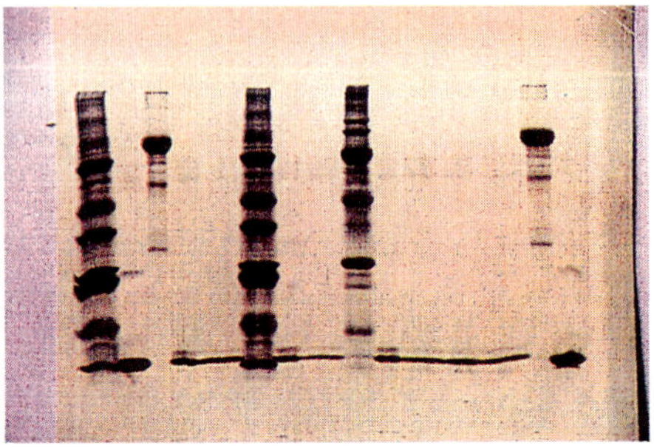

Plate 30 Biotin avidin stained electroblot of the same samples as in Plate 29

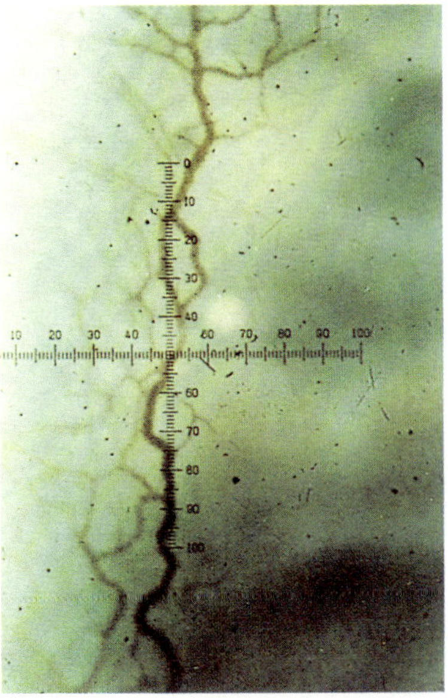

Plate 31. Retroillumination of fine limbral arcades (reproduced by permission of Humphrys, 1982[16])

Plate 32 Slit lamp appearance of infiltrative keratitis (reproduced by permission of Josephson and Caffery, *International Contact Lens Clinic*, 1979[23])

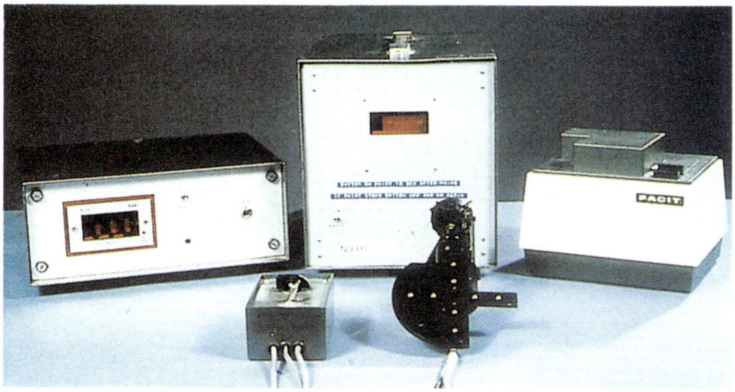

Plate 33 A self-recording pachometer

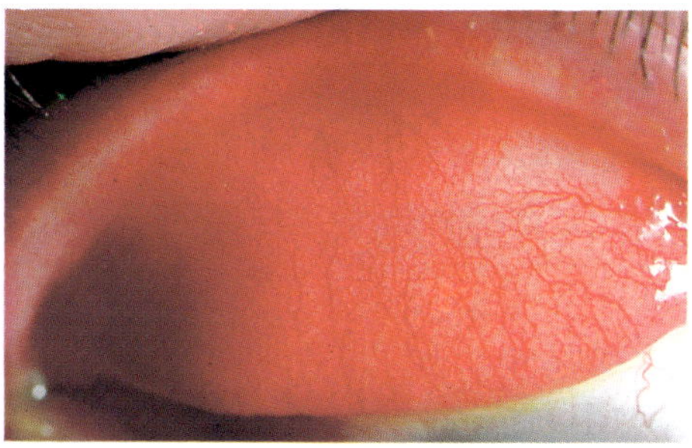

(a)

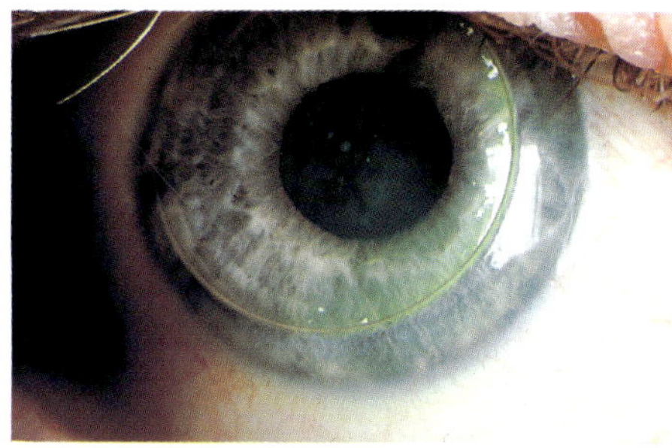

(b)

Plate 34 (*a*) Early contact lens associated papillary conjunctivitis showing hyperaemic, infiltrated and papillary upper tarsal conjunctiva; (*b*) same case showing absence of bulbar conjunctival hyperaemia but mucous deposits on the surface of the contact lens

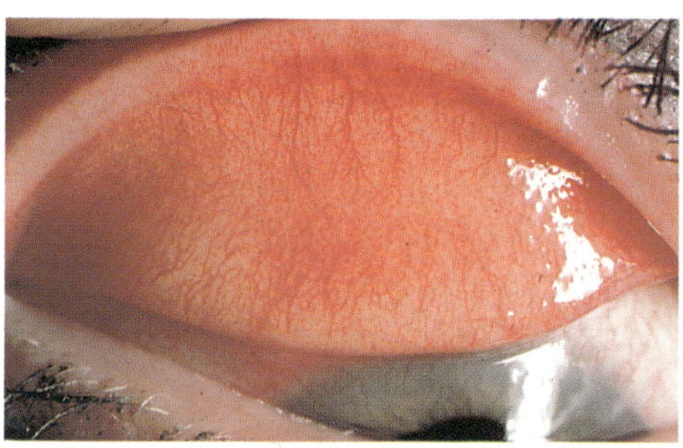

(a)

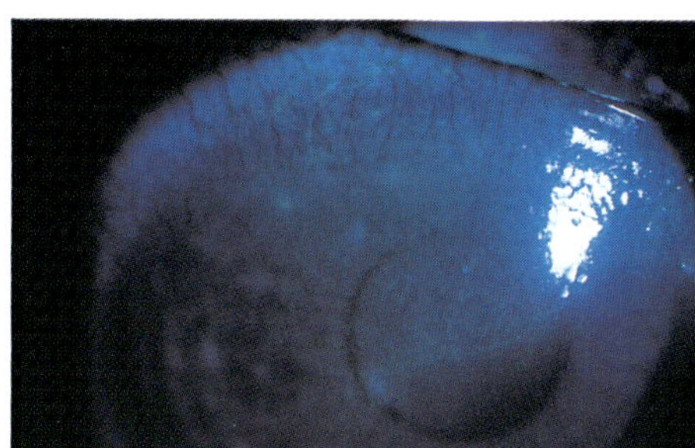

(b)

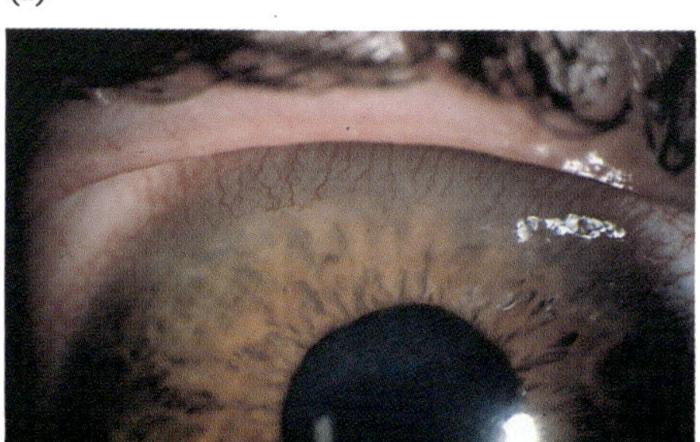

(c)

Plate 35 (*a*) Upper tarsal conjunctiva in thiomersal toxicity showing conjunctival changes indistinguishable from those in Plate 34(*a*); (*b*) and (*c*) corneal changes in moderately advanced thiomersal toxicity with bulbar conjunctival hyperaemia distinguishing it from contact lens associated papillary conjunctivitis. Superior corneal neovascularization is associated with opaque corneal epithelium, staining with fluorescein, in the upper quadrant

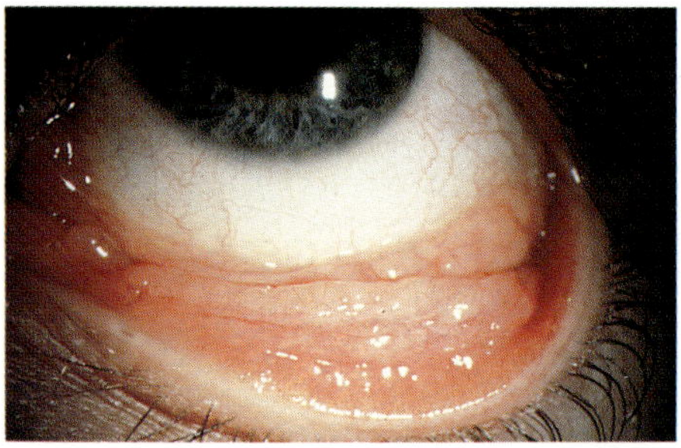

Plate 36 Bulbar and tarsal conjunctival follicles in chlamydial conjunctivitis

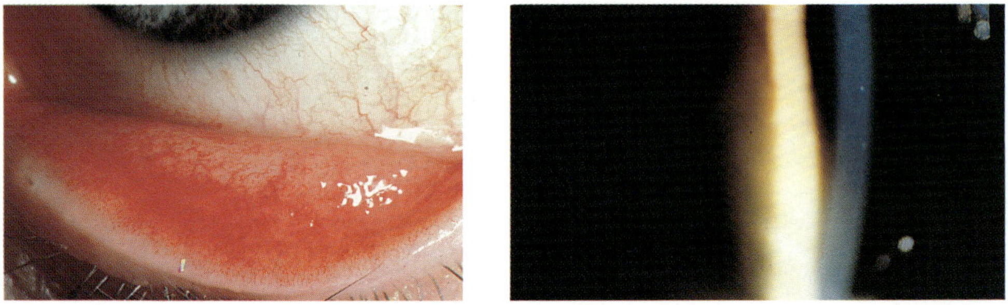

(a) (b)

Plate 37 (*a*) and (*b*) Inferior bulbar conjunctival follicles in early adenovirus conjunctivitis, the larger follicles, growing through the hyperaemic conjunctiva, can be seen by their specular reflection. Early chlamydial conjunctivitis may be identical in appearance. The fine punctate keratitis in adenovirus infection is typical of early viral or chlamydial keratoconjunctivitis

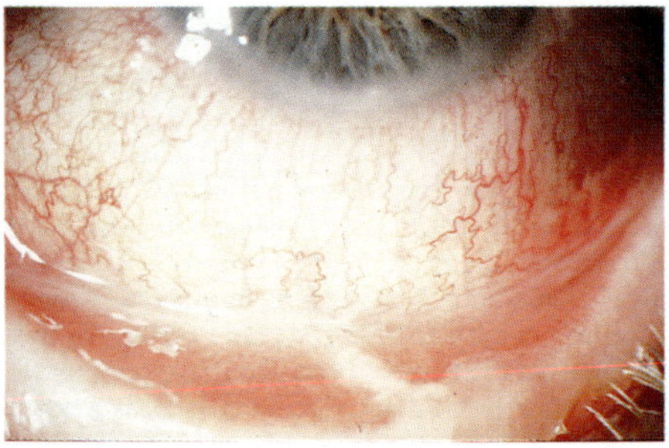

Plate 38 Mucopurulent conjunctivitis, with diffuse bulbar and tarsal hyperaemia and tarsal papillae, in early acute bacterial conjunctivitis

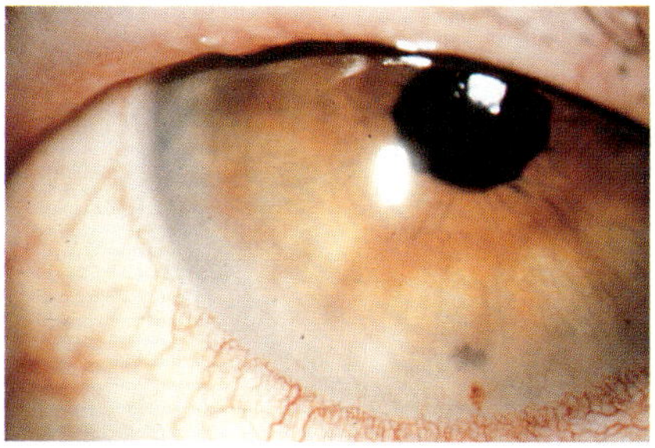

(a)

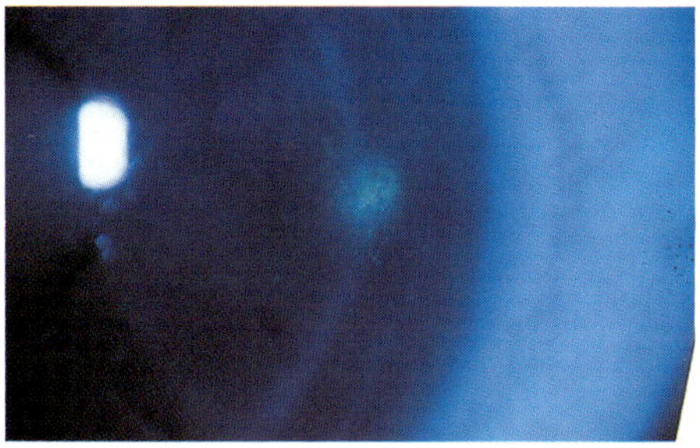

(b)

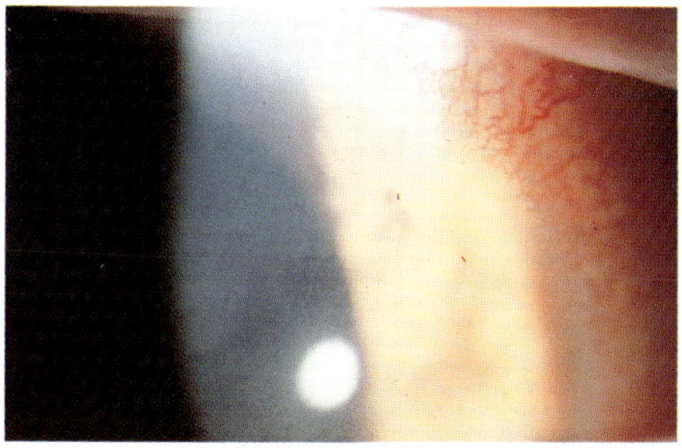

(c)

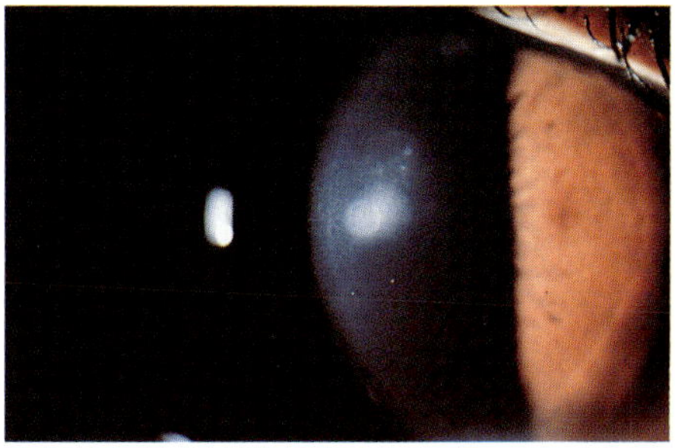

(d)

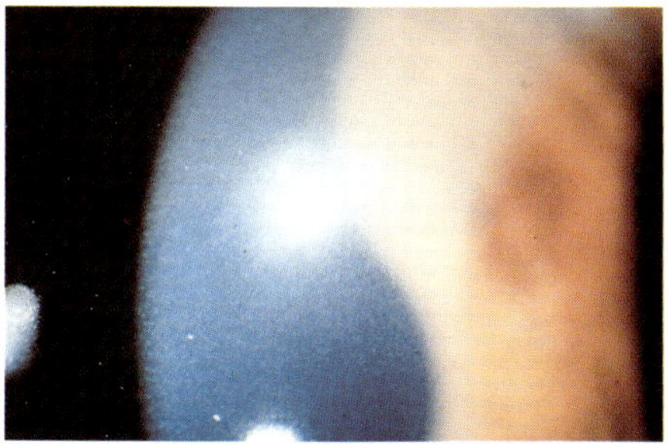

(e)

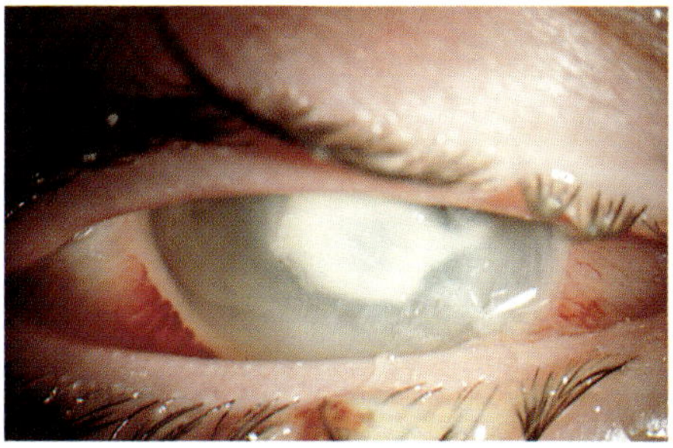

(f)

Plate 39 (*a*) Peripheral aseptic corneal infiltrates, with intact epithelium, in the user of an extended wear soft lens. (*b*) Similar peripheral aseptic corneal infiltrate in a use of disposable soft lenses but with epithelial breakdown over a more intense area of infiltration. (*c*). Intense mid-peripheral corneal infiltrate in a user of a daily wear soft contact lens which may be aseptic or infective. Cultures were negative. (*d*) Early pseudomonas keratitis showing more extensive corneal infiltrate around the principal lesion. Comparison with (*c*) demonstrates the difficulty of differentiating between lesions based on the clinical appearance of the cornea. (*e*) Early staphylococcal keratitis showing a similar appearance to (*d*). (*f*) Severe pseudomonas keratitis like this can develop within 24 hours of onset after starting like the lesion in (*d*)

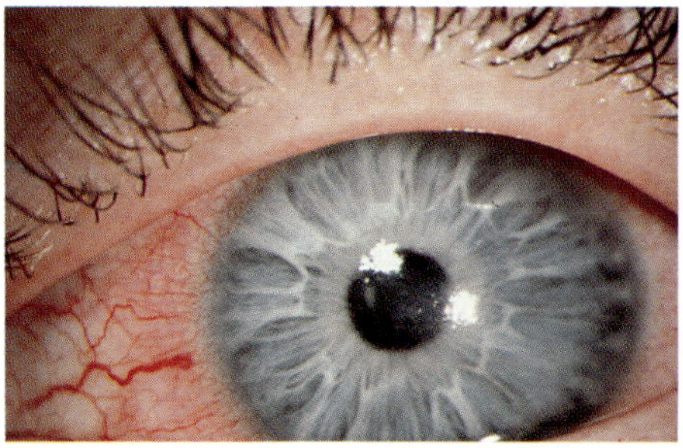

(a)

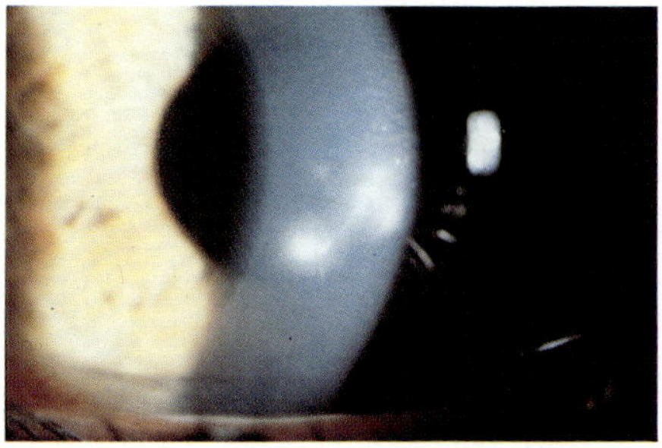

(b)

Plate 40 (*a*) Early Acanthamoeba keratitis showing generalized bulbar hyperaemia which is excessive in relation to the corneal findings showing a slightly irregular corneal epithelium, as demonstrated by the specular reflection, and minimal corneal infiltrate. (*b*) Radial keratoneuritis in early Acanthamoeba keratitis. This is a distinctive characteristic of early infection that is present in 60% of early cases the nature of hydrogel contact lenses and the various extraneous deposits which may impair the optical properties of the lens or produce symptoms of discomfort and often intolerance to the wearer. The reported incidence of lens spoilation in clinical records varies from less than 10% to over 80% of extended wear lenses. Lens spoilation occurs in the majority of cases within 3–6 months of daily or especially extended wear, although it has been observed within 48 hours of wear.

Although it is convenient in an overview to divide the observed types of spoilation into different classes, such a classification is largely artificial. There is considerable overlap between the classes and systematic analyses of the results of spoilation are rarely undertaken in conjunction with clinical reports relating to incidence. The classification is best regarded, therefore, as a grouping of various related types of clinically observed phenomena. An indication is given of the current view of the occurrence, chemical composition and potential aetiology for each clinically observed 'class' of lens spoilation[8,24,30,31,35,61].

Discrete elevated deposits (white spots)

The most chemically complex manifestations of ocular incompatibility are discrete elevated or mucoprotein-lipid deposits, the so-called 'white spots' varying in diameter up to around 1 mm and found on the anterior lens surface. Ruben and others[58] cited the deposition of mucoprotein-lipid deposits on lenses as a major cause of spoilation, with a reported incidence of up to 80% of patients fitted. Such a figure is very much higher than the incidence in current clinical practice, however. This is in part due to the increased emphasis on disposable or frequent replacement lenses in recent years.

There is a considerable variation in the reports of the chemical composition of this group of deposits from patient to patient which has given rise to continued speculation as to their origin. Much of the variation arises from differences in quality and sensitivity of the analytical work. Individual variations do exist, however, especially in the mucoprotein content and in the meibomian secretions, and this may be further influenced by the stimulus of contact lens wear.

Lens coatings

A major manifestation of spoilation involves surface films, coatings and plaques. One group of these, which superficially appeared to be related to the discrete 'white spot' deposits, but are chemically quite different, are the so-called protein films. Such films are characterized by a thin, semiopaque, white superficial layered structure which consists of denatured protein. General accumulation of protein films on the soft lenses leads to an increase in surface haziness and surface rugosity (roughness) and a decrease in visual acuity results due both to lens opacity and to poor lens movement on the eye. Red eye, increased irritation and conjunctivitis are typical patient responses to protein covered lenses[34].

Inorganic films are similar in gross appearance to protein films although their incidence is lower. Heavy inorganic films often cause damage to the lens surface, since the material may penetrate into the lens matrix. These are frequently covered with protein that smoothes the underlying rough inorganic material, which is composed mainly of calcium phosphate. The deposit may well be hydroxyapatite, the thermodynamically stable form of calcium phosphate commonly encountered in biological conditions[7]. Microbial spoilation of lens surfaces is common[25], but generally produces an adverse ocular effect before being physically discernible.

Lens discoloration

Discoloration of hydrogel contact lenses is a major problem in the long-term use of such materials in the eye and this, together with the problems of microbial contamination and poor mechanical durability, has led to the current interest in disposables and planned replacement contact lenses. Discoloration of hydrogels has been linked with several factors including nicotine from cigarettes, topical adrenalin and topical vasoconstrictors, as well as components from the tear fluid. The possible nature of discoloration is described in various papers of which the most noteworthy is that of Kleist[36]. Yellow or brown discoloured lenses have been found to contain granular particles deposited just below the surface of the lens. More recent work has highlighted many of the chemical pathways involved[13,20,57]. The hydrogel acts as an inert matrix for these reactions; discoloration reactions involving the lens polymer are extremely rare.

From this brief overview certain obvious conclusions may be drawn. The chemical composition of lens deposits is extremely complex and nearly all chemical components found to be present in lens deposits are contained within the tear film. This raises analytical problems that have required detailed study, some of which are described in a subsequent section. It has been noted by several workers that differing hydrogel polymeric compositions appear to highlight relatively specific deposit types. Another variable in what appears to be a multifactoral problem is the composition of the tear film – great differences in component concentrations have been noted from one individual to another. It is now clear that hydrophilic soft lens spoilation results primarily from the interaction of the polymer with the microenvironment of the eye. Differing degrees of spoilation from one polymeric composition to another result not only from difference in surface and bulk chemistry of the material but also differences in the patient tear film, together with the design and fit of the lens. For this reason its mechanism of formation is extremely instructive in understanding the underlying problem of hydrogel interactions with tears.

Tears and the white spot phenomenon: the structure and composition of white spot deposits

One of the most fascinating problems in contact lens spoilation is the mechanism of formation of white spots. These have parallels in other body sites and are similar to deposits encountered on heart valves, bile-duct prostheses and ureteral and urethral implants. Whatever other forms of spoilation take place on a given material, white spot formation is the inevitable consequence of long-term wear of all the generic materials listed in Table 4.1. Work in our laboratories has for some time been concerned with the detailed morphology and chemical composition of these deposits on lenses of different materials and with different surface characteristics.

There is a considerable variation in the reports of the chemical composition of this group of deposits from patient to patient which has given rise to continued speculation as to their origin. Much of the variation arises from differences in quality and sensitivity of the analytical work. Tear solutes include proteins (principally albumin, globulin, lysozyme, but many others), amino acids, mucin, glycoproteins, glucose and lipids (phospholipids, neutral fats, fatty acids, cholesterol and its esters), calcium, potassium, chloride, bicarbonate, phosphate and urea. Individual variations do exist, however, especially in the mucoprotein content and in the meibomian secretions, and this may be further influenced by the stimulus of contact lens wear. To this, however, must be added the products of normally desquamating epithelial cells, and in pathological conditions, necrotic tissue as well as altered tear components.

The literature concerned with hydrogel lens spoilation is expansive and has been reviewed elsewhere[8]. It is evident, however, that the bulk of previous communications are simply concerned with reports of the clinical manifestations of the phenomena while those few studies in which chemical analyses were employed, are concerned with the detection of the principal components rather than their detailed structure and origin. Although many other types of deposits such as films and plaques are encountered during lens wear, these are frequently influenced greatly by extrinsic factors such as sterilization and storage conditions. White spots, on the other hand, are not only widely encountered and troublesome but result directly from the interaction of the polymer and the ocular environment. As a result this type of deposit is frequently encountered in extended wear.

Structural studies: visible light and electron microscopy

Deposit morphology may be conveniently assessed using optical microscopy. Lenses are first mounted on pre-cleaned glass slides, concave surface down on a drop of preserved saline and flattened with a coverslip.

Optical microscopy is, however, limited by its lack of resolution and inability to obtain simultaneous sharp focus through a reasonable image depth. Because scanning electron microscopy uses electrons rather than light to 'illuminate' the sample it does not suffer from this restriction, which originates in the fact that the wavelength of visible light is of the order of 0.5μm. As a consequence the normal resolution limit of conventional optical microsopy cannot be better than 0.5 μm (permitting achievable magnifications of a few hundred), whereas electron microscopy enables magnification factors of several tens of thousands together with sharp focus throughout the depth of field.

Sample preparation is a critical aspect of scanning electron microscopy studies and the preparative protocols have a marked effect on deposit morphology. The procedures generally used are very aggressive in modifying deposited lipoidal material and the high vacuum involved frequently causes reticulation of smooth areas of film-like deposits. In our own studies[9,10], a type of fixation protocol which achieves the balance of minimal disturbance of sample morphology coupled with the maintenance of optimum resolution and detail. Final dehydration is achieved with the aid of a critical point dryer before the dried lenses are mounted on aluminium stubs and coated with gold/palladium.

Detailed optical microscopy shows that the discrete elevated deposit has a complex and characteristic architecture which is constructed from three distinctive, but interactive sub-layers. This is visible in Plate 4. The primary deposit layer (i.e., that which interfaces with the hydrogel matrix) is characterized by a flattened, rounded shaped plateau, whose dimensions indicate that it must stand proud of the tear film. Upon this plateau appears a secondary layer, an ellipsoid dome-shaped structure, that significantly contributes to the physical dimensions of the deposit. Darkfield and phase contrast studies reveal this layer to be composed of numerous lobular subunits (see Plates 4, 5, 6). The most anterior, tertiary, layer is devoid of such lobular components, but instead appears to be composed of a complex, multi-nodulated, transparent film-like coating. Autofluorescence indicates that the deposit contains substantial quantities of fluorescent lipoidal material; the wavelengths involved are characteristic of cholesterol and cholesterol esters.

This basic architecture was confirmed by scanning electron microscopy studies. The size of the deposit was recorded to range from 40 μm in diameter to over 160 μm. In many cases, several deposits were found in close proximity to one another, to form complex deposit subunits. Scanning electron microscopy studies suggest that the primary deposit layer is an essential requirement for the latter development of the ellipsoid dome structure since discrete plateaux were detected on many lenses without further deposit development, yet in no case were deposits observed without a primary basal unit.

Comparison of deposit morphologies on spoilt lenses derived from various sources shows that there is little variation in deposit morphology or structural arrangement from one lens to another. Furthermore, deposits on spoilt aphakic lenses are extremely similar in structure to deposits detected on cosmetic lenses. Gross deposit morphology was found to remain constant regardless of patient identity and variations in the wear protocol of the lens had little effect on deposit morphology; deposits on lenses that had been worn on a weekly basis being largely identical in structure to those on lenses worn continuously for 3 months. From comparison of deposit morphologies on spoilt lenses worn in left eye–right eye combination studies it was evident that variations in bulk and lens chemistries did not lead to any significant alteration in deposit structure. Furthermore, when lens combinations were reversed (i.e., the left eye lens material was fitted in the right eye and vice versa) deposit morphology was observed to be largely unaltered.

Even in the absence of more specific chemical information these structural studies suggest that the nature, as distinct from the occurrence, of deposits is a function of a common initiation and growth process. Although the lens surface properties appear to play a negligible role in determining gross deposit morphology, however, they do significantly affect the rate of the common interfacial conversion events.

Chemical composition: X-ray probe techniques

Qualitative and semiquantitative elemental studies of the principal deposit-imbibed inorganic deposit components and the construction of X-ray elemental maps may be performed both on lenses and on lens sections. Typical studies have been using a link system autoanalyser mounted on the stereoscan scanning electron microscope. These techniques enable the concentrations of inorganic components at the deposit surface and through the deposit section to be measured. In addition, they enable the relative concentrations of elements to be visualized in the form of 'elemental maps'[9,10].

These elemental maps demonstrate the presence of the elements used to prepare the samples (osmium, gold) together with calcium, potassium, and chloride ions within the hydrogel matrix of deposit-bearing lenses. The levels of these elements are much greater in the deposit material.

An additional element, silicon, which is not detected in the deposit structure often occurs in appreciable levels at the hydrogel-matrix deposit interface. Further studies of the non-deposit-bearing areas of the lens matrix frequently revealed a random distribution of this element, although, when detected, it has been found to be present at significantly lower levels than that recorded immediately adjacent to deposits. This is clearly not a universally applicable observation, but it does suggest that hydrophobic areas produced by silicon-containing media in lens polishing operations may have an influence on deposit formation.

Studies on sectioned lenses: histochemical techniques

Although a great deal may be deduced from studies on whole lenses, more specific structural information is obtained from thin slices, or sections, through deposited lenses. In a typical procedure lenses were first fixed in 10% buffered formaldehyde (pH 7.4) for 12 hours at room temperature. Fixed lenses are washed thoroughly in distilled water and either embedded in agar, which gives better preservation of lipid, or prepared for resin embedding, which improves the preservation of the deposit architecture and the structural integrity of the deposit-hydrogel matrix interface.

Those lenses embedded in agar (1% w/v phosphate buffered saline) are frozen and sectioned with a freezing microtome. Typically, sections, 10 μm thick, are cut from the frozen block with tungsten carbide knives and floated out on distilled water. Sections are examined using an optical microscope prior to histochemical staining. Alternatively, lens samples may be infiltrated with embedding resin, sealed in gelatin capsules and thermally polymerized. Specimens of this type are cut on the microtome at 25°C. Sections, 2–3 μm thick, are floated out on 30% acetone, on a hot plate and allowed to dry. In all cases normal dehydration procedures should be replaced by the use of critical point drying since this technique minimizes shrinkage and distortion. The procedure for preparing sections for electron microscopy is similar[9,10].

The unstained sections examined optically show a distinctive difference in uniformity (see Plates 7 and 8). Use of fluorescence shows a characteristic of the lipid fraction which is clearly not uniformly distributed throughout the deposit. The primary layers of the deposit structure display the most intense autofluorescence, while that of the outer, tertiary, region is negligible in comparison. This type of autofluorescent pattern was found to be typical of all deposits examined. From studies of the autofluorescence and polarization patterns displayed by deposits derived from a range of patients, it was evident that differing patient identities, lens materials and wear protocols did not significantly alter the intensity or location of autofluorescing components.

A range of stains is employed in the identification and the location of components of discrete elevated deposits[43]. To assess the selectivity of stains employed, control sections of unworn lenses are treated in an identical fashion to spoilt lenses.

White spot deposit sections stain positively and intensely with Oil Red O in a consistent and uniform fashion throughout the deposit (see Plate 9). This shows the presence of fatty lipoidal material throughout the deposit mass. Although staining was noted to be limited to the deposit material and the hydrogel matrix beneath the deposit structure remained unstained, this is more an indication of a difference in lipid concentration and material texture than a demonstration that lipid is absent in the lens material. Indeed, lipid penetration into the lens matrix is undoubtedly an important process in contact lens wear. This point will be amplified later.

Silver nitrate also stains the deposit structure intensely and apparently uniformly. Here again the intensity of the stain in the deposit matrix and the difference in texture of the lens and deposit matrices give a false impression of the uniformity and boundaries of the unsaturated lipid location (Figure 4.3). Positive staining of deposits is also recorded with the other lipid stains, digitonin and PFAS. In these cases staining is weaker but noticeably more intense at the deposit-hydrogel matrix interface. This is consistent with, but scarcely overwhelming evidence for, a

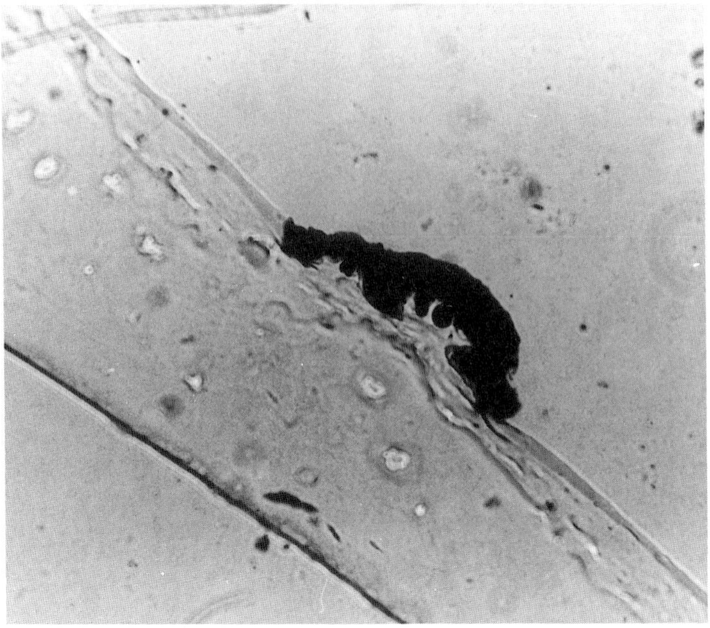

Figure 4.3 Longitudinal section (silver nitrate stained) of a discrete elevated deposit. Phase contrast ×260

gradation in lipid concentration through the matrix. There is also much weaker deposit staining with PAS and mucicarmine, while deposit response to Millon's reagent is more variable than that of the other stains.

These results when taken together indicate that the structure of discrete elevated deposits is complex and is not predominantly composed of protein as has sometimes been suggested in the past. Perhaps, not surprisingly, all the major components of the tear film are represented in the deposit structure. However, of greater significance is that a distinct internal stratification of the deposit structure exists in which a flat basal layer appears to be the primary interfacial region between the deposit structure and the lens matrix.

Although protein is undoubtedly present, the proteinaceous interface does not appear to form the basis of the interfacial process that eventually leads onto the deposit formation. Furthermore, the fact that the primary basal layer does not exhibit a particularly high level of calcium deposition suggests that the formation of discrete deposits of the type discussed here does not result from the development of an inorganic calcareous layer upon which an organic layer is overlain. This type of process does, however, explain the formation of the inorganic film deposits[1] which may be formed under exceptional conditions as will be discussed later.

Histochemical studies suggest that the deposit is predominantly composed of lipid species as indicated by the uniform staining of Oil Red O, a general lipid stain. Staining of the deposit suggests the presence of cholesterol together with cholesterol esters and unsaturated lipids respectively. Furthermore, the positive silver nitrate reaction further suggests the presence of unsaturated lipids.

The combined results of histochemical and autofluorescence studies together with the morphological information provided by scanning electron microscopy studies, suggest that unsaturated lipoidal material is concentrated at the interface and appears to form the basis for deposit formation.

Supporting evidence for this hypothesis is found from scanning electron microscopy and elemental studies where small patches of predominantly lipoidal material have been located on the lens surface. These elevated plateaux, varying is size from 20 to 200 μm, are too small to be noticeable to the naked eye. These regions appear to form the basis on which white spots develop and upon which, once initiated, they grow quickly. The existence of these lipoidal patches correlates with the primarily lipoidal basal layers which were found to be common to all complex elevated white spot deposits. Prior to these studies[9,10], the existence of these structures had not been reported. This is because in conventional scanning electron microscopy specimen preparation techniques, rather than those designed to protect lipoidal material, there will inevitably be removal of deposit material to a greater or lesser extent.

The complex role of lipids in lens spoilation, together with the way in which techniques such as high performance liquid chromatography, fluorescence spectroscopy and confocal scanning laser microscopy, show their penetration into the lens matrix will not be considered.

The role of lipids in white spot formation

These results indicate that the structure of the discrete elevated deposits or white spots is complex and not predominantly composed of a single component as previously suggested. Perhaps not surprisingly, all the major components of the tear film are represented in the deposit structure. However, of greater significance is the fact that a distinct internal stratification of the deposit structure exists, in which a flat basal layer appears to be the primary interfacial region between the deposit structure and matrix. Although protein is undoubtedly present, the proteinaceous interface does not appear to form the basis of the interfacial process that eventually leads to deposit formation. Furthermore, the fact that the primary basal layer does not exhibit a particularly high level of calcium deposition suggested that the formation of discrete deposits of this type does not result from the development of an inorganic calcareous layer upon which an organic layer is overlain. The histochemical studies described above suggest that the deposits are predominantly composed of lipid species such as cholesterol, together with cholesterol esters and unsaturated lipids. The morphological studies showed that the unsaturated lipoidal material is concentrated at the interface and appears to form the basis for deposit formation by the successive laying down of globular structures tightly packed together as a complex multilayered structure consisting of three distinctive yet interactive sublayers.

Additionally, small patches of predominantly lipoidal material have been located on the lens surface even before deposit formation has occurred. These elevated plateaux, varying in size from 20 to 200 μm are too small to be noticeable to the naked eye and appear to form the basis on which white spots develop and grow. The existence of these lipoidal patches correlates with the primary lipoidal basal layer that was found to be common to all complex elevated white spot deposits. They offer an explanation for the common deposit composition and morphology encountered on soft contact lenses and the fact that they appear to be little affected by bulk-lens chemistries, wear protocol or lens application.

Figures 4.4 and 4.5 represent simple members of the lipid family. One of the basic

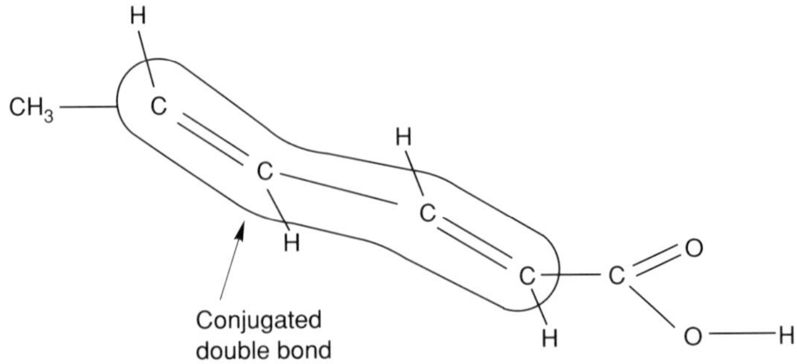

Figure 4.4 Schematic representation of an unsaturated fatty acid molecule

structures is the fatty acid, shown schematically in Figure 4.4. Fatty acids can vary considerably in the number of carbon atoms that they contain and may or may not have double bonds within the chain. Alternating (so-called 'conjugated') double bonds are particularly important because they can react with a variety of chemical species including oxygen. Table 4.2 lists some important saturated (no double bonds) and unsaturated fatty acids. The fatty acids are found in combination with glycerol, as shown in Figure 4.5. These compounds are referred to as mono-, di-, or triglycerides depending upon the number of fatty acid molecules combined with each glycerol unit. Fatty acids can also combine with the cholesterol molecule, also illustrated in Figure 4.5, to form the family of cholesterol esters.

Table 4.2 Some important saturated and unsaturated fatty acids

Acid	*Carbon atoms*	*Double bonds*
Typical saturated fatty acids		
Caproic	6	
Caprylic	8	
Capric	10	
Lauric	12	
Myristic	14	
Palmitic	16	
Stearic	18	
Arachidic	20	
Behenic	22	
Lignoceric	24	
Cerotic	26	
Typical unsaturated fatty acids		
Oleic	18	1
Erucic	22	1
Linoleic	18	2
Elaeostearic	18	3
Linolenic	18	3
Arachidonic	20	4
Clupanodonic	22	5

The literature on the subject of lipids in contact lens deposits is variable and therefore not reliable. Even with white spots which are large enough to give reasonable quantities of material for analysis, variations in quoted compositions are

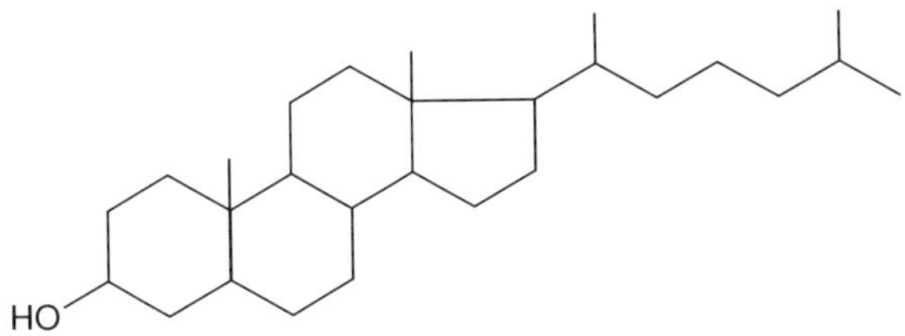

Figure 4.5 Triglyceride formation from glycerol and fatty acid units and the cholesterol molecule

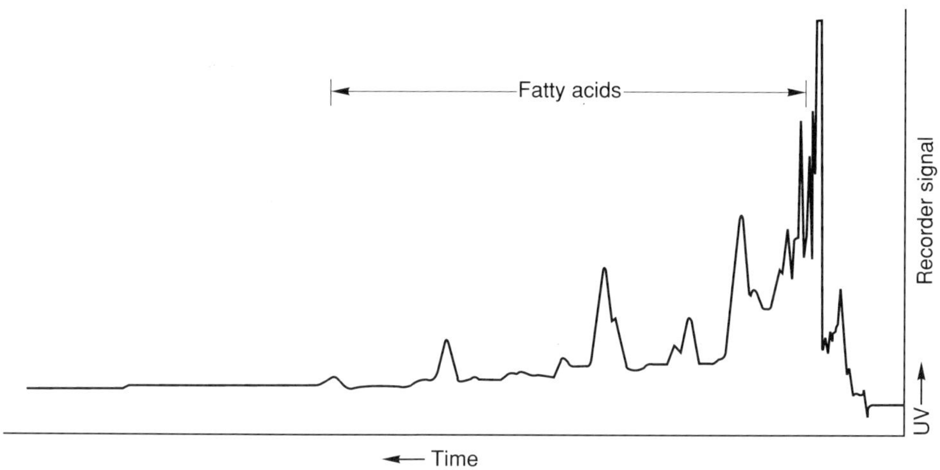

Figure 4.6 HPLC trace showing the lipid profile obtained by solvent extraction of a polyHEMA lens

found. This arises from differences in the quality and sensitivity of the analytical techniques used. Thus, expected lipoidal species in tear deposits include cholesterol, cholesterol esters, monoglycerides, diglycerides and triglycerides, fatty acids and fatty alcohols, although the presence of triglycerides, cholesterol and cholesterol esters was not detected by some workers[44] and that of fatty acids by others[26]. We have shown, however, that by the use of sensitive high performance liquid chromatography techniques it is possible to detect all the previously mentioned lipid classes.

Separation and identification of lipids

An extraction procedure was developed in the laboratories of Aston Biomaterials Research Unit which enables the lipids and protein to be extracted separately from a single contact lens. The lipids are extracted from the contact lens using methanol, which is then evaporated off by bubbling nitrogen over the surface of the solvent. The resulting lipid extracts are then analysed by high performance liquid chromatography (HPLC). Previously untreated spoilt lenses were placed in glass vials, covered with 5 ml of methanol and shaken for 30 minutes, the extract was then examined by HPLC[1]. Methanol was first evaporated off by passing nitrogen over the

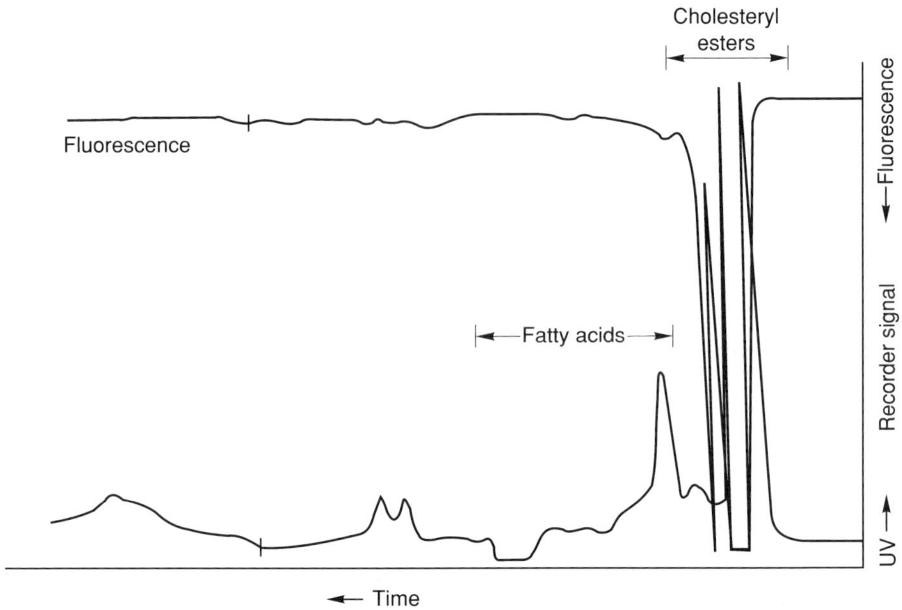

Figure 4.7 HPLC trace showing lipid profile obtained by solvent extraction of a white spot

surface of the solvent. The residue was taken up in 300 μl of mobile phase and then analysed with a Knauer high pressure liquid chromatograph equipped with a Rheodyne 7125 injector and a Sperisorb S5 OD 5 μm reverse phase column (250 mm × 4 mm ID) or a Lichrosorb 5 μm (250 mm × 4 mm ID) SI 60 normal phase column. The eluent was detected using a Perkin-Elmer LC-75 UV detector and Perkin-Elmer Filter Fluorescence detector in series. The pumps were driven by and the data collected by an Apple 11e microcomputer.

A typical spread of fatty acids laid down on a polyHEMA lens during daily wear is best illustrated in the chromatograms obtained with a reverse phase C18 octadecyl silane column and acetonitrile/water (99 : 1 v/v) mobile phase, and shown in Figure 4.12. This reveals the spread of deposited fatty acids, some 20 in number, together with triglycerides and cholesterol esters. Use of these chromatographic conditions maximizes separation of fatty acids. Calibration of the system by measurement of the retention times of fatty acid standards enables the identification of individual tear components. In Figure 4.6 esters and residual traces of solvent used in the initial extraction are rapidly eluted followed by the fatty acids in order of ascending molecular weight: arachadonic (20 : 4), arachidic (20 : 0), linoleoic (18 : 3), linoleic (18 : 2), oleic (18 : 1), stearic (18 : 0), palmitoleic (16 : 1) and palmitic (16 : 0) are readily identified. A small cluster of lower molecular weight components is also present. This is typical of the fatty acid distribution accumulated on soft lenses daily wear. It is the interaction of the unsaturated fatty acids with the lens matrix that provides the first step in the chemistry of conventional 'white spot formation'[57].

More effective separation of the individual non-polar triglycerides and cholesterol derivatives is obtained with normal phase columns and hexane : propan-2-ol : acetic acid (1000 : 5 : 1 v/v) mobile phase. This solvent system separates the lipids into groups based on the polarity of their functional groups. The sequence of elution is cholesterol esters, triglycerides, diglycerides, fatty acids, monoglycerides and cholesterol. The chromatograms are compared to a series of calibrated lipid standards for the column used. When the alternative (normal) phase column separations are used, a good separation of ester components is obtained, immediately followed, in this case, by the cluster of fatty acids. The use of dual u.v. and fluorescence detection enables identification of cholesterol esters and cholesterol itself, although the concentration of these under normal wear conditions is usually outweighed by that of the non-fluorescent components.

The elevated portions of white spot deposits show some differences from this deposition pattern, however (Figure 4.7). This is a chromatogram obtained with the normal phase column and solvent system described above. The feature that sets Figure 4.7 apart from tear fractions laid down directly onto soft lenses is the dramatically greater intensity of the fluorescent components and the lower intensity of the fatty acid components. The clear conclusion is that the deposited layer is dominated by meibomian gland secretion as a result of the interaction of the deposit with the eyelid. This correlates with the distribution of fluorescence found in sectioned lens deposits[16].

Fluorescence spectroscopy

Although HPLC is an excellent technique for identification of the many individual members of the lipid family, it can only measure material that has been extracted from the lens surface. The same is true of electrophoresis in protein analysis. Fluorescence spectroscopy of intact lenses is particularly useful as it is non-destructive and allows the study of the efficiency of the extraction procedure together with the nature of the unextracted layers. We have developed surface spectrophotofluorimetry of hydrogels into a highly sensitive and reproducible technique that quantifies fluorescent species at levels substantially below their detection by fluorescence microscopy. It is a technique which enables the non-destructive analysis of the biological fluorescent components present. Due to the autofluorescent nature of some lipids and proteins it is possible to study their presence on the surface of a contact lens or in the solvent used to extract them from that surface. The technique is routinely used by us to determine the following:

1 Whether fluorescent material has been deposited on the surface of the contact lenses and at what level
2 The extractability of these deposited materials from the contact lens surface with solvents, surfactants and commercial lens cleaning systems (e.g., methanol, sodium dodecyl sulphate)
3 The presence of the fluorescent materials within the extraction solvents used for deposit analysis (e.g., by high performance liquid chromatography or electrophoresis) and the amount of unextracted material remaining on the lens surface
4 The difference between surface deposited species and material that has penetrated into the lens matrix.

Two specially modified spectrophotofluorometers are used to determine the autofluorescent nature of the deposited biological material on the contact lens, which is reproducibly mounted on a block in a quartz cell[2]. The orientation of this cell within the instrument is important, in that only a single surface should be in the light beam and perpendicular to it. Two types of spectra were run, excitation and

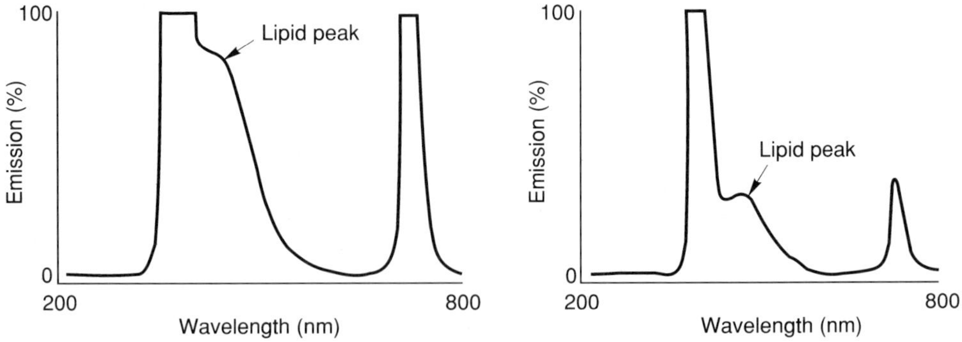

Figure 4.8 Fluorescence spectra of a polyHEMA lens prior to (left) and after (right) extraction

emission. An excitation spectrum is the dependence of the emission intensity at a single wavelength upon the excitation wavelength. An emission spectrum is the wavelength distribution of the emission, measured at a constant excitation wavelength. An excitation wavelength of 360 nm is routinely used for recording the emission spectra in which maximum lipid sensitivity is required. An excitation wavelength of 280 nm is additionally used when distinguishing between protein and lipid contribution to the deposited layer. Figure 4.8 shows the lipid peaks for a typical worn polyHEMA lens before and after extraction. It is clear that an appreciable amount of material is tenaciously bound or has penetrated into the lens matrix.

Confocal scanning laser microscopy

Confocal scanning laser microscopy is a recent development which combines the ease of sample preparation of conventional optical microscopy with some of the investigative advantages of electron microscopy[49]. It has not, as yet, received great attention in the biomaterials and contact lens field, largely because of the cost and rarity of instrumentation. In this technique the three-dimensional structure of a white spot can be determined without extensive sample preparation as in scanning electron microscopy. The confocal scanning laser microscope, by means of laser illumination and the positioning of various apertures in the optical path, collects reflected or fluorescent light from a very shallow depth of field, with little or no out of focus blur. White spots are ideal subjects as they autofluoresce and reflect light while the contact lens material does not. The images shown were collected in reflectance mode.

A large number of X Y images are collected for a sample and then stored on a computer and a composite image can then be formed. The data are then manipulated to give an apparent Z section through a deposit. Pseudo colour can be overlayed to make the deposit morphology more apparent. This is illustrated in Plates 10 and 11. By means of this technique it is possible for the first time to view the 3D morphology of white spots in their hydrated state on the lens. Because the lens is laid onto a microscope slide the deposit in Plates 11 and 12 appears to have a flat upper surface. Two pits are visible in Plate 10 and Plates 11 and 12 (cross-sectional reconstructions at two different points) show that beneath these cavities the deposit has continued to grow down into the lens matrix. Small scale reproduction of two images in this way fails to do justice to the sheer bulk and detail of information that the technique provides. It shows quite clearly that lipid penetration into the lens matrix occurs as an integral part of white spot formation.

Why do lenses dissolve lipids?

Because the interaction and subsequent chemical reactions of lipids with the hydrogel matrix are of such importance in the spoilation chemistry, the underlying reasons for their interaction with hydrogels must be considered. One mechanism is simply the interaction of the carboxyl groups of fatty acids with hydrogen-bonding sites at the dynamic hydrogel interface. Both the polarity and total surface energy of these hydrogels are appreciably higher than those of natural tissue. The other mechanism is similar to that occurring in discoloration reactions, where penetration arises because molecules that have some solubility in water but greater solubility in the polymers are taken into the lens matrix. Many species do this but they usually remain undetected unless the molecules involved are coloured. In some cases their presence leads specifically to deposit formation, which usually appears to be quite unconnected with the primary penetration process, i.e., the true culprit remains undetected, as is certainly the case with lipid penetration and the problems that this produces. Fluorescence spectroscopy used in conjunction with a novel analytical method, plasma etching and emission monitoring system (PEEMS), shows quite clearly the substantial proportion of lipid that penetrates the lens matrix[50,51] and which non-destructive extraction techniques cannot remove. The combined picture produced by various techniques is clear and consistent. The reality of this migration process is illustrated by the fact that relatively hydrophobic steroids, such as progesterone, are some two hundred times more soluble in polyHEMA hydrogel than is a water soluble sugar molecule of similar size such as sucrose.

It may seem surprising that organic chemical species can actually dissolve in polymers. It is, however, this fact that makes RGP materials so permeable to oxygen. The term *Dk* for oxygen permeability simply implies diffusion rate (*D*) multiplied by solubility (*k*). The term *k* is the partition factor – it indicates the proportion of oxygen that is dissolved (or partitioned) out of the atmosphere into the lens material. In the case of hydrogels the oxygen is no more soluble in the water in the lens than it is in the bulk water or tear film. It has virtually no solubility in the polymer part of the hydrogel at all. This is why the *Dk* of hydrogel lenses is governed by the water content and explains the current interest in silicone hydrogels. Here, an attempt is made to give the polymer in the hydrogel some oxygen dissolving power. This would increase its *k* value and thus its *Dk* value.

Although the polymer segments of conventional hydrogels have a low *k* value for oxygen, they have a much higher *k* value for organic molecules. This is because the polymer chain is itself organic. For this reason dyes really prefer the organic environment of the polymer to the aqueous environment of the solution, i.e., the *k* value for the dye and polymer is higher than the *k* value for the dye and water. In the same way, lipids with some water affinity and many other organic species are taken up into hydrogel and RGP networks. They cannot be seen because they have no light-absorbing or chromophoric groups. They do, however, have implications for spoilation processes. Although this discussion is concerned primarily with hydrogels, the arguments extend to RGP materials. Figure 4.9 shows the lipid profile obtained by extraction of an RGP lens that had been worn over a period of 18 months. This lipid represents only part of the story, however. Fluorescence spectroscopy used at

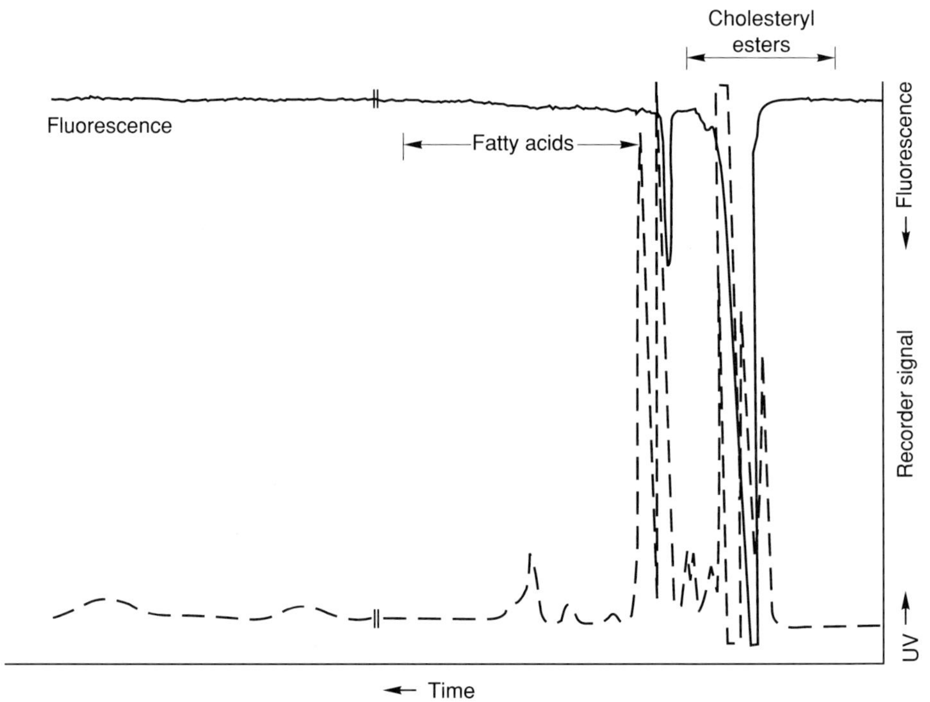

Figure 4. 9 HPLC trace showing the lipid profile obtained by solvent extraction of siloxymethacrylate itaconate copolymer lens

various stages of the extraction process, shows quite clearly the substantial proportion of lipid that had penetrated the lens matrix and which non-destructive extraction techniques cannot remove. The combined picture produced by the various techniques is clear and consistent.

It is essentially the interaction of unsaturated fatty acid lipids with the lens surface that preconditions the lens to the formation of discrete elevated deposits. This mechanism, arising from the regular collapse of the tear film, is independent of protein adsorption which will be an ongoing interfacial process. The mechanism of immobilization of the fatty acids at the lens surface is one of polymerization. This is a well known process and is identical to the 'drying' of early linseed oil-based paints in the presence of air and sunlight. Linseed oil, just like the tear film, contains unsaturated fatty acids. Once formed, these small (50–100 μm in diameter) lipoidal 'islands' with free fatty acid groups can interact with calcium. Indeed, the role of calcium appears to be more important than that of protein since calcium functions as a deposit stabilizing component. A schematic representation of the process is shown in Figure 4.10.

These studies show that lipid interactions with the polymer surface and penetration into the polymer matrix modifies the polymer–host interface and changes the course of the biological conversion process. One sobering outcome of these observations can be summarized in the statement, 'you can affect the rate but not the fate'. In essence, changes to material chemistry, within the hydrogel family, produce changes in the rate at which the various spoilation processes occur, but do

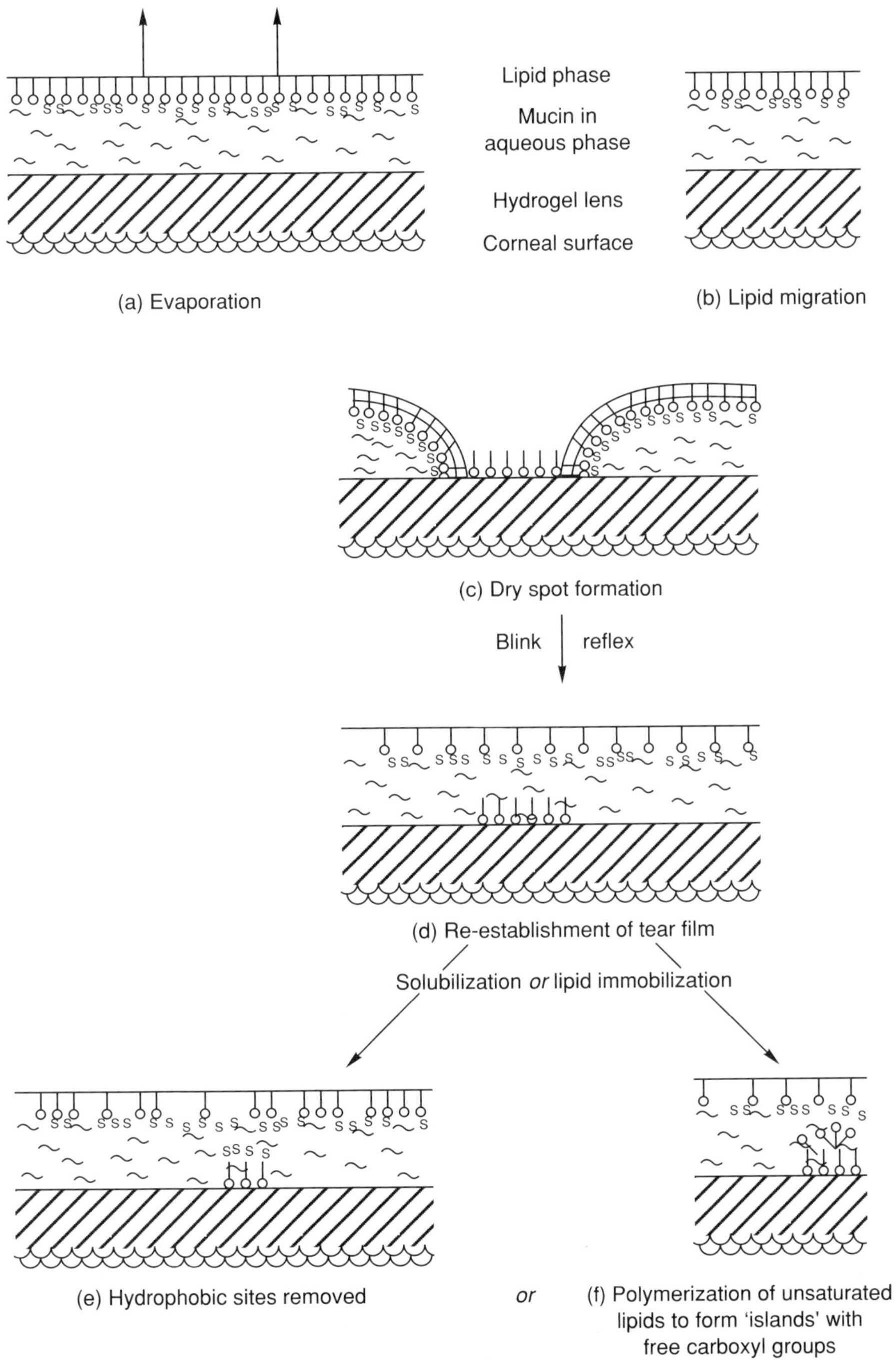

Figure 4.10 Initiation of white spot formation. Schematic representation of lipid immobilization in the form of discrete elevated 'islands' at the lens surface

not inhibit them. There is clearly a great deal to be done in understanding the nature of the initiating steps in order to effect more marked changes in spoilation resistance.

Calcium films and surface plaques

Another clinical manifestation of hydrogel contact lens spoilation is the occurrence of surface films, lens coatings and surface plaques which, characteristically, cover a significant area of the lens surface. Two forms of this type of hydrogel contact lens spoilation are the occurrence of a milky white lens coating that characteristically covers a significant area of the lens surface, and the surface located lens plaque[8]. Although several workers have suggested that the calcium film results from the deposition of inorganic salts[4,5,36,37,46,60], the aetiology and causative mechanisms still remain unclear, as are the roles of the lens surface chemistry and wear protocol in the formation of this type of spoilation. The same is true for the surface located lens plaque with the precise chemical composition and the role of the bulk and lens surface properties, together with the method of lens fabrication in determining the aetiology of the deposit remaining unclear. Furthermore, the relationship between the formation and chemical composition of the calcium film and the discrete elevated deposit, both of which contain calcium, remains to be clarified. The morphology and structural architecture of these surface plaques is apparent under the optical microscope. Using phase contrast illumination the structurally heterogeneous nature of the film with its discrete elevated crystalline structure and overlying transparent film which is characteristic of this type of coating is clearly observed (see Plate 13). This deposition is unaffected by lens chemistry and wear regimen, but the formation is much greater in extended wear regimens.

The lens plaques are surface oriented, morphologically complex, highly rugose deposits. Although this is consistent for all lens types examined, the thickness of the deposit varies. Multiple layers are apparent with this type of deposit and a characteristic autofluorescence pattern is observed, particularly at the periphery and subsurface layers (see Plate 14).

Sections of spoilt lenses stain positively with the Von Kossa (calcium) stain. Plate 15 shows a section perpendicular to the optical zone of the lens, and Plate 3 a section cut parallel to the lens surface. These sections show that black silver particulate deposits are located throughout the lens matrix, although their density is greater at the anterior lens surface. This corresponds to the air-tear-lens interface. Sections did not stain with Oil Red O or periodic acid Schiff reagent, although there was evidence of positive staining with Millon's reagent and to a less extent Oil Red O, at the most anterior layer of the deposit. This is consistent with the presence of a conventional overlying organic tear film deposit. It is conventional to separate analyses of the total deposited material into work relating to the white inorganic layer and to the overlaid organic layer.

The heterogeneous geology suggested by phase contrast and fluorescence studies was confirmed by histological analysis of the plaque structure. The primary plaque layer, that which interfaces with the hydrogel matrix, stained strongly with Oil Red O while a positive PAS reaction was recorded with the more anterior layers of the plaque indicating the presence of carbohydrate species. A limited positive response was recorded at the most anterior layer of the deposit when stained with Millon's reagent indicating the presence of tear proteins in this area of the deposit. However, from the intensity of the stain coloration, it was evident that proteins are only a

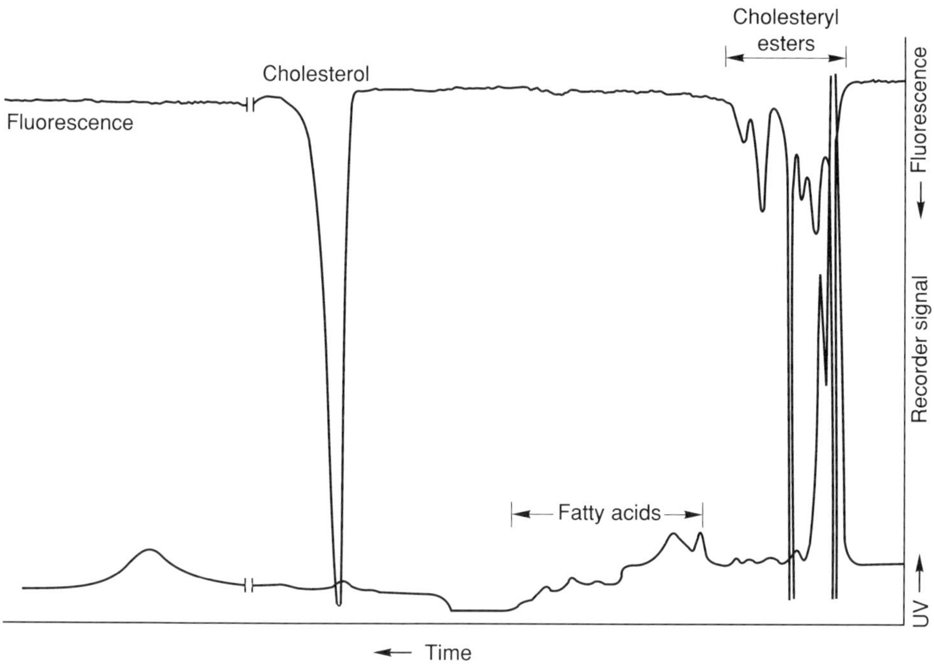

Figure 4.11 HPLC trace showing lipid profile obtained by solvent extraction of a single 'calcium film' lens. Chromatographic conditions: LiChrosorb SI 60 normal phase column, 1000 ml hexane/5 ml propan-2-ol/ 1 ml acetic acid mobile phase, flow rate 2 ml/min. Dual u.v. and fluorescence detection

minor deposit component. This stain response was found to be constant from one lens to another and was unaffected by the patient identity of the lens or the length of lens wear.

Scanning electron microscopy studies using a Cambridge Stereoscan electron microscope and energy dispersive X-ray analysis (EDXA) determination of the elemental composition of the crystalline deposits was undertaken with a link system autoanalyser mounted on the Stereoscan[10]. Both the surfaces of 10 μm sections of the lenses have been examined after coating with gold-palladium. These studies confirmed the surface-located crystalline deposits which are rich in calcium and phosphorus particularly at the deposit-hydrogel interface.

Qualitative elemental studies of the lens plaque demonstrated that calcium, potassium and chloride ions were present in the plaque. It was also noted from elemental studies of cross-sections through the deposit material hydrogel matrix interfacial region that osmium was particularly concentrated in this area of the plaque.

In order to study the deposit formation further dissolution studies were carried out. The inorganic layer was unaffected by methanol, but the organic layer was removable and using HPLC, u.v. light and fluorescence spectroscopy this layer could be profiled. All the lenses with particulate surface calcium films showed an interesting deviation from this deposition pattern, however, illustrated in Figure 4.11. The striking features that sets this apart from tear fractions normally laid down on soft lenses are the dramatically greater intensity of the fluorescent components and the relatively low intensity of the fatty acid components. The clear conclusion is that the deposited layer is dominated by meibomian gland secretion as a result of the interaction of the rugous calcium film with the eyelid. The contribution of non-meibomian derived lipids is relatively small.

After removal of this organic layer, the inorganic layer of the deposit could be removed[1] using a combination of SDS (sodium dodecyl sulphate; a detergent that is routinely used to solvate proteins and lipids) and EDTA (a divalent chelating agent). When the samples were pre-treated with SDS and then EDTA almost complete removal of the crystalline discrete deposits is achieved in a single treatment. Total removal was attained by increasing the intensity of treatment, regardless of lens composition, patient identity, or the length of wear time. Complete plaque removal was observed when lenses were treated with SDS at 70°C for 24 hours.

This type of inorganic deposit can be simulated *in vitro* by combining the calcium and phosphate ions found in phosphate buffered saline with added calcium and exposure to carbon dioxide. Lenses treated in this manner produce a crystalline milky white surface coating. It is likely that crystalline lens deposits similarly result from the imbibition and interaction of buffer-derived ionic species with the hydrogel matrix during lens storage. This then enables nucleation site development on insertion into the eye producing the crystalline deposits at the lens surface. The carbon dioxide content of the atmosphere together with the partial anterior lens surface dehydration causes the solubility product of the calcium-phosphate-carbonate to be exceeded. This effect does not occur at the lens posterior as, although the carbon dioxide content may be higher, the net solubility product is lower due to the lack of the dehydration effect.

Although these inorganic films have low levels of lipid and protein species, the primary interfacial layer is unsaturated lipid, e.g., fatty acids which are characterized by their high autofluorescence and osmium interaction. This primary layer is also likely to be covered by tear mucin-lipid complexes produced as the eye attempts to rewet the lipid modified layer. In addition, these inorganic films are often overlaid by an organic layer. This is due to the stimulation of the meibomian glands by the rugose surface of the inorganic film and this in turn will affect the composition of the lipid component.

The discrete elevated deposit and lens plaque/surface film all contain similar tear derived species, but represent the extremes of the deposition process. This process is governed by the interaction of the causative effects. The surface film being produced where the calcium levels exceed a critical level and are enhanced by concurrent increases in phosphate concentration. Whereas under normal conditions the ocular environment is dominated by the lipid adsorption rate and composition with the calcium playing a secondary deposit stabilizing function.

Discoloration and staining processes within the lens matrix

Hydrogel contact lenses undergo a number of changes in their physical properties and dimensions during wear and care procedures. Discoloration is one of these changes. It is a form of spoilation that has over the years been a major drawback in both daily and extended wear programmes. It has been noted that the appearance of the discoloration occurs over variable periods. Although the frequency of its appearance is not well documented, an increased rate of discoloration of high water content lenses as compared to those of low water content has been noted by several

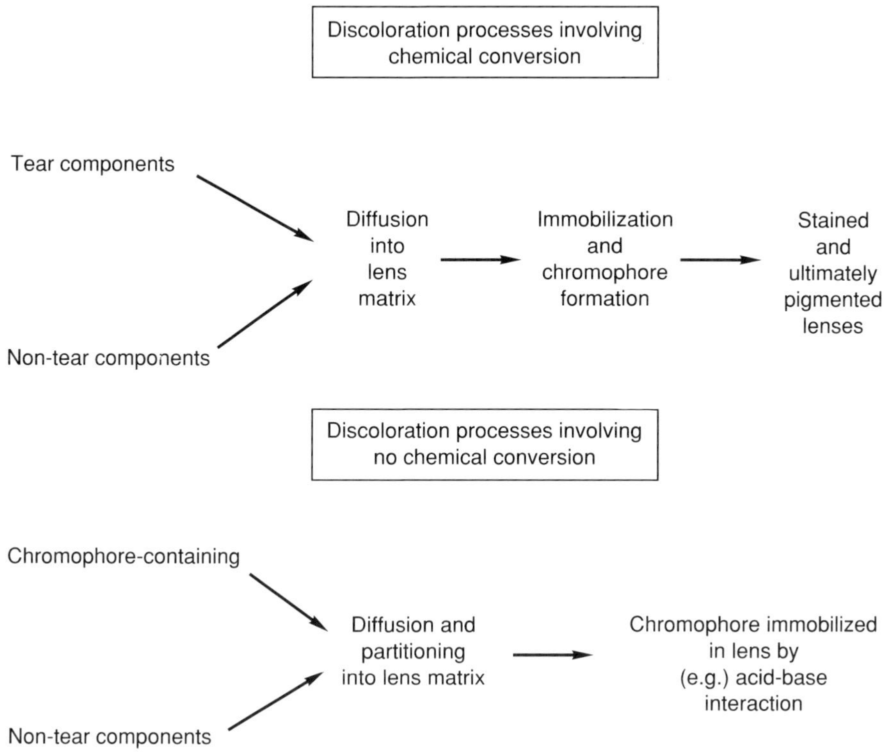

Figure 4. 12 Classification of discoloration processes

workers. In addition, discoloration is more common when the lenses are disinfected thermally as opposed to chemically.

Discoloration and staining of soft contact lenses results in the loss of lens transparency and has been attributed to a number of factors both exogenous, i.e., they are caused by substances originating outside the eye, and endogenous, originating within the ocular environment. These factors include calcium deposition, nicotine from cigarettes, foreign bodies with metallic aetiology, degradation of materials with optical non-homogeneity, diffraction effects at both ends of the spectrum, selective absorption of preservatives and dyes from solution (e.g., chlorhexedine, thermerosal, topically applied eye medications), make up products, biological components of skin etc., mucus and cells, microorganisms, pigments, absorption of coloured metabolic solutions (e.g. tyrosine-like compounds) and side products of metabolites present in tears. A number of different colours have been reported including yellow-brown, orange, amber, blue, grey, pink and green. Some systematization and explanation can be offered of the ways in which discoloration arises. This is not a comprehensive catalogue but a classification with illustrative examples. Different routes to lens staining may conveniently be summarized in the form shown in Figure 4.12. This will be used as a basis for the information contained in this discussion.

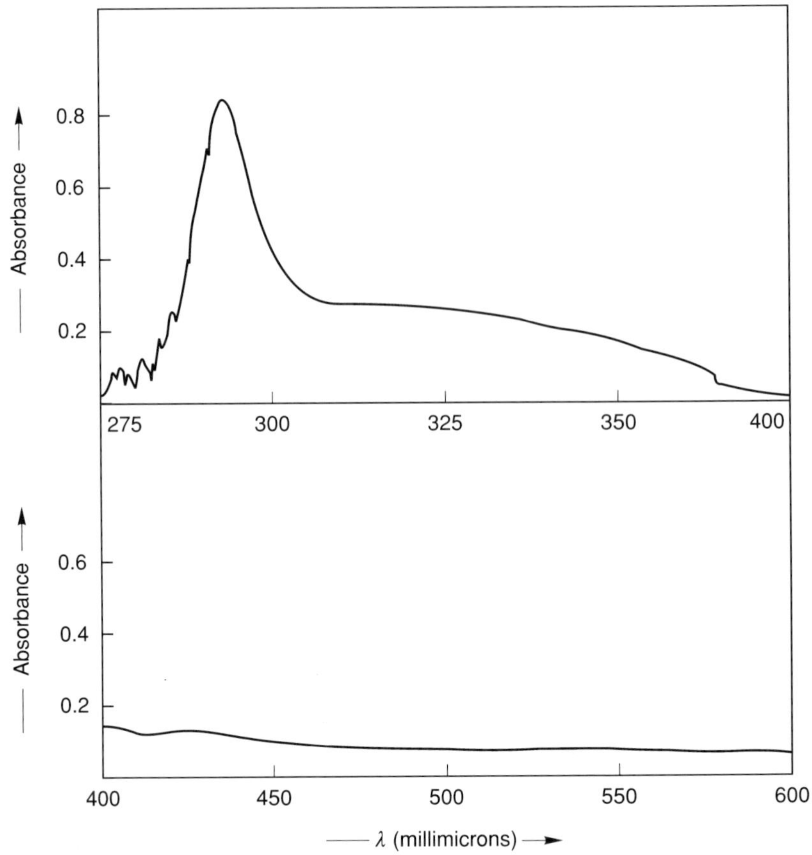

Figure 4.13 U.v. and visible spectrum of a yellow-brown discoloured Permalens

Discoloration processes involving chemical conversion: yellow-brown discoloration

Yellow-brown discoloration is a progressive process which may begin at the edge of a lens and gradually builds up until the entire lens is affected. Lenses affected in this way vary dramatically in the intensity and colour of the lens matrix, between pale yellow and deep brown. In cases of severe discoloration a marked reduction in the elasticity of the lens can be detected. Plate 16 shows three worn lenses illustrating various relatively early stages of the discoloration process. A variety of factors has been proposed in the literature to account for yellow-brown discoloration, some without any supporting evidence. It is certainly true that the occurrence of yellow or brown discoloured lenses has diminished in recent years largely due to the decrease in popularity of thermal disinfection regimens.

Although discoloration of this type has been long known and is perhaps one of the best identified examples of lens spoilation the underlying chemistries are complex, varied and not clearly understood. Almost inevitably, the discoloration results from the diffusion into the lens matrix of water soluble species that are not, in themselves, coloured. These species undergo chemical reaction which gradually reduces their mobility, introduces chromophores (colour-forming groups) and increases their

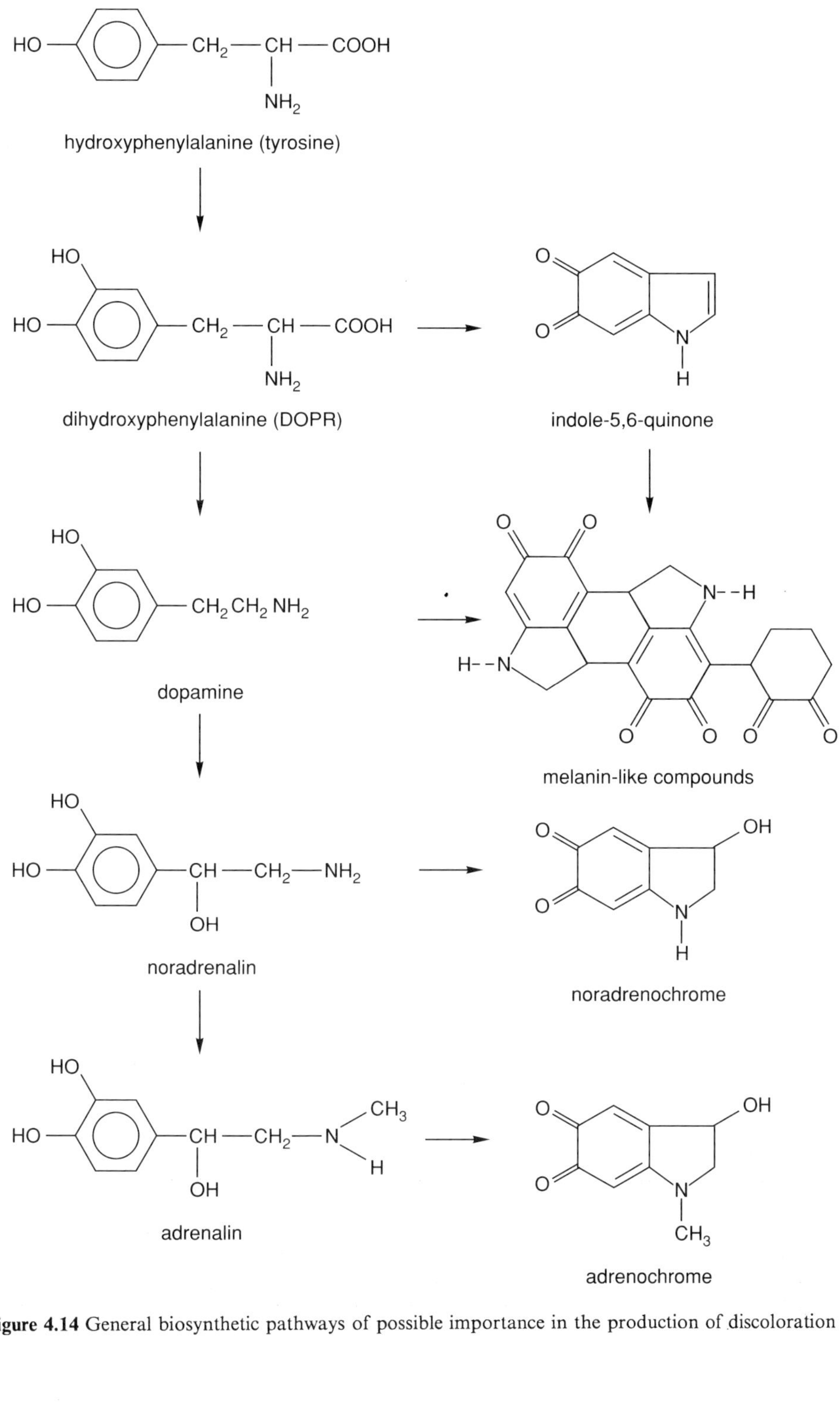

Figure 4.14 General biosynthetic pathways of possible importance in the production of discoloration

optical density. Particulate materials are thus gradually formed which become immobilized in the lens matrix. It is important to note, however, that lenses can become quite yellow in the early stages of such processes before individual particulate deposits are formed. It is convenient to consider reactions of this type in two separate groups. The first involving native tear components and the second involving species that are foreign to the external eye.

It was recognized many years ago, notably by Kleist[36], that yellow-brown discoloration of lenses was associated with the appearance of a melanin-like pigment within the lens matrix. A great deal more work has been carried out in the intervening years that has provided substantiating detail. The progress of the discoloration is associated with increase in size of the individual particles and the distribution of the particles through the lens matrix becomes more uniform in extended wear as compared to daily wear regimens. Plate 17 shows an optical micrograph of a typical yellow-brown lens viewed normally to the surface and showing clearly the individual pigment deposits. Plate 18 shows a section, or slice, through the lens (the microtome knife marks are clearly visible) illustrating the even distribution of the pigment throughout the lens. This is an example of a high water content lens following 3 months extended wear.

The evidence for the chemical identity of the dispersed pigmentary material is quite varied. The u.v. and visible light absorbance spectra are shown in Figure 4.13. These are certainly consistent with complex melanin structures and the peak at 280 nm is consistent with the presence of aromatic groups.

The broad absorption in the visible light region corresponds to the indefinite colour – other colours show defined absorption in the appropriate region of the visible light spectrum. The use of chemical identification reactions derived from histology is also of help. Although the conventional and very specific Masson-Fontana for melanin identification does not give good results, the lenses do react to the Schmorl reagent which stains melanins containing sulphydryl groups blue. Plates 19 and 20 show a conventional phase contrast picture of a section of a yellow-brown lens together with a section stained (blue) with Schmorl reagent. The pigmentary material is extremely difficult to remove from the lens matrix. It cannot be dissolved and can only be destroyed by strong oxidizing agents of the alkaline perborate family. This evidence, taken together, provides strong evidence for the presence of particulates of the melanin family. These vary from diffuse yellow particles (phaeomelanin) which contains sulphur to the brown or black (eumelanin granules).

Yellow-brown discoloration: role of tear components

As with the actual structure of melanin, there is quite a lot of doubt about the details of melanin production, although there is almost general agreement about the key points of the synthesis. The compounds adrenochrome and noradrenochrome are also considered here as they may play a part in the discoloration.

The basic biosynthetic pathway is shown in Figure 4.14: tyrosine (an amino acid), can be oxidized enzymatically to dehydroxyphenyl alanine (DOPA) which can be converted to the hormones, noradrenalin and adrenalin. Alternatively, the DOPA may be converted to various intermediates and eventually melanin. Normally, this conversion takes place in melanosomes (organelles in melanin producing cells). However, it is known that enzymes, such as occur in the melanosomes, are not necessary for melanin production as DOPA darkens rapidly when exposed to oxygen.

Many experiments have been carried out with possible melanin precursors and their oxidation to coloured pigments. One of the most important precursors is believed to be indole-5,6-quinone. It appears that in the actual lens these low molecular weight precursors diffuse into the lens and then are oxidized to produce the high molecular weight coloured pigments in the lens matrix. These precipitate on formation and are thus unable to diffuse away.

The reason why epinephrine (adrenalin) and other similar compounds used in eye medication may be important in lens discoloration is that they can be taken up by the lens, then chemically changed to adrenochrome (see Plate 20) which absorbs in the u.v. and visible spectra and so is coloured. Again, this effect can be demonstrated *in vitro* by incubation of an adrenaline solution. Additionally, adrenochrome is believed by some to be a possible precursor of melanin so the 'natural' production of melanin may be enhanced if adrenalin is in eye medication.

The incidence of this type of yellow-brown discoloration has also been said to be much higher in smokers than non-smokers. This increase is attributed to the stimulation of melanin production by nicotine or other polycyclic aromatic compounds in tobacco smoke. The handling of the lens during cleaning may also contribute to the discoloration due to staining of the fingers as a result of smoking. Thus, the effect of smoking is both direct and indirect as a nicotine-stimulated biochemical mechanism.

Yellow-brown discoloration: extrinsic factors

A good example of an extrinsic factor which is capable of causing yellow-brown discoloration of contact lenses is sorbic acid. This is one of a number of antimicrobial agents used in contact lens solutions either as the free acid or in the form of its potassium salt. When used in solutions in which the lens is soaked (such as saline) rather than simply in limited contact solutions (such as cleaners) this agent can diffuse into the lens and lead to discoloration, particularly in conjunction with thermal sterilization and/or high environmental levels of u.v. radiation. Although this does not currently present great problems in the UK it is a useful illustration of the way in which selection of solution components for one particular attribute, can lead to problems in unforeseen ways.

Plate 21 shows examples of yellow-brown discoloration produced by sorbic acid preserved salines in conjunction with thermal sterilization. The spectral characteristics of these lenses are similar but not identical to those of the melanin pigmented lenses. Fluorescence spectroscopy is a valuable technique, probing those differences which are not apparent in the visual spectrum.

This low toxicity and large usage throughout the food industry, cosmetics and pharmaceutical industries facilitated governmental approval of ophthalmic products containing this material in the USA, and has contributed to its recent preference over other undoubtedly more toxic chemicals such as thiomersal and chlorhexidine gluconate.

Some indication of the evidence which has been used to argue of sorbic acid's low toxicity, may be gleaned from its oral LD_{50} which, in rats, is 10 g/kg, compared with 5 g/kg for common salt (NaCl). As a result of the favourable toxicological and physiological characteristics of sorbic acid, the World Health Organization has allowed it the highest acceptable daily intake figure for all food preservatives.

Sorbic acid and lens discoloration processes

The usage of sorbic acid in the contact lens field has not apparently given rise to major eye care problems. Its chemical nature, however, indicates that in common

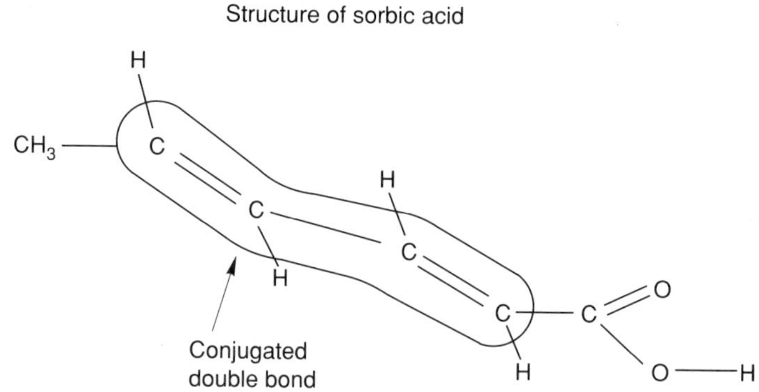

Figure 4.15 Structure of sorbic acid

with certain other chemicals in ophthalmic solutions it will be concentrated within the matrix of soft contact lenses, particularly those of high water content, with which it can interact. As the subsequent discussion will show, these interactions are very weak in HEMA-based materials, but greater with the more polar groups used in extended wear materials. It is this interaction combined with chemical reactivity of sorbic acid that provides the basis for accelerated lens discoloration in certain situations. The structure of sorbic acid is shown in Figure 4.15.

The mechanism by which sorbic acid may be absorbed into the lens matrix is well understood. Hydrogels, which are used to make high water content lenses contain highly polar groups such as carboxyl, amide and the lactam ring. The carboxylic acid group, present in sorbic acid, can form hydrogen bonds or Zwitterion complexes with such polar groups and therefore be bound to the network. The best characterized example of this process is found in polymers which contain *N*-vinyl pyrrolidone as a co-monomer.

The sorbic acid molecule then, like the molecular and ionic components of the tear fluid and other ingredients in ophthalmic solutions, is of a sufficiently small size to diffuse into hydrogel contact lenses (especially those of a high water content). Thus, it can be taken up and concentrated within the lens matrix when the lens is left in a soaking solution for a prolonged period.

Although sorbic acid is a relatively non-toxic substance it is a very versatile chemical reagent. Ironically it contains the very type of structure (i.e., residual conjugated olefinic unsaturation) that polymer chemists seek to avoid in polymers if they wish them to be stable and non-coloured. This unsaturation is linked to a polar carboxyl group that facilitates the retention of the molecule within the lens structure. The conjugated double bonds result in the molecule absorbing very strongly in the u.v. range of the electromagnetic spectrum; the peak of the absorption occurs at 256 nm. This absorption of u.v. light by absorbed sorbic acid molecules within the matrix of the lens could well be a mechanism for introducing the energy necessary for a variety of photochemical reactions with tear fluid components.

Another consequence of the molecule possessing two conjugated double bonds is that it can take part in a group of chemical processes known as Diels–Alder and Michael type reactions. An example of the type of reaction that can occur is the self dimerization of sorbic acid, which leads to the formation of larger less soluble molecules (Figure 4.16). This has obvious similarities to the early stages of melanin formation. This is only one of a large number of potential reactions of the Diels–

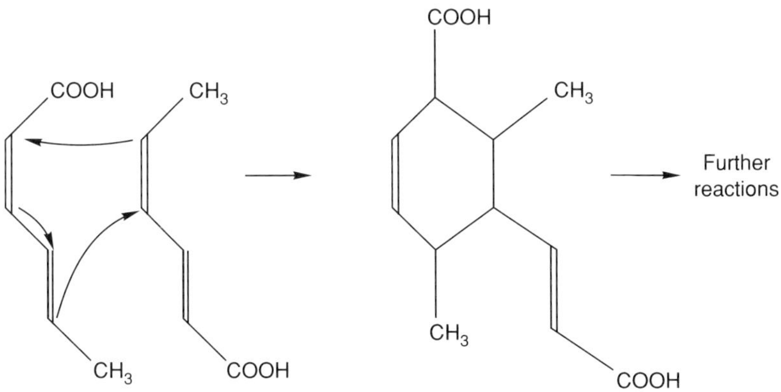

Figure 4.16 Dimerization reaction of sorbic acid

Alder type which could occur not just with other sorbic acid molecules, but with actual components of the tear fluid itself which have diffused into the lens matrix. Photochemical activation and the heat disinfection process would certainly help to accelerate some of these reactions, all of which will lead to increasing concentrations of immobilized coloured species within the lens matrix.

Discoloration by direct uptake of coloured species

There exists a wide variety of observations and reports, some well documented and some anecdotal, that seem to suggest that hydrogel lenses are capable of taking up and holding coloured species within the gel matrix. The factors that are responsible for this group of spoilation reactions are outlined here.

In the group of reactions considered in the previous section, small water-soluble molecules were taken up and released from the lens matrix and only immobilized in coloured form when chemical chain reactions made them too large and insoluble in water to leave the matrix. At the same time these immobilization reactions led to formation of chromophores – light-absorbing groups usually characterized by the presence of multiple double bonds. In the category of discoloration reactions considered in this section the problems usually arise because molecules are taken into the lens matrix that have some solubility in water but more in the polymers. Many species do this but they remain undetected unless the molecules involved are coloured. The group of molecules that cause discoloration are those whose chemical structures contain chromophores – the multi-unsaturated groups previously described. The troublesome molecules, then, have three characteristics:

1 Chromophoric groups to render them coloured
2 Substantial hydrophobic organic segments to give them solubility in, or affinity for, the polymer
3 Hydrophilic groups to render them water soluble – these groups also bind to hydrophilic sites in the polymer.

Molecules that possess characteristics 1–3 are found in the families of synthetic or vegetable dyes. Some examples are shown in Figure 4.17. Although the names may

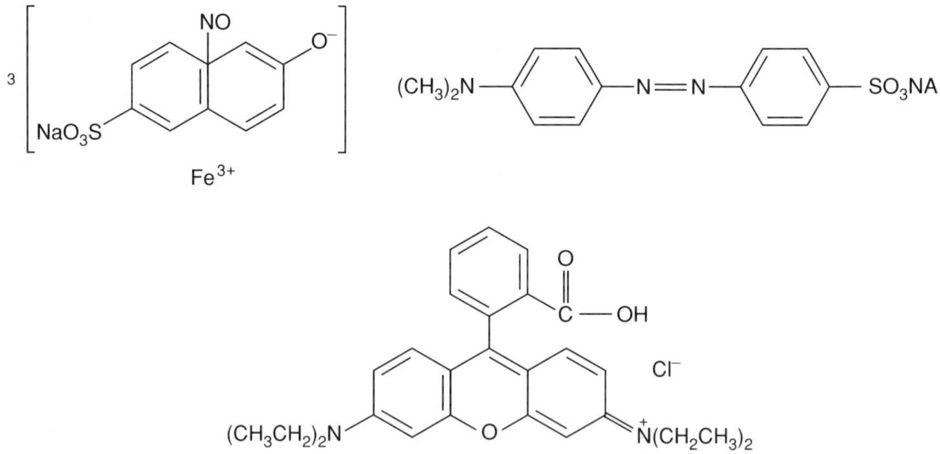

Figure 4.17 Characteristics of dye molecules (left to right) naphthol green B, methyl orange and rodamine B respectively

seem obscure, their structures are typical of the wide range of such compounds encountered in daily life.

It may seem surprising that chemical species such as those shown in Figure 4.17 can actually dissolve in polymers. It is this fact that makes RGP materials so permeable to oxygen. The term *Dk* for oxygen permeability simply implies diffusion rate (*D*) multiplied by solubility (*k*). The term *k* is the partition factor – it indicates the proportion of oxygen that is dissolved (or partitioned) out of the atmosphere into the lens material. In the case of hydrogels, the oxygen is no more soluble in the water in the lens than it is in the bulk water or tear film. It has virtually no solubility in the polymer part of the hydrogel at all. This is why the *DK* of hydrogel lenses is governed by the water content and explains the current interest in silicone hydrogels. Here an attempt is made to give the polymer in the hydrogel some oxygen dissolving power. This would increase its *k* value and thus its *Dk* value.

Although the polymer segments of conventional hydrogels have a low *k* value for oxygen they have a much higher *k* value for the molecules in Figure 4.1. This is illustrated in Plates 22–25 which show, in each case, a 40% polyHEMA lens and a 70% VP-based lens that has been exposed to a very low concentration dye solution for a period of time and then placed in saline for several days. The colour of the lenses after exposure was more intense than the colour of the solution to which they were exposed. This is because the dyes really preferred the organic environment of the polymer to the aqueous environment of the solution, i.e., the *k* value for the dye and polymer is higher than the *k* value for the dye and water. In the same way, lipids with some water affinity and many other organic species are taken up into hydrogel networks. They cannot be seen because they have no light-absorbing or chromophoric groups. They do, however, have implications for other spoilation processes.

Factors affecting uptake, retention and ultimate colour

It is clear that the combination of lens materials and dyes in Plates 22–25 have not all behaved in the same way. Although both HEMA and VP-based lenses took up dye, they were not equally effective at retaining the dye. Similarly, not all dyes were taken up or retained to the same extent by a given lens type. VP contains nitrogen and is more basic (less acidic) than HEMA (which is fairly neutral). Similarly, some dyes are dominated by acidic SO_3H or COOH groups and some by basic *N*-containing groups (N^+ is especially basic). Some, such as pH indicator molecules, switch structure, and thus colour, with pH change.

The factors influencing uptake, retention and colour stability of dyes are summarized below:

1 Water content or pore size of hydrogel
2 Presence of acidic or basic groups in hydrogel
3 Size of dye molecule
4 Sensitivity of pH change of dye molecule (this will not necessarily be the same in solution and when bound in the gel matrix).

It is clear that a higher water content lens allows more rapid uptake of larger dyes. More importantly, however, higher water content lenses almost always contain basic VP which attracts dyes containing acidic groups such as SO_3H or COOH. These groups are very commonly found on dye molecules that have some water solubility. This acid–base attraction plays a powerful role in the partitioning process and gives the dye a high affinity for the polymer. The figures show this point clearly and illustrate the propensity that high water VP-containing lenses have for becoming stained. Plate 25 shows lenses that had not been extracted for the same length of time as those in Plates 22–24. This illustrates that if the basicity of the dye is appropriate, however, polyHEMA lenses will retain stains very effectively. Dyes with pH sensitivity are typified by phenophthalein which switches from colourless to pink, stains basic hydrogels and is also a common laxative ingredient. A trial to establish the relationship between oral ingestion and tear concentration would be interesting if the necessary volunteers could be assembled!

Given the ease with which the high water content lenses take up certain organic components it is perhaps surprising that there are not more reports of irreversible contact lens staining. There is a variety of potential stains of synthetic and vegetable origin that are capable of staining lenses. Some of these, such as beetroot dye (which although intensely coloured is only weakly bound) are commonly found around the home and, given the horrendous tales that practitioners tell of patient non-compliance, it is not difficult to imagine close encounters of the nth kind that would result in lens staining! It is certainly not surprising then, given the strength of interaction between many organic dyes and contact lens polymers, that the lenses do not completely release stains once they are imbibed. Plate 26 shows two high water vinyl pyrrolidone-containing lenses (Lunelle) submitted to the Optician 'Contact Us' column. Comparison of these with Plates 22–25 illustrates how relatively pale they are and therefore how relatively little of the active colourizing species is present.

An overview of this type would not be complete without reference to manganese in tears. The work of Willaim Frey has highlighted the fact that manganese levels in tears are some 30 times greater than in plasma from the same subject. He concluded that 'the lacrimal gland does concentrate and excrete manganese', and that the manganese level is equally high in irritant and emotional tears! Because it is possible to detect manganese in worn lenses and because some manganese salts (potassium permanganate) are highly coloured it is tempting to make connections which may have no real foundation. It would be tempting for example to equate the enhanced tear flow in emotional patients with enhanced uptake of manganese by the lens and to suggest this as an origin of lens discoloration. The shortcomings of this argument include the fact that colours of manganese salts are very dependent upon valency state and are much less intense than those of organic dyes at similar concentrations. Because manganese can be oxidized or reduced by simple chemical reagents, its coloured states would not be expected to be stable to lens care regimens. Although, as Plate 27 shows, it is possible to induce artificially colour in lenses with relatively low levels of manganese, these do not appear to be representative of the generality of discoloured lenses; they are also more difficult to produce than are, say, simple beetroot stains!

Tear proteins and proteinaceous films

In addition to the surface calcium films and organic plaques described earlier, another form of surface coating occurs. This surface coating is related to discrete elevated deposits, although somewhat more geographically disperse, and is the so-called protein films. Such films are characterized by a thin, semiopaque, white superficial layered appearance. These layers appear to consist of denatured protein[34]. The films vary in the extent of lens coverage, ranging from small patches to complete covering of the lens surface. The general accumulation of protein films on soft contact lenses leads to an increase in surface haziness and rugosity. A decrease in visual acuity results due both to lens opacity and to poor lens movement on the eye. Red eye, increased irritation and conjunctivitis are typical patient responses to protein covered lenses. These deposits have been variously attributed to mucoproteins, albumin, globulins, glycoproteins and mucin[4,5,60].

Karageozian, with the aid of an amino acid analyzer, has reported that protein films consist mainly of denatured lysozyme. Since lysozyme was said by the author to comprise only 18% of the total tear protein, in comparison with 60% albumin and 22% globulin, he concluded that it was selectively adsorbed and denatured on the lens surface[34]. Other workers have come to different conclusions, however, and Hathaway and Lowther have reported that albumin, as well as lysozyme, forms marked deposits in a short period of time[27]. Furthermore, it was found that ionic solutions, such as calcium and sodium chloride, enhanced the rate of and degree of deposit formation of organic tear components.

Kleist subsequently reported that protein films are found on both thermally and chemically disinfected lenses[36]. Not surprisingly, the level of proteinaceous films was higher on thermally disinfected lenses. Young and Hill suggested that lens surface coatings are more likely to occur in patients who have a higher level of phosphatase, lactic acid dehydrogenase and cholesterol. Conversely, patients with low plasma creatinine levels are more likely to show coatings on the lens[63]. Hathaway and Lowther found that there was no correlation between protein concentration and the rate of deposit formation. However, a correlation was found between the rate of deposition and tear break up time. Short break up times were found to correlate with rapid deposit formation[28]. Several workers report that drying out the lens surface due to poor blinking or low tear volume may also enhance deposit formation.

As a point of reference, one should note that break up times and lens drying are not synonymous. Tear films break-up time can occur in a matter of seconds and therefore cannot be a function of drying alone, since it has been estimated that it would take approximately 10 minutes to eliminate the entire tear film by evaporation[38]. Briefly, break up time is caused by the migration of polar lipids from the superficial tear film layer, since when the lids open, the new tear–air interface has a high surface tension. When the mucous layer has become sufficiently contaminated it ruptures, producing a 'dry spot' or a discrete area of hydrophobicity on the lens surface. Our own work suggests that these dry spots provide a favourable environment for deposit formation and throws light on the mechanism of subsequent growth processes.

Keotting reported that the time before the detection of visible protein is made decreases drastically when the lenses are rubbed and rinsed in saline before disinfection[38]. There are conflicting reports in the literature on this subject. Several workers indicated that the regular use of surfactant cleaners reduces the incidence of spoilation, while others suggested that their use makes no difference at all. The formation of protein films may apparently be inhibited by the use of strong oxidizing agents such as persulphates, perborates and even hypochlorite bleaching agents. Oxidative reagents may indeed remove protein films, however, Eriksen pointed out that in many cases irreversible damage to the lens may result from their use[15,16]. The use of enzymes such as papain, in soaking solutions provides a safe and effective method of film removal[16,52]. Heavy white visible films may be removed by the enzyme but at this stage the lens may have other types of deposits that are unaffected by the cleaner.

Tear fluid proteins

The techniques used to identify and quantify the different protein components present in normal human tears include electrophoresis, immunochemistry and enzymatic assay. By far the most widely used analytical techniques are based on electrophoresis, but no single technique has been used on all proteins. Furthermore, the collection methods used to obtain tears are often traumatic to the eye, resulting in reflex tearing, and it is now well established that different types of tear (e.g., basal, stimulated, emotional) have different compositions. For example, greater quantities of serum proteins such as albumin and immunoglobulins are present in tears collected by Schirmer filter strips which cause reflex tearing, than are found in unstimulated tears collected by microcapillary pipette. The Schirmer-strip method is believed to abrade the conjunctival tissue and cause leakage of serum proteins into the tear fluid. As would be expected if this is the case, a similar increase in serum proteins is found in tears of patients with inflammatory diseases[33]. Tear fluid collected following nasal stimulation with irritants such as ammonia gas or onion vapour also differs from non-stimulated (basal) tears[21,52]. The major serum proteins, albumin, transferrin and IgC, were shown to be present at significantly higher concentrations in non-stimulated tears[53].

Other variations in particular tear component concentrations have been reported and attributed to age, sex, health and contact lens wear. The concentration of lysozyme and lactoferrin, for instance, show a gradual decline with age, while IgC tends to increase[21,40]. Tear osmolarity, and the concentrations of some tear proteins, have been found to be higher in contact lens wearers than in non-wearers[17]. Another factor not normally taken into account is the sex of the person contributing the tears. Tapaszto reported significant differences between male and female subjects for a number of tear components, including some of the major tear proteins[54]. Serum albumin in female tears was found at concentrations almost twice those occurring in tears from male subjects, while the concentration of lysozyme was lower in tears from females. Tapaszto also reported higher concentrations of lipids in the tears of women than in men[50]. Age also exerts an influence as mentioned above as, of course, do eye infections and the general health of the person. Thus, the figures quoted in the literature for any particular protein concentration are highly variable and not absolute.

The proteins, lysozyme, lactoferrin and tear-specific pre albumin, are secreted by both the main and accessory (Wolfring's glands and the glands of Krause) lacrimal glands, so their concentrations should remain reasonably constant in both stimulated and non-stimulated tears. Thus, the wide range of values quoted for the concentration of these proteins in normal tears must be largely due to the different sensitivities of alternative analytical tests. For example, enzymatic assays of lysozyme, which are the most commonly used technique to quantify this protein, may overestimate the concentration of this bacteriolytic enzyme since the tear fluid has been shown to contain factors which may enhance lysozyme activity. Gel electrophoretic methods and other techniques which made use of stains such as Coomassie brilliant blue, make the assumption that the intensity of protein stain is independent of protein type, but this has been shown not to be the case. For the majority of tear proteins, however, their concentrations are reported greater in non-stimulated tears than in stimulated tears.

There is frequently a large range between the highest and lowest values quoted for the tear components due to the techniques used to assay and the number of studies conducted[11]. For example, values for lysozyme range from 65 mg/100 ml[33] to 555 mg/100 ml[59]. The source of these large errors lies in the collection methods and analytical techniques used. The ratios of some of the proteins (serum albumin, lysozyme and lactoferrin) obtained in different studies remains fairly constant for tears collected atraumatically. For tears collected by the Schirmer strip method, the concentration of serum albumin is dramatically increased[3]. It would, therefore, make sense to consider tear protein ratios in addition to actual concentration values when interpreting the importance of tear analyses. This would eliminate any differences in sensitivity between the various techniques used to quantify the tear components.

In producing the average values for this chapter, these factors were ignored, although only values for 'normal' and 'healthy' and, where specified, unstimulated tears were used.

Also questionable is the interpretation of tear analyses. For instance, although lysozyme is widely assumed to be by far the most abundant tear protein, the range of values quoted by those who have analysed tears hardly supports this. Indeed, the fact that analytical studies of deposited lenses frequently show lysozyme as the major protein may rather reflect the strong adsorption of proteins such as lactoferrin to the lens surface, making them difficult to remove.

Conventional electrophoresis studies of tear proteins

Electrophoresis is the most widely used technique for identification of proteinaceous material extracted from a lens surface. Electrophoresis is the separation of a mixture of molecules according to their charge, size and, to a lesser degree, shape. This process is facilitated by the application of a voltage across the system which induces the mobilities we witness. The process is normally carried out on an inert gel support matrix which stabilizes the separation and acts as a filter medium for the molecules. The gels commonly used include agarose, polyacrylamide and starch.

Wedler[61] carried out extensive studies on which chemicals give the desired extraction, both singly and in combination, to yield samples suitable for gel electrophoresis. The optimal extraction was observed with a combination of sodium dodecyl sulphate (SDS), heat and the thiol reagent, dithiothretitol (DTT). The other solubilization agents investigated included the chaotropic reagents urea, gutanidine hydrochloride, potassium thiocyanide, potassium perchlorate hydroxylamine and ethylenediaminetetra-acetic acid (EDTA); all proved less effective than SDS and DTT. The result of this study suggests that apolar interactions and disulphide bonds may be important in stabilizing the deposit structure. Using this extraction procedure, Wedler found that a single lens contained 5–10 mg lens protein, 1–1.2 mg lens carbohydrate and 0.01–0.05 mmole lens phospholipid.

Wedler[61] also analysed the proteins extracted by SDS-page using a slightly modified extraction procedure (i.e., 2% SDS, 5 mM dithiothreitol and 1 mM EDTA in a total volume of 1.5 ml for 10 minutes at 95°C) and found all proteins that are present in the lens deposit are present in human tear fluid.

Sack *et al.*[48] carried out extraction from various lens types, which were classified as non-ionic and anionic depending on their declared monomer composition. On non-ionic polymers, the lens-bound protein layer was invariably thin and largely insoluble. The extractable protein layer proved to be devoid of active lysozyme, amino acid analysis showed a variable composition. On the anionic polyHEMA co-polymer lenses, the lens bound protein layer was much thicker and composed primarily of loosely bound protein which, on electrophoresis, was shown to be lysozyme. The activity of the lysozyme proved to have been retained. Amino acid analysis partly supported the hypothesis that the layer was made up of lysozyme. The specificity of deposition was attributed to ionic affinity of lysozyme, the retention of activity is due to the stable nature of lysozyme under extreme conditions. Sack *et al.* in further studies[47] found that the white cloudy deposits found on high water content hydrogels lenses was lysozyme, the published electrophoretograms were far from equivocal to this. This study by Sack *et al.* also involved the use of amino acid analysis to confirm this result; thus a doubt is cast on its validity.

In a general study of the protein adsorption properties of the groups of polymers that make up the FDA system of contact lens material classification, it was found that high water content ionic lenses adsorbed the highest amount of protein[41].

Bilbaut *et al.*[6] and Lin *et al.*[39] both reported lysozyme as the major component of the deposits found on worn contact lenses. Lin *et al.* also reported that the other proteins detected did not increase after longer periods, while lysozyme did. Bilbaut *et al.* found again that lysozyme was present, but also large numbers of proteins or degraded peptides.

Recent studies by Payor[42] quantified total protein deposited on human worn soft contact lenses using visible light scatter, electrophoresis and amino acid analysis to demonstrate the varying levels of proteins taken up by different lens materials.

Mucin, when studied after extraction[48], was found only on heavily deposited lenses, and not on normally or lightly deposited lenses. Alcian blue/periodic acid Schiff reagent was used to stain the gels to show mucins. This stain has a relatively low sensitivity and this could explain the apparent absence of mucin on normal and lightly deposited lenses. The mucin proved to be a complicating factor in electrophoresis as it causes smearing and formed elemental silver mirrors on silver stained SDS-page gels.

Wedler's study[61] makes an interesting comparison with Castillo's work using Fourier-transform infrared (FTIR) on mucin, with which he found that mucus formed a complex three-layered structure that quickly built-up after the lens was placed in the eye. Castillo *et al.*[12] and Holly[29] both suggested that mucin adsorption

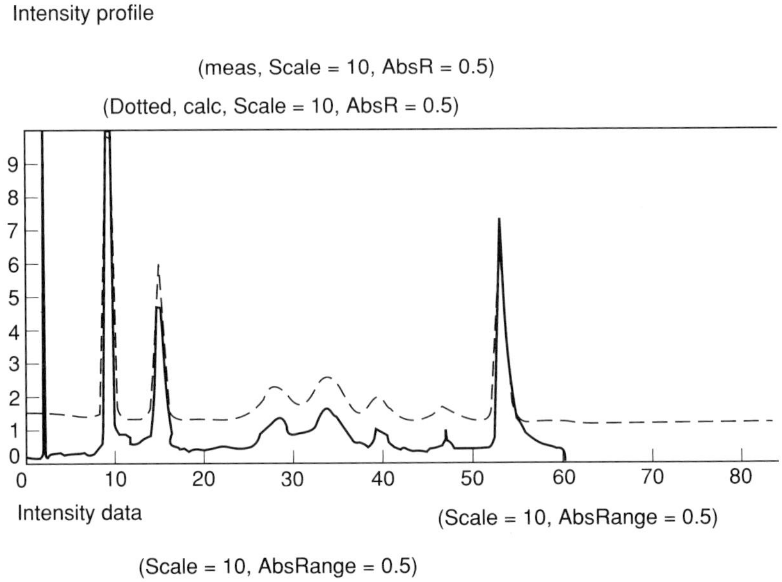

Figure 4.18 A densitometry trace as an intensity versus time graph

to the lens was advantageous in that it aided wettability and biocompatibility. Wedler suggested that mucin only builds up on heavy deposits and only then is it a problem. He found a high correlation between heavily irritating lenses and deposition of mucin components on top of the tear protein aggregate. Wedler even suggested that a mucin removal component should be included in lens cleaning fluid. This subject of mucin's role needs further study before it can be decided whether its adsorption is beneficial or not.

We employ two main electrophoretic techniques, isotachophoresis and polyacrylamide gel electrophoresis. Isotachophoresis is a little used, but potentially powerful, method of analysis. In these laboratories we use a sodium dodecyl sulphate- polyacrylamide gel electrophoresis (SDS-page) system. The use of the detergent SDS masks the native charge that proteins possess and as all proteins are given a charge proportional to their size their mobilities can be assumed to be a function of size alone. This treatment also denatures the protein and considerations of molecular shape become less important.

Although SDS-page is an excellent technique for identifying proteins it does have some limitations. These include its ability to identify the components present is dependent on the sensitivity of the extraction technique used to remove the proteins from the lens' surface. In addition the quantification of the gels using densitometry is limited by the relatively short concentration range of Beer Lamberts law, being linear. The staining efficiency of the proteins also varies between gels, thus assumptions as to the optical density and concentration between gels are not necessarily true. These problems may be surmounted by the inclusion on each gel of a number of standard proteins to ensure reproducibility.

There are then, several available techniques for 'visualizing' the protein components separated by electrophoresis. Plate 28 shows a conventional Coomassie blue stain. Figure 4.18 is a densitometry trace in which stain intensities have been converted to peaks on an intensity versus time graph. Plate 29 shows the result of a silver stain on SDS-page gel electrophoresis samples extracted from lenses worn for 2 weeks at a concentration approximately 10-fold less than that used in Plate 28. A much more sensitive staining technique, electroblotting (where the proteins are transferred to a nitrocellulose membrane by means of a small current and stained with biotin avidin), is shown in Plate 30, which relates to the same samples as in Plate 29 and demonstrates the enhanced sensitivity. Although the biotin avidin technique (which is experimentally more sophisticated and demanding) has not yet been adopted by researchers in the contact lens field, it has clear advantages in terms of sensitivity.

Current trends in protein evaluation

The essential problems that are being assessed in these laboratories at the present time go beyond the simple question of 'which proteins and how much?'. Topics of current interest are summarized below:

- How much protein penetrates the bulk of different contact lens materials, and how much deposits as surface film?
- Is the protein in different locations still biologically active?
- How is the protein composition at the surface stratified?
- Which proteins are strongly bound and denatured at the interfacial regions of the lens surface?

In tackling these questions an array of techniques has been assembled. These include gas plasma etching[50,51] coupled with probe techniques and a variety of immunological assays.

One such technique involves electroblotting of the electrophoresis gels and total protein assay using biotin avidin followed by lysozyme and lactoferrin characterization using the antibodies method. These techniques have been used in protein analysis employing a range of additional electrophoretic systems including isoelectric focusing, immunoelectrophoresis and gradient electrophoresis[14,23,32], but not effectively applied to the denatured question associated with protein behaviour at the lens surface.

An interesting sideline in these studies relates to the commonly used method of cleaning soft contact lenses using proteolytic enzymes to digest the adsorbed protein. The role of these agents in the build-up or removal of adsorbed protein is open to debate and the effectiveness of the enzyme cleaners varies greatly from protein to protein in the deposited layer. A cocktail of enzymes does not overcome this problem, in that if the enzymes are derived from different sources it is likely that they will digest one another as opposed to the adsorbed tear proteins. Additionally, the effect of the part digested proteins around, on and in the lens matrix may themselves contribute to the spoilation process. It is clear that problems associated with protein and lens materials are complex and require careful study with sophisticated techniques.

Short-term tear interactions – disposable and frequent replacement lenses

It is more important in these cases to understand the primary interaction of protein as there is not a great deal of time for dramatic tear interactions and changes in conformation. These short-term wear periods demonstrate the patient variability

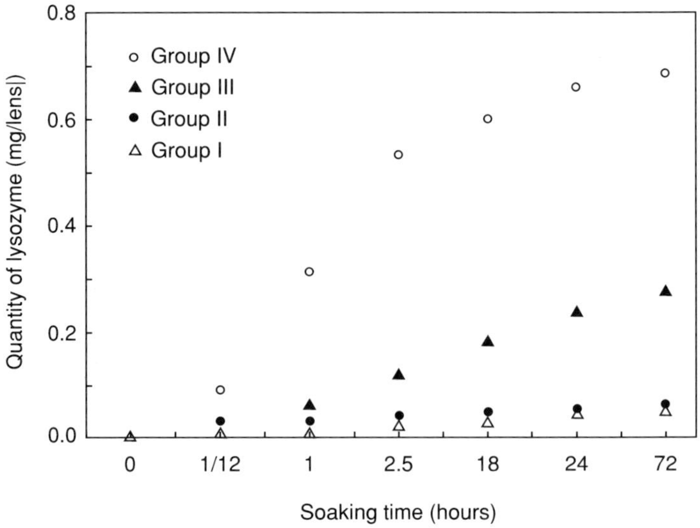

Figure 4.19 Lysozyme uptake by lenses in FDA Classes 1–4

better than longer term studies, where the observed spoilation pattern variability is usually averaged.

The adsorption of protein at an interface is followed rapidly by adsorption of secondary and tertiary protein layers and the competitive adsorption of other biochemical species. Additionally, some components, such as lipids, begin to diffuse into the lens matrix and are held within it.

The advent of disposable and frequent replacement lenses has not overcome the problems associated with lens–tear interactions, Indeed, the widespread use of high water content ionic lenses (e.g., FDA Group 4; Etafilcon and Vifilcon) has meant that the problem is more acute. Although it is widely accepted that proteins such as lysozyme interact strongly with group 4 materials, no systematic study has been made of the relative interaction of tear proteins with these lenses, the subsequent mobility of the proteins and the effect of interaction on their biological activity. This section addresses these three questions.

A series of lenses from each of the four FDA groups (low water content non-ionic (1); high water content non-ionic (2); low water content ionic (3); high water content ionic (4)) were examined in conjunction with individual tear proteins and with a range of additional proteins (riboflavin, ribonuclease, myoglobin, ferrodoxin, insulin) which enabled effects of size and charge to be identified. Protein concentrations were measured by u.v. spectroscopic and capillary electrophoresis techniques. The activity of lysozyme was measured by measuring the decrease in the turbidity of a solution of *Micrococcus lysodeikticus*. Comparative studies were carried out with *ex vivo* lenses.

Figure 4.19 shows the rate of deposition of the three major tear proteins which indicates the influence of charge and water content of the substrate polymer on the rate of protein accumulation. Subsequent studies enabled the relative quantities of surface adsorption and absorption into the lens matrix to be established, together with the influence of protein size and charge on these two processes. Although lysozyme was most readily absorbed into the lens matrix, lactoferrin was also found

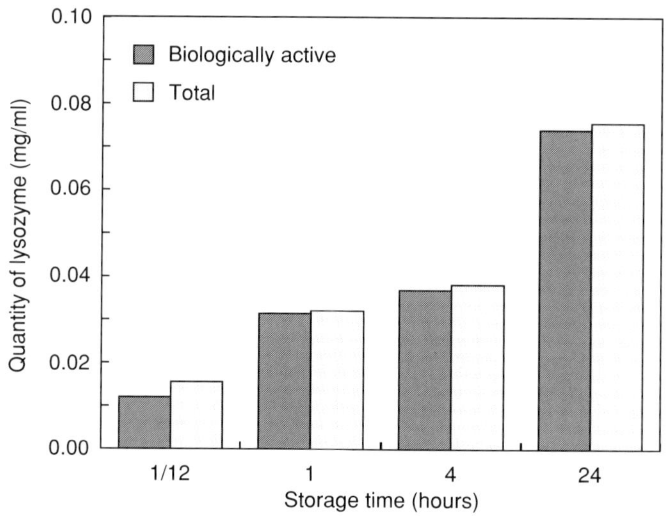

Figure 4.20 Retained biological activity of desorbed lysozyme

to penetrate the matrix of group 4 lenses.

Both absorbed and adsorbed lysozyme proved to be extremely mobile and were readily desorbed in substantial quantity from both surface and bulk of the lenses. The process of adsorption and desorption was found not to affect the biological activity of lysozyme. This is illustrated in Figure 4.20. Similar retention of activity was observed with protein absorbed into and desorbed from the lens matrix of both *in vitro* spoiled and *in vivo* worn group 4 lenses.

Extrinsic contaminants and surfactant cleaners

The processes that occur when a contact lens is placed in the eye are examples of biological interfacial conversion processes. It is quite instructive to think of the various ways in which contact lens spoilation processes can be subdivided. They do not all involve tear components, i.e., compounds that are intrinsically involved in the functions of the ocular environment. Some of them are extrinsic factors. The various chemical and biochemical processes involved can be subdivided as shown in Table 4.3, in which features of both intrinsic and extrinsic processes are shown. It is worth noting that the features of intrinsic and extrinsic spoilation are not mutually exclusive.

Examples of extrinsic contaminants that are encountered in contact lens spoilation include:

- Skin (especially finger) lipids
- Cosmetics
- Care solution components (e.g. sorbic acid)
- Coloured organic contaminants (e.g. dyes and stains)

Examples of the last two named categories were referred to previously[20]. Attention now turns to the group of organic materials traditionally called oils, fats and waxes.

They have in common their insolubility in water due to the fact that they contain substantial hydrocarbon components, often joined by ester linkage. The lipids that are so common in our bodies fall right into the centre of this group of compounds. Here we will look at some of the ways in which they come to contaminate contact lenses.

Table 4.3 Example of the different ways in which spoilation processes may be subdivided

A	*B*
Processes that involve ocular components (*intrinsic*)	Processes that involve non-ocular components (*extrinsic*)
Processes that involve biological components	Processes that involve synthetic components
Processes that involve water-soluble components	Processes that involve water-insoluble components
Processes that involve inherently coloured species	Processes that involve non-coloured species
Processes that produce discoloration	Processes that do not produce discoloration
Processes that involve chemical reaction	Processes that do not involve chemical reaction
Processes that occur on the lens surface	Processes that occur within the lens matrix

Finger lipids: transfer to contact lenses

The purpose of lipids in the body is sometimes described as being to keep the water out and keep the water in. They are certainly commonly associated with most of the external surfaces of the body.

Digital manipulation of contact lenses by the wearer provides considerable potential for contamination of the lens by skin lipids. The analysis of this type of contact transfer of such skin lipids is very difficult. It was possible to do it in our laboratory with the highly sensitive high performance liquid chromatography system developed for studying tear lipids involved in ocular spoilation.

In order to study the effect of contact transfer of skin lipids, a range of volunteers, both lens wearers and non-wearers, took part in a study where a number of lenses were handled for varied periods of time. The volunteers washed their hands prior to handling the lenses and once the lenses were returned to the vial they were not handled again.

After the lenses had been rinsed briefly in sterile saline they were removed using tweezers and extracted with an appropriate solvent prior to the HPLC analysis. A typical chromatogram is shown in Figure 4.21. The traces obtained were similar to, but not identical with, those deposited on a lens after insertion into the eye. In particular the fatty acid fraction was enhanced. Several conclusions were drawn from the study.

- Lipids are effectively transferred to the lens by finger contact
- The area of contact is more important than the time of contact
- There is an observable patient to patient variation

For a given area of finger–lens contact, lipids are transferred immediately on contact. The quantity transferred only increases appreciably if the contact is increased (e.g., as when the lens is rolled between the fingers).

One of the most important factors in contact transfer, other than the question of sterility, lies in the transfer of unsatruated fatty acids to the lens surface. These can

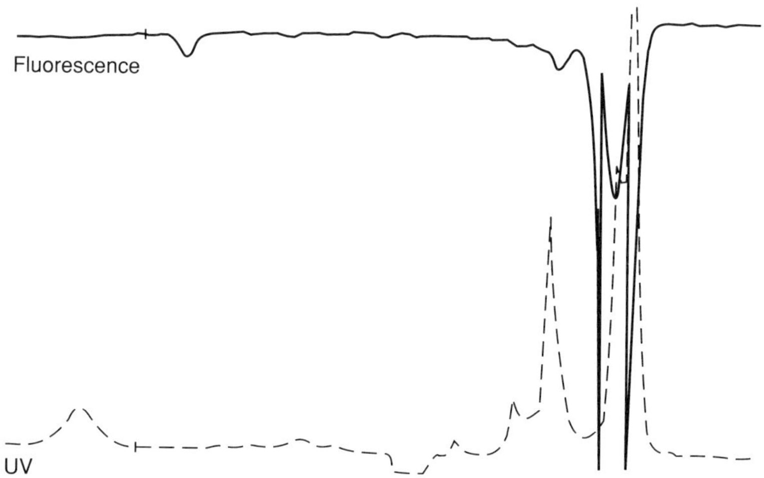

Figure 4.21 Typical chromatogram of skin lipids transferred to a polyHEMA lens by finger contact

then migrate into the lens matrix by the partitioning process described earlier. Although their involvement in discoloration processes is limited by their low concentration and mobility, they can contribute to spoilation in other ways. One particular role of the fatty acids is the creation on the lens surface of localized hydrophobic regions which will then permit deposition and migration into the lens matrix of tear lipids. This migration process can be easily illustrated by the fact that relatively hydrophobic steroids (e.g., progesterone) are some 200 times more soluble in polyHEMA than a water soluble sugar molecule of similar size, e.g., sucrose.

It is quite clear that finger lipids are readily transferred to lenses. These unsaturated finger lipids if not removed, increase the lipid burden on the lens and thus, ultimately the formation of insoluble white spots localized at and within the lens surface.

Cosmetics and lens contamination

The extent of any complications caused by cosmetics is difficult to assess in a quantitative and objective fashion. There is no quantitative information available to permit clinicians to assess objectively the relative effects of the different types of cosmetic agents and lens care systems.

Taking a representative made-up eye (mascara, eye shadow, eye liner) brings the ocular environment into contact with an astonishing number of constituents. These are listed in Table 4.4. It is clear that conventional cosmetics are a prime source of oils, fats and waxes!

Currently available cosmetics are based on very old principles of formulation. Many are still a natural oil, fat or wax emulsified with water in the presence of an emulsifying agent which 'carries' the solid particulate colouring agent or pigment. The texture of the make-up varies dependent on which of the range of waxes and softening agents are incorporated into the composition.

A typical eye make-up preparation will contain at least 15 constituents including surfactants and preservatives in its formulation. Fortunately, the majority of these oils and waxes used as binding agents are almost always based on saturated compounds, as distinct from the unsaturated fatty acids, esters and alcohols. This means that they do not possess the reactive double bonds present in the unsaturated tear lipids. This lack of double bond does, however, mean that these compounds are very difficult to detect using standard u.v. spectroscopy which will only detect the residual coloration caused by the cosmetics.

Analysis of cosmetic contamination

The techniques routinely used to analyse spoilation are all highly sensitive and able to detect the range of chemical and biochemical components which are frequently present in minute quantities and intimately involved with the contact lens matrix. The lack of availability of this type of technique has led to the commonly held expectation that commercial surfactant cleaners can remove all lipoidal contamination from the lens surface. Quite simple studies shown here illustrate: the relative abilities to contaminate the lenses in the case of cosmetics and the relative abilities to cleanse the lens in the case of lens care systems.

Table 4.4. Typical constituents of mascara, eye shadow and eye liner

Beeswax
Carnuba wax
Hydrogenated palm kernel oil
Microcrystalline wax
Ozokerite
Paraffin hydrocarbons
Butylated hydroxy anisole
Cetostearyl alcohol
Stearic acid
DEG stearate
Propylene glycol
Butylene glycol
PVP
Carbopol
Lecithin
Triethanolamine
Phenoxyethanol
Magnesium aluminium silicate
Potassium octoxynol phosphate
Sodium lauryl sulphate
Methyl para amino benzoic acid
Propyl para amino benzoic acid
Cyclomethicone
Dimethicone
Oleamide
Quaternium-15
SD alcohol 1
Various pigments
Water

Useful information can be obtained by contamination of the lenses by direct cosmetic application and indirect application of the cosmetic in an appropriate carrier solvent. This enables the examination of the contribution of the following features of the contamination:

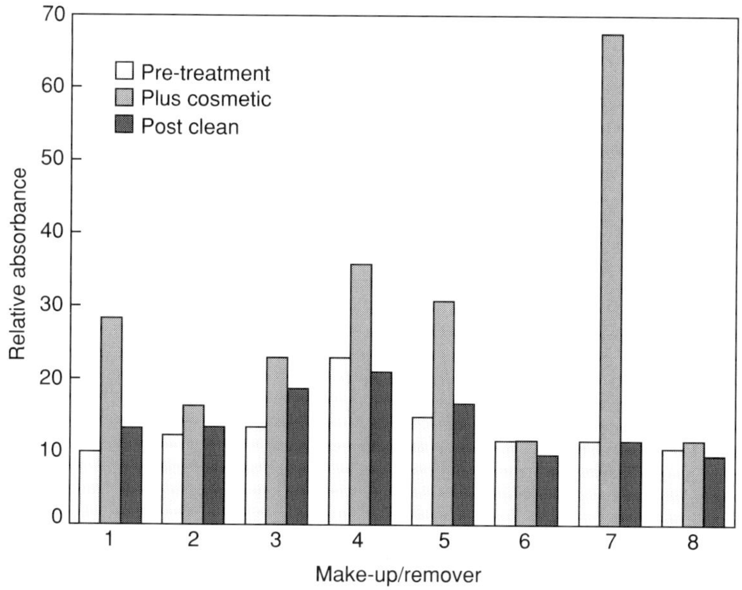

Figure 4.22 Relative absorbances of polyHEMA lenses after use of cosmetics and make-up removers and after these have been removed by a surfactant cleaner (1–3 mascara; 4–5 eye shadow; 6 eye pencil; 7–9 make-up remover)

- Contamination of the surface by the pigment particles
- Discoloration of the lens matrix
- contamination of the surface and matrix by contact transfer and migration of non-coloured components

In addition, the effect of the eye make-up removers, as both contaminants and cleaners of the lenses was assessed.

The effects of the first two factors described above can be checked using visible and u.v. spectroscopy. The results, together with the effect of a surfactant cleaner in removing the contamination, are shown in Figure 4.22. Residual analysis of the non-coloured components demonstrated the presence of esters from the oil–water carriers. The oil-based eye make-up removers cause the most pronounced contamination of the lens surface-matrix. The pigmentation in solvent suspension did not cause matrix discoloration, but did attach residual pigment particles to the lens (Figures 4.23 and 4.24). In addition to these observations, it was also noted that all the cosmetics produce non-coloured contamination of the lens surface which is not easily removed by simple cleaning procedures. Relatively small differences were detected between those make up formulations designed for contact lens wearers and the 'standard' cosmetic preparations.

Our studies have highlighted the complexity of the compositions of apparently simple make up formulations. Not only does the contamination remain on the lens after all visible traces have been removed, the eye make-up removers themselves can cause marked residual lens contamination. Thus, it is important that such products should not be used on soft contact lenses. The best method of removing any make-up

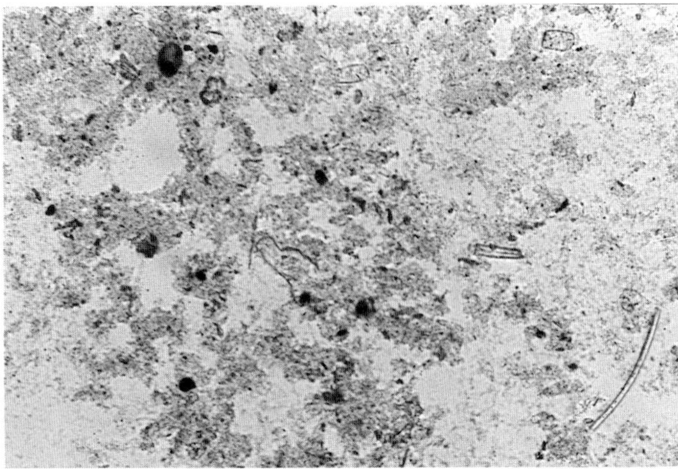

Figure 4.23 Mascara pigment particles on the surface of a polyHEMA lens. Brightfield ×125

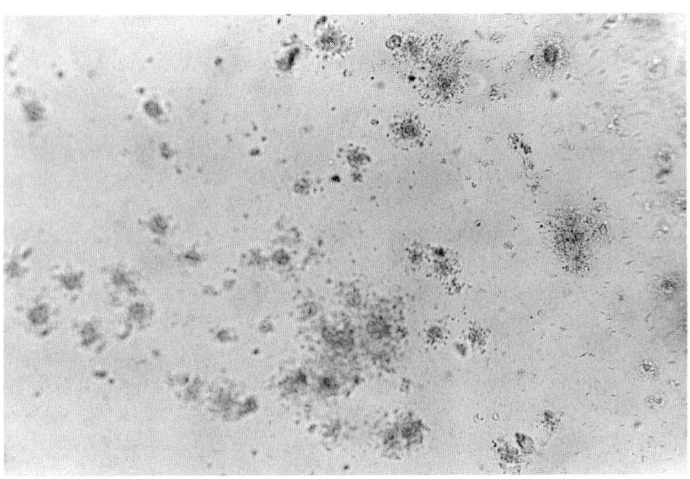

Figure 4.24 Eye shadow pigment particles on the surface of a polyHEMA lens. Brightfield ×125

contamination is to use a surfactant cleaner. These may, however, give a false impression of how clean the lens surface is, as they cause a coherent layer of water to be retained by the lens surface. To date, these studies have been concerned with polyHEMA lenses, but the initial ongoing studies have so far shown very little variation with types of lens material.

Wetting, cleaning and surfactants

Wetting solutions and cleaning solutions have in common the need for a reduced surface tension to enable them to wet the lens surface more effectively than does water. To achieve this surfactants are commonly used in both cases. The function of the surfactant or surface active agent is, however, somewhat different in the two cases.

The removal of deposited biological material from contact lenses is achieved by 'solubilization' rather than by a conventional dissolution process. This is achieved in a similar way to that encountered with washing powders, thus individual particles of dirt are removed from the solid surface and held in solution. In order to do this, rather more sophisticated behaviour than simple reduction of surface tension is required.

The requirements of the surfactant in an effective cleaning solution might be simply stated as follows: to remove the deposited material from the surface; the suspension of the deposited materials in solution; and the provision of sufficient surfactant to enable all deposited material to be removed and 'solubilized' in this way.

The efficacy of commercial lens cleaners

The differences in cleaning ability of soft lens cleaners has been measured in our laboratories. PolyHEMA lenses were for spoiled for 28 days using a total *in vitro* tear model developed at Aston University, Birmingham. The quantity of lipoidal material on the lens surfaces was measured by fluorescence spectroscopy. The lenses were then subjected to a series of cleaning steps with different cleaners and the residual lipoidal material monitored after each step. In each case the lens was finally cleaned twice with a very effective surfactant to bring it to a common level.

The Aston tear model enables controlled spoilation of various contact lens materials to be carried out *in vitro*[18,19]. The model mimics the biochemistry of the ocular spoilation process and may be modified to mimic the extremes of deposition. It avoids the problems of patient-to-patient variation.

After 28 days of *in vitro* spoilation, lenses were removed from the tear model, rinsed with saline, disinfected with hydrogen peroxide and their fluorescence spectra recorded. These lenses were then treated according to the steps of the protocol and their fluorescence spectra re-recorded at each step. Triplicate spectra of each lens/tear model/cleaner combination are obtained. In addition, three separate readings were taken each time a spectrum was recorded: the lens being assessed and then relocated between readings. The quantitative peak maximum is read directly in each case from an optical density meter. The height of the peak maxima of the spoiled lenses is normalized to 100 units on the optical density meter. This gives a quantitative measure of material remaining on the surface.

Extensive work has previously been carried out with both *in vitro* and *in vivo* spoiled lenses using HPLC, electrophoresis and isotachophoresis to identify the nature of spoilation products and the characteristic residual fragments obtained with different types of cleaning regimen. In particular, the correlation of fluorescence emissions in the 400–500 nm region with the nature of proteinaceous and lipoidal species sorbed onto the lens surface has shown the value of fluorescence spectroscopy for studies of this type.

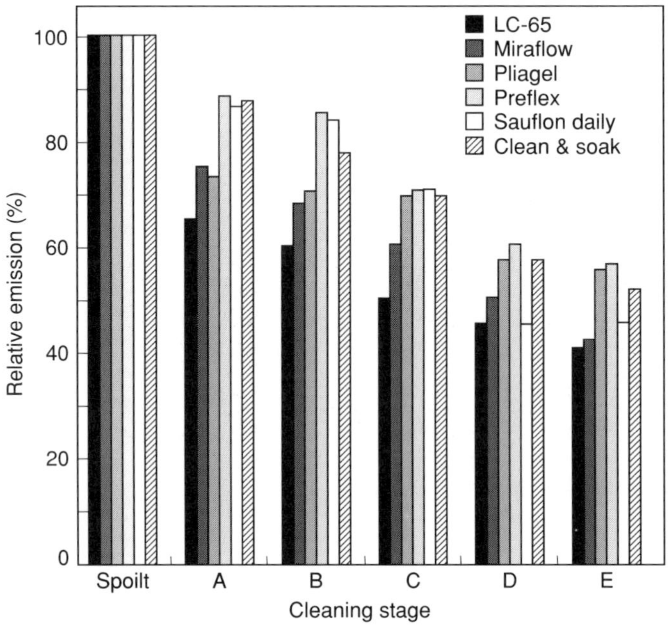

Figure 4.25 A graph to show the progressive reduction in residual spoilation at each stage of the cleaning protocol for the surfactant cleaner on polyHEMA lenses

Five successive steps were used to assess the cleaning ability of individual care products:

A 20 sec mechanical agitation of lens and 5 ml of the cleaner under test in 15 ml vial followed by saline rinse (copious)
B Repeat step A
C 20 sec digital clean with 2 ml of cleaner under test followed by saline rinse (copious)
D Digital clean with standard surfactant followed by saline rinse (copious)
E Repeat step D.

Relative intensity of spoilation peak (fluorescence emission at 480 nm at an excitation wavelength of 360 nm) is measured and recorded at each stage. The initial spoilation peak is normalized to 199 units and the results of stages A–E presented in histogram form. Figure 4.25 illustrates the results for a range of cleaning solutions used in conjunction with polyHEMA.

Relative cleaning efficiency (RCE) is obtained by taking the results of steps A–E in the form:

$$\text{RCE} = \frac{100 - \text{C}}{100 - \text{E}} \times 100\%$$

This relative cleaning efficiency indicates the proportion of surfactant-removable spoilation that is attainable by a given cleaner using steps A–C. Distilled water gives a relative cleaning efficiency of 20–30%, whereas the most effective commercial lens products produce values around 80%.

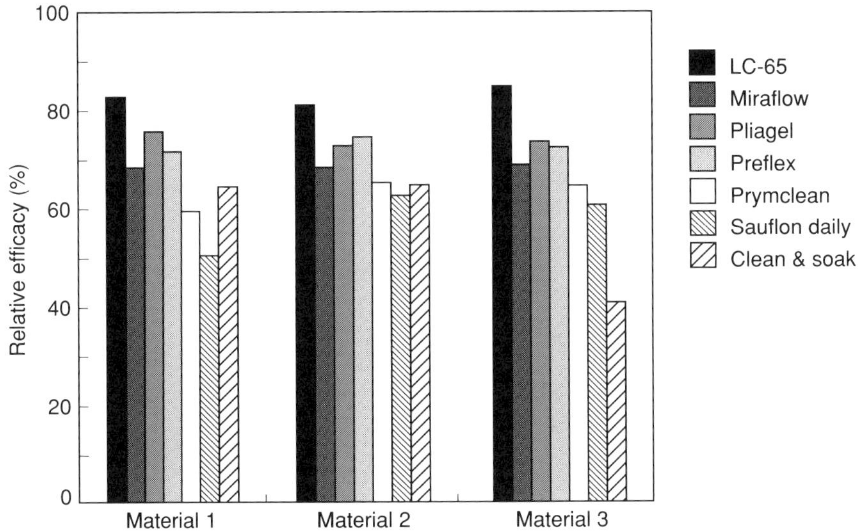

Figure 4.26 A graph showing the cleaning efficacy of soft, soft/RGP or multi-purpose cleaners

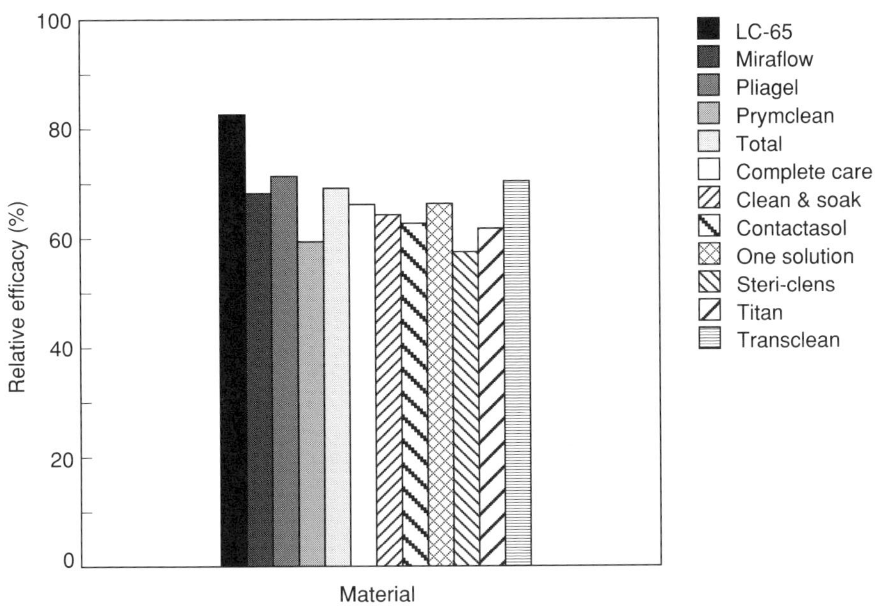

Figure 4.27 A graph showing the cleaning efficacy of RGP, RGP/soft or multi-purpose cleaners

Relative cleaning efficacies for a range of soft lens cleaners, RGP cleaners and multipurpose solutions are shown in Figures 4.26 and 4.27.

These studies clearly demonstrate that all the commercial surfactant cleaners are much more effective in removing sorbed lipid from the surfaces of both hard and soft lenses than is distilled water or saline. Efficacy is not simply related to surface tension or viscosity which are in themselves an inadequate indication of the action of surfactant during cleaning. While it is true that more viscous solutions are easier to maintain in contact with the lens during digital cleaning and that low surface tension indicates the presence of a surfactant, these factors do not in themselves indicate the 'appetite' of the cleaner for the biological debris on a given lens.

Our results show that the available commercial contact lens cleaners differ considerably in their ability to remove lipid from the surface of the lens, but that for rigid gas permeable lenses the cleaning efficacy of different cleaners was much more similar. It is quite clear that soft lenses are generally more difficult to clean than hard lenses.

Another interesting observation is that the soft lens cleaners generally had a similar efficacy when used on RGP lenses, whereas a decrease in cleaning efficacy was observed with RGP cleaners used on soft contact lenses.

These results, when taken with other studies in our laboratories demonstrate the following:

1 Spoliation is rapid with respect to both protein and lipid deposition on the lens surface
2 Cleaning may reduce this deposited layer, but it is rapidly re-established on reinsertion of the lens
3 The immobilized species (proteins and lipids) will undergo chemical conversion with time following deposition. It is this process which produces problems. As a result cleaning is important in minimizing long-term surface deposition which reduces disinfection efficacy especially for heavy lipid deposition.

Although the surfactant cleaners do remove some of the lipid present on the lens surface they are unable to prevent the build-up of the lipid within the contact lens matrix. Because surfactant clings to the lens surface, a freshly cleaned lens retains a coherent water film that gives an optimistic impression of cleanliness of the lens. The presence of lipid within the lens matrix has been demonstrated using fluorescence spectroscopy and scanning confocal laser microscopy.

Thus, although in the short term the surfactant cleaners remove some of the lipid film and are an essential component of safe disinfection, the lipid layer is rapidly re-established by the tear film. In the longer-term, this lipid is partitioned within the lens matrix and undergoes chemical conversion to form insoluble high molecular weight products. The longer-term effects of all factors of this type on the course of interfacial biological conversion process involving tears leading to hydrogel spoilation are part of ongoing experimental studies.

It is paradoxical that, as techniques for the study of long-term interactions of hydrogels with the eye become more sophisticated, leading to a more complete understanding of these phenomena, emphasis on contact lens wear modality has moved dramatically towards disposability and frequent replacement. This does not remove the need for an understanding of these ocular biomaterials with the eye, but does raise several new issues which will become more apparent as the influence of newer wear modalities achieves maturity. These include the enhanced importance of group 4 lenses, with their ability to reduce dramatically tear lysozyme concentrations in the period following insertion of the virgin lens; the changing pattern of solutions usage and its effect on lipid-protein balance at the lens surface; and the long-term effects of repeated insult to the ocular environment by daily insertion of a new piece of synthetic polymer. It is in the unexplored effects of daily disposability that the greatest degree of uncertainty lies. Strangely enough, there seems to be a general lack of concern about the potential long-term effects of this dramatic change in the use of polymers as contact lenses.

References

1 Abbott, J. M., Bowers, R. W. J., Franklin, V. J. and Tighe, B. J. (1991). Studies in the ocular compatibility of hydrogels (IV) *Journal of the British Contact Lens Association*, **14**, 21–28
2 Abbott, J. M., Franklin, V. J. and Tighe, B. J. (1990). *Analysis of lipoidal spoilation of individual worn contact lenses by an HPLC technique*, Part V. In Press
3 Allansmith, M. (1973) Immunology of the tears. In: *The Preocular Tear Film and Dry Eye Syndromes*, edited by F. J. Holly and M. A. Lemp. Boston: Little, Brown, and Co. pp. 47–72
4 Allen, J., Botting, R., Sharp, A. and Tuffery, A. A. (1978). *Optician*, **8**, 175
5 Bailey, N. J. (1975). *Journal of the American Optometric Association*, **46**, 214
6 Bilbaut, T., Gachon, A. M. and Dastugue, B. (1986). *Experimental Eye Research*, **43**, 153–165
7 Bloomfield, S. E., David, S. D. and Rubin, A. L. (1978). *Annals of Ophthalmology*, **10**, 355–360
8 Bowers, R. W. J. and Tighe, B. J. (1987). *Biomaterials*, **8**, 8–13
9 Bowers, R. W. J. and Tighe, B. J. (1987). *Biomaterials*, **8**, 89–93
10 Bowers, R. W. J. and Tighe, B. J. (1987). *Biomaterials*, **8**, 172–177
11 Bright, A. M. and Tighe, B. J. (1992). *Journal of the British Contact Lens Association*, **15**, 17–24
12 Castillo, E. J., Koeing, J. L., Anderson, J. M. and Jenotoft, N. P. (1986). *Biomaterials*, **7**, 9–16
13 Corkhill, P. C., Hamilton, C. J. and Tighe, B. J. (1990) The design of hydrogels for medical applications. In: *Critical Reviews in Biocompatibility*, Vol 5, edited by D. F. Williams. St Louis: Mosby. pp. 363–436
14 Coyle, P. K., Sibony, P. A. and Johnson, C. (1989). *Investigative Ophthalmology and Visual Science*, **30**, 1872–1879
15 Erisken, S. (1975). *Annals of Ophthalmology*, **7**, 122–135
16 Erisken, S. (1978). Cleaning hydrophilic contact lenses: an overview, Allergan Report series.
17 Farris, R. L. (1985). *Transactions of the Ophthalmic Society*, **83**, 501–545
18 Franklin, V. J., Jones, L. W., Ma, J., Sariri, R., Singh-Gill, U., Evans, K. *et al.* (1994). Reprinted in *British Contact Lens Association Journal*, **17**, 153
19 Franklin, V. J., Singh-Gill, U., Sairi, P. and Tighe, B. J. (1993). Tear deposition on spoilation resistant materials. A preliminary study. Poster Presented at the BCLA Annual Clinical Conference, London, May
20 Franklin, V. J. and Tighe, B. J. (1991). *Optician*, **201**, 16–22
21 Fuchell, R. N., Farris, R. L. and Mandel, I. D. (1981). *Ophthalmology*, **88**, 858–861
22 Fullard, R. J. and Snyder, C. (1990). *Investigative Ophthalmology and Visual Science*, **31**, 1119–1126
23 Gachon, A. M., Verrelle, P., Betail, G and Dastugue, B. (1979). *Experimental Eye Research*, **29**, 539–553
24 Hart, D. E. (1987). *Journal of the American Optometric Association*, **58**, 962–974
25 Hart, D. E. and Shih, K. L. (1987). *American Journal of Optometry and Physiological Optics*, **64**, 739–748
26 Hart, D. E., Tidsale, R. R. and Sack, A. (1986). *Ophthalmology*, **93**, 495–503
27 Hathaway, R. A. and Lowther, G. E. (1976). *International Contact Lens Clinic*, **3**, 27
28 Hathaway, R. A. and Lowther, G. E. (1978). *Australian Journal of Optometry*, **61**, 92
29 Holly, F. J. (1980). *American Journal of Physiological Optics*, **58**, 324–330
30 Hosaka, S., Ozawa, H., Tanzawa, H., Ishida, H., Yoshimura, L., Momose, T. *et al.* (1983). *Journal of Biomedicine and Materials Research*, **17**, 261–274

31 Huth, S. W. and Wagner, H. G. (1981). *International Contact Lens Clinic*, **8**, 19–27

32 Janssen, P. T. and van Bijterveld, O. P. (1981). *Clinica et Chimica Acta*, **114**, 207–218

33 Janssen, P. T. and Van Bijsterveld, O. P. (1983). *Investigative Ophthalmology and Visual Science*, **24**, 623–630

34 Karageozian, H. L. (1976). *Contacto*, **20**, 5–10

35 Kiral, R. M. and Vehige, J. G. (1988). *Contact Lens Spectrum*, **3**, 31–42

36 Kleist, F. D. (1979). *International Contact Lens Clinic*, **6**, 120–130

37 Klintworth, G. K., Reed, J. W. and Hawkins, H. K. *et al.* (1977). *Investigative Ophthalmology and Visual Science*, **16**, 158–161

38 Koetting, R. A. (1976) *Contacto*, **20**, 20

39 Lin, S., Mandell, R. B., Leahy, C. D. and Newell, J. O. (1991). *CLAO Journal*, **17**, 44-50

40 McGill, J. I., Liakos, G. M., Goulding, N. and Seal, D. V. (1984). *British Journal of Ophthalmology*, **68**, 316–320

41 Minark, L. and Rapp, J. (1989). *CLAO Journal*, **15**, 185–188

42 Payor, E. (1992). Quantification of total protein deposited on human worn soft contact lenses using visible light scatter, electrophoresis and amino acid analysis. *BCLA Annual Clinical Conference*, 21–24 May 1992, Harrogate

43 Pearce, A. E. G. (1968). *Histochemistry: Theoretical and Applied.* 3rd edn, Vols I & II, London: Churchill

44 Rapp, J. and Brioch, J. (1984). *CLAO Journal*, **10**, 235–239

45 Refojo, M. F. (1978). Contact lenses. In: *Encyclopedia of Polymer Science and Technology*, Vol. 1. New York: Wiley Interscience. pp. 195

46 Ruben, M., Tripathi, R. C. and Winder, A. F. (1975). *British Journal of Ophthalmology*, **59**, 141–148

47 Sack, R. A., Harvey, H and Nunes, I. (1986). *CLAO Journal*, **15**, 138–145

48 Sack, R. A., Jones, B., Antignani, A., Libow, R. and Harvey, H. (1986). *Investigative Ophthalmology and Visual Science*, **28**, 842–849

49 Shuman, H., Murray, J. M. and DiLullo, C. (1989). *Biotechniques*, **7**, 154–163

50 Singh-Gill, U., Mann, A. and Tighe, B. J. (1994). The use of a novel plasma etching and emission monitoring system (PEEMS) in contact lens spoilation studies. Poster presented at the BCLA Annual Clinical Conference, Torquay

51 Singh-Gill, U. and Tighe, B. J. (1994). The use of a novel plasma etching and emission monitoring system (PEEMS) in contact lens spoilation studies. *11th European Conference on Biomaterials*, Pisa, Italy, September 1994

52 Spring, T. F. (1974). *Medical Journal of Australia*, **1**, 449

53 Stuchell, R. N., Feldman, J. J., Farris, R. L. and Mandell, I. D. (1984). *Investigative Ophthalmology and Visual Science*, **25**, 374–377

54 Tapaszto, I. (1973). Pathophysiology of human tears. In: *The Preocular Tear Film and Dry Eye Syndromes*, edited by F. J. Holly and M. A. Lemp. Boston: Little, Brown, and Co. pp. 119–147

55 Tighe, B. J. (1987). Hydrogels as contact lens materials. In: *Hydrogels in Medicine and Pharmacy*, Vol. 3, edited by N. A. Peppas. Boston: CRC Press. pp. 53–82

56 Tighe, B. J. (1988). Contact lens materials. In: *Contact Lens Practice*, 3rd edn, edited by J. Stone and A. J. Phillips. London: Butterworths. pp. 72–124

57 Tighe, B. J. (1990). Blood sweat and tears: some problems in the development of biomaterials. Nissel Memorial Lecture, Royal Society of Medicine. *British Contact Lens Association Transactions*, **13**, 13–19

58 Tripathi, R. C., Tripathi, B. J. and Ruben, M. (1980). *Ophthalmology*, **87**, 365–380

59 Van Haeringen, N. J. and Thorig, L. (1986). Enzymatic composition of tears. In: *The Preocular Tear Film in Health, Disease, and Contact Lens Wear*, edited by F. J. Holly. Lubbock: Dry Eye Institute. pp. 522–528

60 Wedler, F. C. (1977). *Journal of Biomedical Material Research*, **11**, 525

61 Wedler, F. C., Illman, B. L., Horensky, D. S. and Mowrey-McKee, M. (1987). *Clinical and Experimental Optometry*, **70**, 59–68

62 Wolff, E. (1954). *Anatomy of Eye and Orbit*, 4th edn. New York: Blakiston Co. pp. 207–209

63 Young, W. and Hill, R. M. (1973) *Journal of the American Optometric Association*, **3**, 424

Chapter 5

Anterior limbus

Introduction

The anterior limbus forms the junction between the cornea and sclera and is the site of new vessel growth into the cornea. The reasons for vascular ingrowth in some forms of contact lens wear are not wholly clear.

In haptic and hard corneal lens wear, neovascularization is a rare event that probably arises from inappropriate lens fitting. However, in some forms of soft lens wear as many as 2-in-5 corneas may eventually become vascularized. The incidence of neovascularization in soft lens wear can be reduced by the use of thin carefully fitted lenses and a realistic approach to wearing times. Even so, the potential for vascularization remains and careful examination of the anterior limbal zone is a necessary part of the after care of all soft lens wearing patients.

Anatomy of the limbus

The limbus is not a separate structure of the eye, but rather a junction between two other structures; the cornea and sclera. There is no clear agreement in the literature as to the precise boundaries of the limbus, although for the purposes of the clinician it may be considered to be an annulus extending approximately 1.5 mm between the cornea and sclera. The limbus is shown diagrammatically in Figure 5.1. For the purposes of this chapter the anterior limbus will be regarded as only the cornea/scleral junction, although the limbal area is generally taken to include part or all of the aqueous drainage pathways.

The anterior limbus provides a pathway for the supply of metabolites to the corneal periphery. Although formerly thought to be one of the principal sources of metabolites for the cornea as a whole, it has been clearly demonstrated[23] that it is only the extreme periphery which benefits from this source.

At the limbus, the 5 epithelial cell layers of the cornea increase in number until as many as 10 or 15 layers may be observed; the majority of these cells are wing cells, with occasional goblet cells being found in the extreme limbal/scleral periphery. This increased number of cell layers is only maintained in the limbal zone. As the sclera is approached, the number of epithelial cells again reduces to 5 layers.

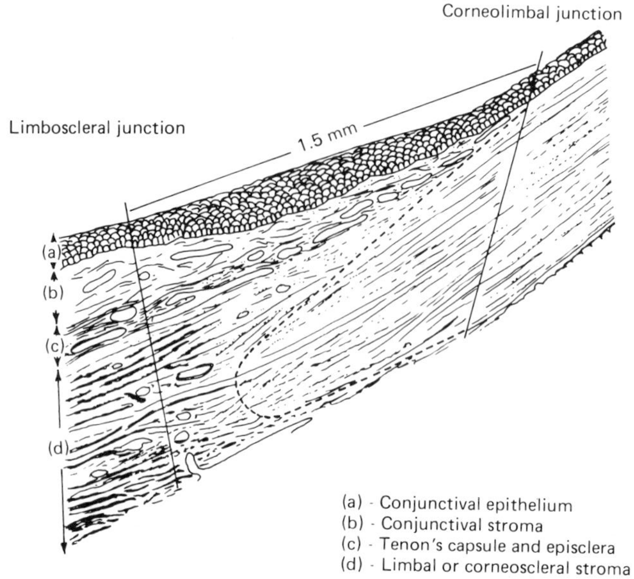

Figure 5. 1 The anterior limbus (based on a drawing in: *History of the Human Eye*, by Hogan, Alvarado and Weddell. WB Saunders, 1971)

The termination of Bowman's layer represents the cornea-limbal junction. Extending from this boundary to the limboscleral junction is a region of loose connective tissue and blood vessels which increases in thickness as the sclera is approached.

Tendon capsule is found immediately beneath the subepithelial stroma, and forms a thin ill-defined region of connective tissue.

The limbal stroma occupies the largest portion of the limbal area and represents the transition between the regularly ordered collagen fibrils of the cornea, and the unordered but, in many respects, structurally similar region of the sclera. For the purposes of this chapter the anterior limbus will be considered to terminate at the posterior limit of this region. Beneath the limbal stroma are found the structures concerned with aqueous drainage.

Blood vessels of the limbus

Arteries

The arterial supply to the limbus is derived from the anterior ciliary arteries. The episcleral branches of the ciliary arteries produce conjunctival and interscleral vessels. The conjunctival vessels form a plexus around the anterior limbus from which is derived:

1 Peripheral corneal arcades
2 Recurrent vessels which run posteriorly in the conjunctiva.

The interscleral branch runs forward to supply the sclerolimbal junction. Both the peripheral corneal arcades and the interscleral vessels are of considerable interest in

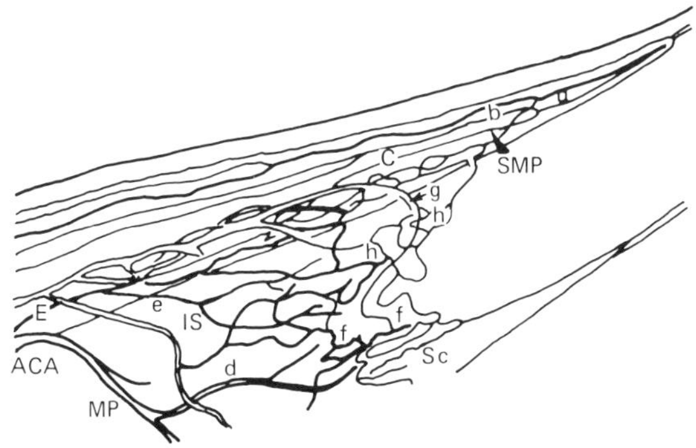

Figure 5.2 Blood vessels of the anterior limbus. ACA: anterior ciliary artery; E: episcleral branch of the major ciliary artery; MP: major perforating branch of the anterior ciliary artery; C: conjunctival vessel; IS: intrascleral vessel; SMP: superficial marginal plexus of the cornea; a: peripheral corneal arcade; b: recurrent vessels (both a and b arise from the superficial marginal plexus); d: a branch from the major perforating passes forward to form the intrascleral arterial channels of the limbus; e: episcleral vessel arising directly from the anterior ciliary artery. Venous channels: f: the deep scheral venous plexus; Sc: Schlemm's canal; g: aqueous vein; h: the intrascleral venous plexus

contact lens practice, as it is from these vessels that neovascularization occurs in various forms of contact lens wear.

Veins

The veins of the anterior limbus follow a similar distribution to the arteries. The peripheral limbal arcades are, in essence, arterial to venous capillaries, and are the only site in the body where this transition may be readily observed. With the improvements in slit lamp biomicroscope design, there must be few contact lens practitioners who have not observed the intermittent passage of groups of blood corpuscles through these fine vessels. After leaving the arcades blood drains via the episcleral vessels. The episcleral veins also receive blood from the large meshwork of vessels in the limbal stroma.

The blood vessels of the anterior limbus are illustrated in Figure 5.2.

Limbus lymphatics

Lymphatic fluid drains from the limbal region by way of an encircling meshwork of fine lymphatic vessels. The meshwork of vessels includes both returning arcades and structures which end blindly in corneal tissue. The periphery of this lymphatic meshwork terminates in a series of radial vessels which drain lymph from the region.

The palisades of Vogt

The palisades of Vogt are found as radial spoke-like structures formed in the limbal conjunctiva and the cornea. They are between 2–4 mm long and are approximately 0.5 mm wide. The palisades are occupied by all of the structures found in the limbal conjunctiva.

The nerves which radiate into the cornea are found along the edges of the palisades, while lymphatic vessels are located towards the centre of the palisades.

The anterior limbus is innervated by branches of the intrascleral and conjunctival nerves, which form networks in the conjunctiva, episclera and stroma.

Mechanisms of corneal neovascularization

Unlike many changes which occur in the various structures of the eye in contact lens wear the limbus is the site of a single but important event; the growth of adventitious vessels from the limbal region into the cornea. The mechanisms by which corneal neovascularization (angiogenesis) is produced in contact lens wear is complex. Neovascularization is essentially a response to a metabolic or angiogenic factor by mature existing blood vessels[22]. New vessels form from the existing vascular endothelium which retains the capacity to revert to primitive vascular mesenchyme[1]. It is from this mesenchyme that the endothelial cells, pericytes, smooth muscle cells and fibroblasts of the new growing vessel are formed. It would appear that the formation of new vessels is not dependent upon other factors such as blood flow or other types of cell[13,25].

The effect of vasostimulatory factor is to initiate new growth by a direct effect on endothelial cells and to determine the direction of growth.

The mechanism by which neovascularization is provoked in contact lens wear has only recently been described[28]. In rabbits, soft contact lens wear stimulates the metabolism of arachidonic acid by an NADPH-cytochrome P450 mono-oxygenase. The two major products are 12(R)-hydroxyeicosatetraenoic acid and 12(R)-hydroxyeicosatrienoic acid, (12(R)-hetre) a pro-inflammatory and angiogenic factor. The synthesis of 12(R)-hetre is increased substantially in contact lens induced hypoxia. 12(R)-hetre has biological actions which include increases in barrier permeability, vasodilation, polymorphonuclear chemotaxis and vascular endothelial cell mitogenesis. *In vitro* experiments utilizing rabbit corneoscleral rims in a micropocket assay, a direct (as apposed to an indirect) angiogenic effect has been demonstrated. Angiogenesis based on this mechanism has been demonstrated for both the cornea and the conjunctiva, although the hypoxic provoked increase in 12(R)-hetre was two- to four-fold more in the epithelium than in the conjunctiva. Due to the proximity of the cornea and conjunctiva, metabolite production by one tissue may potentially influence the physiological state of the other.

New blood vessel growth into the cornea is invariably accompanied by lymphatic excursions[6,7,8,9] and the parallel development in both systems has been carefully examined in animal studies[10,15,27,29].

Contact lens wear and corneal neovascularization

Corneal vascularization as a result of haptic lens wear was observed as long ago as 1929[20]. Since this first report, a number of detailed case histories have been published where neovascularization has resulted from limbal constriction[18,31] or chronic oedema[21,24] provoked by haptic lens wear. However, the incidence of neovascularization among haptic lens wearers is low, and few patients develop the complication[14].

Among corneal lens wearers the incidence of corneal neovascularization is also

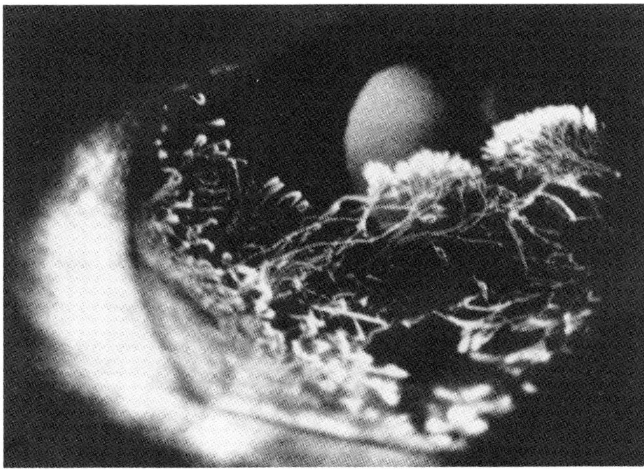

Figure 5.3 Anterior fluorescein angiography in neovascularization due to contact lens wear (reproduced by permission of Bron and Dixon, *Contact Lens*, 1972[4])

low[12]. Reported case histories[2,11] strongly suggest that limbal coverage by an eccentrically riding lens is a common causative factor, as is persistent overwear.

In soft lens wear, the incidence of corneal vascularization is higher than with other types of lenses. This complication is often associated with the use of large (14–16 mm), thick (0.2–0.4 mm) lenses which cover the entire limbal zone. Among wearers of this type of soft lens, as many as 1-in-5 may develop new corneal vessels at some point of lens wear[3,19].

Examining the eye for neovascularization

Examining the human eye for evidence of neovascularization presents a number of difficulties. The limbal arcades may be viewed in retroillumination with the aid of a slit lamp microscope. However, the vascular structure is almost exclusively filled with plasma, rather than whole blood, although red corpuscles may be observed to migrate intermittently through individual vessels. In initial periods of contact lens wear, or indeed with any ocular irritation, the existing vessels dilate and fill with blood to give the appearance of gross change.

Undoubtedly the technique of choice for examining corneal vascularization is that of fluorescein corneal angiography[5]. The evidence gained from fluorescein angiography of both superficial and deep stromal vascularization is superior to other techniques (Figure 5.3). However, this technique cannot be applied to cosmetic lens wearing subjects, even in a research environment, due to the risks associated with the injection of fluorescein. Therefore, the techniques available to contact lens practitioners to monitor the eye for evidence of neovascularization consist of photography or subjective impressions of vascular state.

Photography of limbal vascular structure

High-magnification photographs of the limbal arcades may be taken with the aid of a Holden/Zantos attachment to a conventional photoslit lamp microscope.

Individual conjunctival vessels may be used as a reference point for sequential photography of the same corneal area. Although the conjunctival vessels may be readily displaced in areas away from the limbus, at the sclerolimbal junction they become attached to the surrounding tissue and are relatively immobile. Retro-illumination with a beam width of approximately 1 mm will give successful results (see Plate 31)). Although useful, the technique has considerable limitations:

1 It is only possible to photograph and therefore monitor small limbal areas
2 The contrast of the photographs is very much better on eyes with a blue iris, than on those with a brown
3 A number of photographs have to be taken to ensure a good probability of one photograph being clearly in focus.

Subjective records of limbal structure

Subjective impressions of limbal vascular structure are of value in monitoring patients, but only when the same observer is used. The earliest clinically detectable stage of neovascularization occurs when 'unlooped' or 'non-returning' vessels are seen as extensions of a pre-existing arcade. This observation may be coupled with the general limbal appearance to develop categories both for the ratios of blood filled arcades and the presence of new vessels:

1 Eye normal. Majority of limbal arcades (> 9-in-10) not filled with whole blood. No 'unlooped' arcades. No suggestion of congestion in the perilimbal plexus of vessels
2 Limbal congestion. More than half the limbal arcades filled with whole blood. No 'unlooped' arcades, but vessels apparently distended
3 Apparent early neovascularization. One or more 'unlooped' arcades extending less than 1 mm into the cornea
4 Apparent neovascularization. Vessels extending more than 1 mm into the cornea.

Clinical implications of corneal vascularization in contact lens wear

Haptic lenses

Corneal vascularization in haptic lens wear is the most widely documented instance of neovascularization reported in the literature. However, in all the reported cases the lenses were fitted as part of the treatment of a pre-existing ocular disorder, and it is not possible to attribute the growth of new vessels to the presence of the lens alone. Among wearers of haptic lenses fitted for sport or cosmetic reasons, corneal vascularization is a very rare event, and usually indicates insufficient limbal clearance[26].

Corneal lenses

The occurrence of neovascularization in corneal contact lens wear is very uncommon[11]. Except in those instances where a corneal lens overlies the limbal area, or where unusually large lenses are being used, it is doubtful if the stimulus to new vessel growth exists.

Soft lenses

Vascularization is a frequent complication of at least some forms of soft lens wear[16,17,23] and the observations made by Bron and Dixon in 1972[4] bear repeating:

> We cannot yet report if the gel lens itself represents a stimulus to corneal neovascularization compared to the microcorneal lens. However, the gel lens has many characteristics which could stimulate neovascularization. The entire cornea is covered and the tear flow beneath the lens is minimal, because of the relatively tight fit which is needed to keep the lens in position. This encourages hypo-oxygenation of the superficial cornea, which is not completely relieved by the somewhat greater permeability of the gel lens to oxygen compared to the methacrylate lens.

Among wearers of extended wear soft lenses there is a sustained increase in the apparent luminal diameter of the limbal vessels, at least in the first 6 months of wear[16]. It is likely that similar changes occur in some types of day wear soft lenses and that a proportion of these will eventually lead to new vessel growth.

The practical steps which may be taken to at least reduce the incidence of neovascularization among soft lens wearers include:

1. The use of thin (0.04–0.08 mm thickness) lenses to improve oxygen transmission values
2. Limitations on wearing times
3. Careful fitting to encourage the maximum amount of lens mobility consistent with stable vision.

Even if these measures are taken it is likely that some patients will present at aftercare with neovascularization. Careful monitoring of limbal vascular state is a very necessary part of soft lens patient care, particularly in long-term wearers.

References

1 Ashton, N. (1967). In: *Vascular Complications of Diabetes Mellitus*, edited by C. Kimura and A. Caygil. St Louis: Mosby

2 Ben Ezra, D. (1978). *American Journal of Ophthalmology*, **86**, 455

3 Ben Ezra, D. (1981). *Documenta Ophthalmologica*, **25**, 125

4 Bron, A. J. and Dixon, W. (1972) *Contact Lens*, **3**, 16

5 Bron, A. J. and Easty, D. L. (1971) *British Journal of Ophthalmology*, **55**, 671

6 Collin, H. B. (1966). *Investigative Ophthalmology*, **5**, 1

7 Collin, H. B. (1966). *Investigative Ophthalmology*, **5**, 337

8 Collin, H. B. (1970). *Experimental Eye Research*, **10**, 207

9 Collin, H. B. (1971). *Journal of Pathology*, **104**, 99

10 Collin, H. B. (1974). *Experimental Eye Research*, **18**, 171

11 Dixon, J. M. (1967). *Transactions of the American Ophthalmological Society*, **65**, 333

12 Dixon, J. M. and Lawaczeck, E. (1963). *Archives of Ophthalmology*, **69**, 72

13 Folkman, J. and Haudenschild, C. (1980). *Nature*, **288**, 551

14 Fonda, D. A. (1962). *Southern Medical Journal*, **55**, 126
15 Fromer, C. H. and Klintworth, G. K. (1975/76) *American Journal of Pathology*, **79**, 537; **81**, 531; **82**, 157
16 Humphrys, A. J. (1982). Doctoral Thesis. University of Aston in Birmingham
17 Kaufman, H. E. (1979). *Ophthalmology*, **86**, 411
18 Kori, C. (1979). *Folia Ophthalmologica*, **30**, 154
19 Larke, J. R., Humphrys, J. A. and Holmes, R. (1981). *Journal of the British Contact Lens Association*, **7**, 105
20 Lauder, H. (1929) *Klinische Monatsblätter für Augenheilkunde*, **83**, 535
21 Mandelbaum, J. (1964). *Archives of Ophthalmology*, **71**, 633
22 Manschot, W. A. (1983) *Documenta Ophthalmologica*, **55**, 113
23 Maurice, D. M. (1960). *American Journal of Ophthalmology*, **49**, 1011
24 Momose, T. (1978). *Japanese Journal of Clinical Ophthalmology*, **32**, 957
25 Polverini, P. J., Cotran, R. S., Gimbrone, M. A. and Unanue, E. R. (1977). *Nature*, **269**, 804
26 Sabell, A. G. (1980). Personal communication
27 Schanzlin, D. J., Cyr, R. J. and Friedlaender, M. H. (1983). *Archives of Ophthalmology*, **101**, 472
28 Schwartzman, M. L., Webb, S. C., Rosenberg, J., Dunn, M. W., Abraham, N. G. and Conners, M. S. (1983). *Investigative Ophthalmology*, **4**, 1405–1406
29 Sidky, Y. A. and Auerbach, R. J. (1975). *Journal of Experimental Medicine*, **141**, 1084
30 Slatt, B. and Stein, H. A. (1979). *Contact and Intraocular Lens Medical Journal*, **5**, 82
31 Strebel, J. (1937) *Klinische Monatsblätter für Augenheilkunde*, **99**, 30

Chapter 6

The cornea

S. Hodson

Introduction

The cornea – the window of the eye – fulfils three special roles. Together with the sclera, it forms the physically robust outer layer of the eye, which acts to protect the fragile tissues within the eye. The cornea also forms, at its outer surface, a high quality optical surface over which the thin tear film is spread. (The tear film/air interface, supported on the cornea, provides most of the dioptric power of the visual system.) The third function of the cornea is to be transparent; after light is carefully refracted at the tear film/air interface it is essential that the tough underlying tissue of the cornea should be transparent and allow the refracted wave front to be transmitted smoothly on towards the crystalline lens.

This chapter is about corneal transparency (although it touches slightly upon corneal toughness) and, in particular, about how corneal transparency is maintained, because the cornea must expend metabolic energy in order to keep itself transparent. A simple experiment illustrates this need. If a whole eye is refrigerated at just above its freezing point, the metabolism of its tissues (including the cornea) is effectively switched off and the cornea slowly but progressively loses its transparency, starts to scatter significant quantities of light and becomes opaque. The really interesting observation arises on the reversal experiment, when the eye is warmed back up to body temperatures. The cornea slowly but progressively, as its metabolism is switched back on, reverts and becomes more transparent.

We shall see that this reversible change in transparency is related directly to a reversible increase (and then decrease) of fluid within the cornea, and so our interest in the mechanisms regulating corneal transparency develop naturally into an interest into understanding the mechanisms which regulate the amount of fluid in the cornea.

The anatomy of the cornea with special reference to its transparency

The cornea has different layers. The outer cellular epithelium is bathed in the tear film; the middle layer is the (mainly) non-cellular corneal stroma and the inner layer is the cellular corneal endothelium bathed in the aqueous humour. Corneal epithelium consists of several layers of cells progressing in shape from the basal mitotic columnar cells to the apical squamous flattened cells, which gradually desquamate into the tear film and are continuously replaced by cell division in the basal cells and migration. Optically, the most important property of the epithelium resides in the outer surface of the squamous superficial cells over which the tear film is spread. Perhaps surprisingly, the regulation of the shape of this important surface has rarely been investigated. The multilayered epithelium provides a permeability barrier to prevent (very efficiently) the penetration of the tear film fluid into the underlying corneal stroma. The epithelium secretes Bowman's membrane which provides the first few microns of the connective tissue of the corneal stroma.

Most of the middle layer, the stroma, is connective tissue secreted by the cellular components of the stroma which are called keratocytes. The corneal stroma is mainly an extracellular matrix whose predominant component is collagen. Collagen molecules (synthesized by the keratocytes) condense into the very much larger collagen fibrils. Each fibril is a long but flexible rod which lies parallel to the upper and lower surfaces of the cornea and each fibrin is thought to span the whole corneal arc. Each fibrin has the capability of scattering light (because of its size and refractive index of 1.6 immersed in an aqueous solution, the stromal fluid, of refractive index of 1.34). The fibrils give the cornea its mechanical strength.

The cornea has solved the problem of light scattering by the collagen fibrils by adopting the following strategy. Each collagen fibrin is just about the same diameter, although the diameter varies in different species (32 nm, human; 36 nm, ox; 40 nm, rabbit). Electron microscopy suggests that the diameter is 13 nm but there could be artefacts associated with the preparation of the specimens. Crystallography gives ambiguous results depending upon how the data are interpreted. The control of stromal fibril diameter, i.e., what stops fresh collagen molecules combining with the fibril to enlarge it, is currently of great interest. A number of mechanisms have been proposed and are being investigated. Whatever the regulatory mechanism, the uniform size of the fibril diameter means that each individual collagen fibril scatters light in the same fashion. David Maurice in 1957[4] suggested that if the fibrils are uniformly spaced then there will be total destructive interference between the scattered wave fronts from all the fibrils (the optical analogy is a diffraction grating – the novelty was that Maurice's proposed diffraction grating is three dimensional) and therefore only the central maximum (corresponding in geometrical optics terms to the incident ray) is transmitted. All the scattered light vanishes by destructive interference. The theory has the requirement that the collagen fibrils should not only have a uniform size, but should also pack into a regular lattice. Many years later, crystallographic investigations proved that there is a nearest neighbour distance, or order, in the packing of the collagen fibrils. The order is not as high as in a crystal but Farrell and Hart[2] had already indicated that corneal transparency did not require perfect order in the packing of the collagen fibrils.

Corneal transparency requires that the collagen fibrils should be of uniform diameter and that there should be an ordering force between nearest neighbours. (A fuller understanding of the relationship between corneal transparency and collagen fibril spacing would probably arise from an analysis using the methods of quantum electrodynamics.) Meanwhile, the interfibrillar ordering force has been the subject of much investigation because it has considerable physiological impact. If left to their own devices, the interfibrillar ordering forces will push the fibrils apart and the

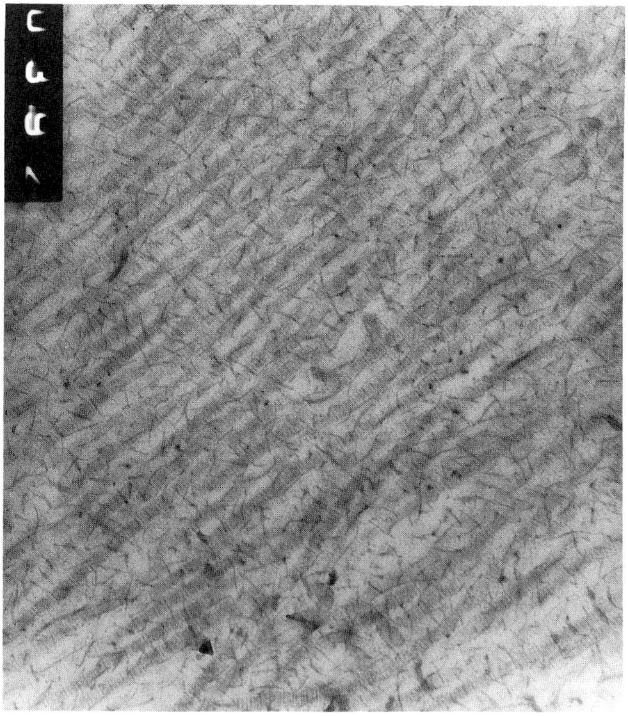

Figure 6.1 The collagen fibrils of corneal stroma which, in each bundle or lamella, lie parallel to each other have associated glycosaminoglycans which tend to orientate radically outwards from each fibril (×110 000; courtesy of Dr Keith Meek)

corneal stroma will swell. The intrafibrillar forces will then become weaker, the ordering force between the collagen fibrils will diminish, order in the fibril lattice will decrease, and the cornea will scatter light and lose its transparency.

The ordering force between the fibrils cannot be supplied by the collagen molecules which make up the fibrils. Collagen is essentially an electrically neutral molecule (at physiological pH) and any collagen associated van der Waal's forces would create an attractive not a repulsive force. The repulsive forces ordering the optical array of collagen fibrils have to be electrical (i.e., electrostatic) and they are supplied by other large, negatively charged molecules which are weakly attached to the collagen fibrils. Some of these negative charges are provided by the sugar chains of the glycosaminoglycans (GAGs) keratan sulphate and chondroitin sulphate. The repeating disaccharide units of the glycosaminoglycans contain carboxylic and sulphonic acid groups which are ionized at physiological pH. The distribution of the glycosaminoglycans is shown in Figure 6.1.

Bounding the posterior surface of the corneal stroma is a monolayer of cells, the corneal endothelium, which secretes its own (rather peculiar) basement membrane called Descemet's membrane (Figure 6.2). The endothelial cells are packed together on Descemet's membrane. Each cell at its apical surface is roughly a hexagon of side 12 μm and there are consequently about 2600 cells/mm^2. In cross-section, it is seen that between each pair of neighbouring cells is an extracellular space which opens at its anterior side into Descemet's membrane and is characterized at its posterior

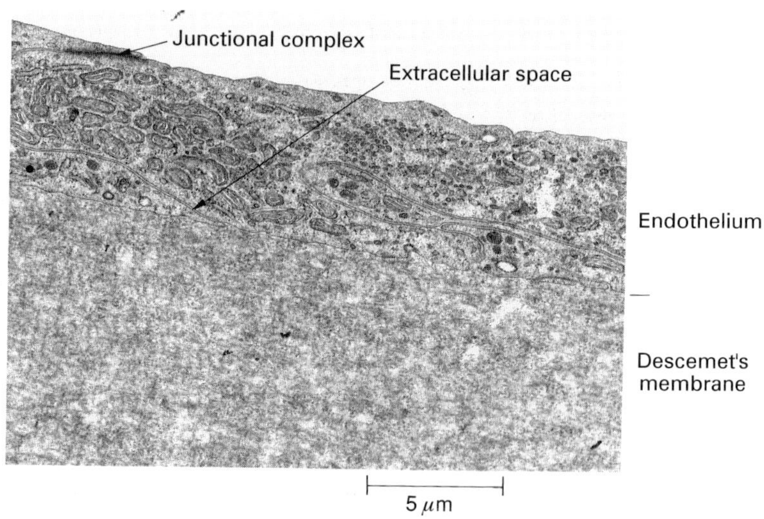

Figure 6.2 The corneal endothelium. The corneal endothelium is a monolayer of cells which secretes its own particularly thickened basement membrane called Descemet's membrane. Cells are separated by an extracellular space which provides the paracellular route for passive diffusion across the monolayer. At its apical end, the paracellular route terminates in a junctional complex.

surface by a junctional complex. The junctional complex pins the cells together. When materials passively cross the endothelium by diffusion, exchanging between the aqueous humour and the corneal stroma, then, unless they are very special (water itself is the best-known example), they must travel through the paracellular route (this narrow passage between neighbouring cells), and the length (the tortuosity) and the narrowness of the paracellular route determine the ease of passage. The junctional complex at the aqueous humour side of the endothelial paracellular route does not impede this diffusional exchange, as it often does in other epithelia. Otherwise, the endothelial cells have the normal complement of organelles, mitochondria, Golgi complex, a little rough endoplasmic reticulum and a nucleus (or sometimes two). The endothelial cells do not appear to undergo mitosis much after the age of 17 years (in humans) which is a pity from the point of view of their survival after intervention. As their numbers diminish naturally, through ageing or unnaturally after intervention, then the mosaic remains intact by neighbouring cells spreading to cover the region of cellular loss. Eventually, there comes a time when if the cell density decreases from its average value of 2600 cells/mm^2 to below around 400 cells/mm^2, compensation no longer takes place and the endothelium loses its barrier properties and 'holes' appear in the mosaic. It has been estimated that we would need to live to 300 years old before this decompensation would occur by natural means.

Corneal transparency, corneal hydration and corneal thickness

When an isolated cornea is chilled, it begins to lose its transparency, as in the whole eye experiment described above, and on temperature reversal, provided that the cornea is irrigated with a suitable balanced salt solution which mimics the nutritional requirements of native aqueous humour, corneal transparency is fully restored. It is observed that increasing opacity of the cornea associated with chilling corresponds with an increase of corneal stromal hydration and regain of corneal transparency (on re-warming the cornea) corresponds with corneal stromal dehydration. In general, the amount of water in the cornea (its hydration) corresponds with its ability to transmit light, and so, many years ago, it was realized that the study of the metabolic regulation of corneal transparency corresponds with the study of corneal stromal hydration (and its metabolic regulation). The two facets, transparency and hydration, are regulated by the same set of mechanisms. There is a further simplification which applies to the study of the hydration of rabbit corneas (human corneas behave in a slightly more complex fashion): hydration is linearly related to thickness because when isolated rabbit (and ox) corneas swell, they do so in only one direction which is along the optic axis. Consequently, by observing optically the changes in thickness of an isolated cornea, it became possible to determine several of the features which collectively regulate corneal hydration and, of course, transparency.

Optical observations on the thickness of isolated corneas: the pump-leak model of corneal hydration control

If a non-metabolizing cornea is immersed in a balanced salt solution, the corneal stroma will swell slowly, at a rate of about 40 μm/h, but if the corneal stroma is denuded of either its epithelium or its endothelium covering respectively the front and the back surfaces of the corneal stroma, the cornea will swell at a much faster rate, of the order of 1000 μm/h, and the preparation very soon becomes opaque. These simple experiments illustrate two properties important for an understanding of the regulation of corneal hydration. First, the corneal stroma has an innate tendency to imbibe fluid and swell if it is exposed to aqueous solutions. Second, both the epithelium and the endothelium slow the innate swelling rates of the corneal stroma by acting as permeability barriers to the passage of aqueous fluid into the corneal stroma. And so one set of mechanisms – the set which generates the movement of fluid into corneal stroma – is revealed. The passive rate of swelling of corneal stroma, driven by its gel pressure (see later), is modulated by the permeability barriers offered by the endothelium and the epithelium which act to slow the rate of swelling of the stroma. The slowing factor is considerable but different between the two layers. In balanced salt solution, denuded stromas swell at about 1000 μm/h; passive flow into the stroma across the endothelial barrier is reduced to 40 μm/h, but passive flow across the epithelial barrier is even less at around 1 μm/h. Corneal epithelium is a very much more effective barrier to flow than corneal endothelium and so, in life, most of the potential leakage of fluid into the stroma would be through the corneal endothelium.

For the cornea to be stabilized, it must take appropriate actions to counter the leak by an outward (from the stroma) directed pump. It is easy to show, by optical examination of the corneal thickness, that the pump which balances the leak is located in the endothelial cells rather than in the epithelial. Figure 6.3 illustrates three classic scenarios of how pre-swollen corneas thin back to near their physiological thickness in: (*a*) the presence of the endothelium and epithelium; (*b*) the absence of the epithelium; and (*c*) the absence of the endothelium. These experiments (and many others) were used to demonstrate that the hydration

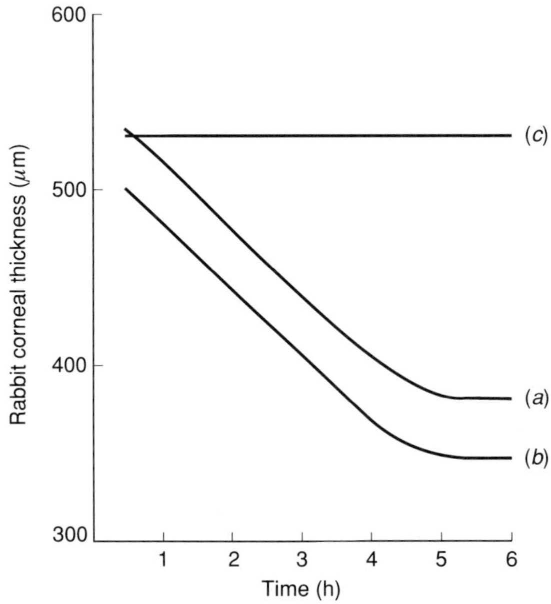

Figure 6.3 The pump is in the endothelium. Rabbit corneas were refrigerated for 1 day (when they swelled) and then re-warmed to 35°C and had their thickness alterations monitored under three different conditions: (*a*) in the presence of the endothelium and epithelium; (*b*) without epithelium (when the de-epithelialized side of the cornea was blocked with non-toxic silicone oil); (*c*) without endothelium (when the de-endothelialized side of the cornea was blocked with non-toxic silicone oil). The presence or absence of epithelium (curves (*a*) and (*b*)) was irrelevant (except for its own thickness of 45 μm) indicating that the 'pump' which restores the cornea to its physiological thickness is in the endothelium. (Contrast with curve (*c*) where the endothelium is absent and negligible fluid movement is seen)

regulating pump resided in the endothelial cells lining the posterior surface of the corneal stroma.

Both the pump and the leak occur (in opposite directions) across the corneal endothelium. The pump leak model is illustrated in Figure 6.4.

Other conclusions were possible after optical observation of the corneal thickness. The classic one is that the endothelial pump is driven by Na-K-ATPase, because inhibition of this membrane enzyme by the specific inhibitor 10^{-5} M ouabain led to a total cessation of pump activity and the corneal stroma swelled at 40 μm/h, which is numerically the same rate at which stroma sucks fluid across a metabolically inhibited but structurally intact endothelium.

A peculiar observation made in substitution experiments, where individual ions were substituted out of the bathing fluid, indicated also that the endothelial pump was dependent for its operation on the presence of bicarbonate. Omission of bicarbonate inhibited the pump and the reversal experiment, when bicarbonate was re-introduced, restored the pump.

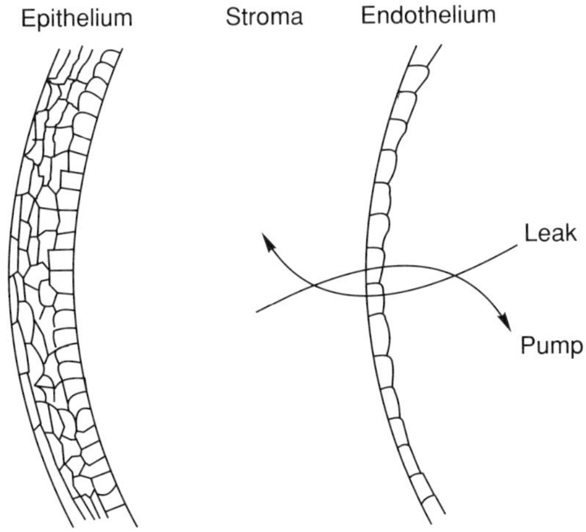

Figure 6.4 The pump-leak model of corneal hydration. The hydration of the cornea is in dynamic balance. The fluxes of the leak and the pump pass across the endothelium lining the posterior surface of the stroma

Conclusions
Optical examination of corneas established that corneal hydration is in dynamic balance. The passive swelling tendency of cornea is modulated by the permeability barrier of the endothelium. The two properties together constitute 'the leak'. Balancing 'the leak' is 'the pump' which is located in the endothelium. The 'pump' is driven by Na-K-ATPase. The 'pump' is activated only in the presence of bicarbonate ions. Further understanding of the 'pump–leak' balance (which maintains corneal transparency) requires an independent investigation of the several components of the equation.

The endothelial pump

The endothelial pump acts by lowering the osmotic pressure of the corneal stroma by actively removing ions from it. The removal of any ion would do the job of offsetting and balancing the swelling tendency of the stromal gel pressure but, in fact, the endothelium pumps bicarbonate ions alone out of the stroma and into the aqueous humour (Figure 6.5). The active removal of bicarbonate ions from the stroma by the corneal endothelium is the major metabolic event, in terms of energy expenditure, in maintaining corneal transparency.

The corneal endothelium does this in a series of four consecutive steps.

Step 1: the exit of sodium
Located in the basolateral membranes of the corneal endothelium, i.e., the side touching Descemet's membrane, but absent from the apical membranes of the cell, is the enzyme Na-K-ATPase. This interesting enzyme exists in every cell of the body and consumes an estimated 70% of whole body metabolic energy and 80% of ocular metabolic energy, i.e., almost everything except the energy consumed by muscular contraction. For each cycle of the enzyme, energy is liberated by the hydrolysis of

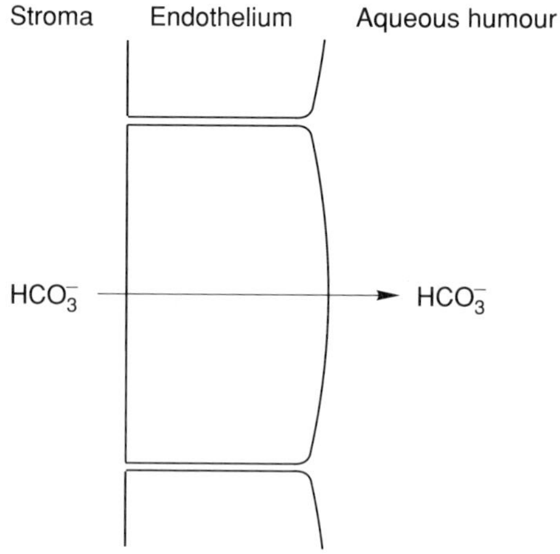

Figure 6.5 The endothelial pump is a current of bicarbonate ions. Bicarbonate ions are continuously pumped from the stroma to the aqueous humour. The bicarbonte ion current is driven through each cell of the endothelium by the expenditure of metabolic energy. In an equilibrated cornea *in vivo*, the pump is neutralized by an equal passive flow of bicarbonate ions through the paracellular route in the opposite direction, into the stroma. The net effect of the two flows is to lower the osmotic pressure of the stroma and back off the stromal gel pressure (equation (**13**), in the text)

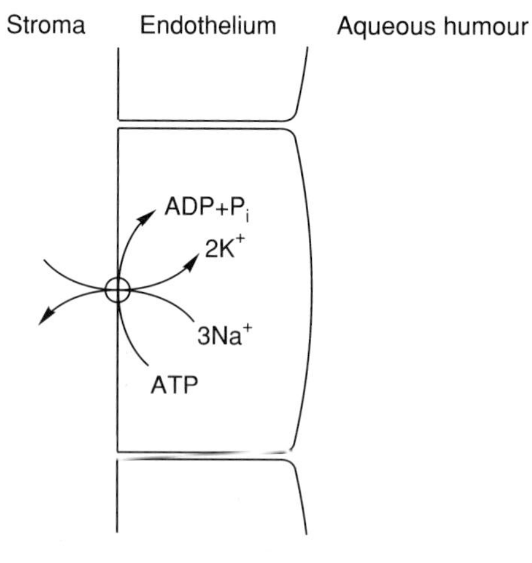

Figure 6.6 The exit of sodium. The plasma membrane enzyme Na-K-ATPase is located in the basolateral membranes of corneal endothelium. It acts to reduce the sodium concentration in the cell and helps to generate a membrane potential or around -30 mV

one molecule of ATP to ADP and free phosphate and the energy is donated to the expulsion of $3Na^+$ out of the cell and $2K^+$ into the cell (Figure 6.6). Let us concentrate our attention on the expelled sodium ions. The consequence is that the Na ion concentration within the cell diminishes about ten-fold, from Na outside equals about 154 mM to Na inside equals about 14 mM. Na ions therefore have a passive tendency to drive back into the cell, promoted not only by their ten-fold chemical gradient but also by the negative membrane potential of the corneal endothelium of -30 mV – equivalent to a further three-fold chemical gradient.

At steady state, the rate of exit of any ion from the corneal endothelium must equal the rate of entry of that ion. In the case of the Na ion, the exit is forced by the metabolic energy resulting from the hydrolysis of ATP by Na-K-ATPase, whereas the entry of the Na ion back into the endothelium is vigorous and filled with energy.

There are two major routes for Na re-entry into the corneal endothelium (and a number of very minor ones) but the re-entry route which results in the osmotic bicarbonate pump, which regulates corneal transparency, will be described.

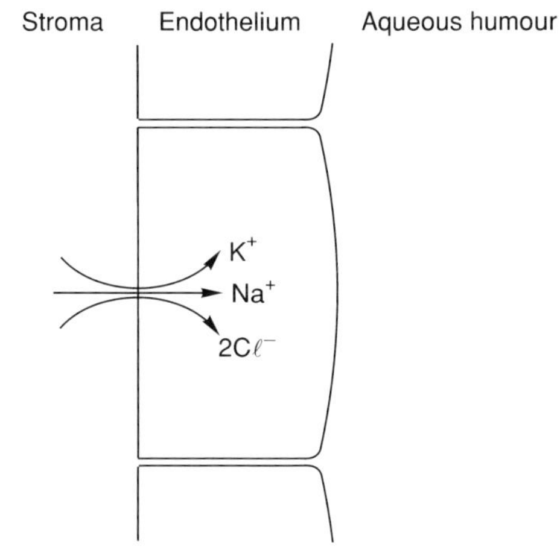

Figure 6.7 The re-entry of Na: the entry of Cl. Sodium re-enters the cell via two membrane traffic proteins but the important re-entry route for the bicarbonate pump is via the co-transporter located in the basolateral membranes. For each action of its cycle, the co-transporter allows one Na^+, one K^+ and two Cl^- to enter the cell. It is therefore electrically neutral. The energy of the downhill re-entry of Na is coupled to an (uphill) accumulation of Cl within the cell

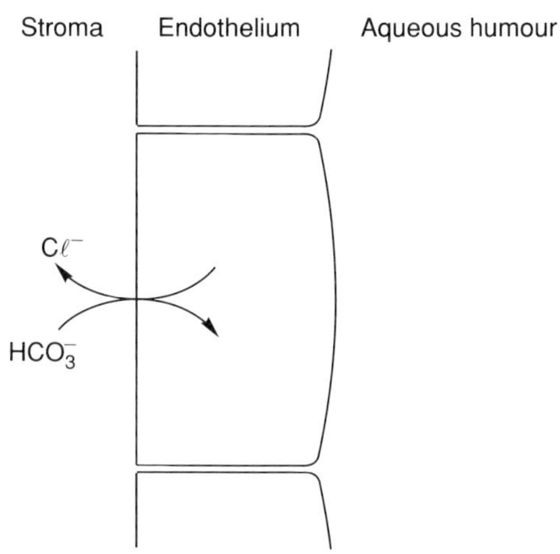

Figure 6.8 The exit of chloride; the entry of bicarbonate. Band III traffic protein, located in the basolateral membranes of corneal endothelial cells, exchanges Cl for HCO_3. The downhill flow of Cl from the cell energizes the uphill intracellular accumulation of HCO_3

Step 2: the re-entrance of sodium and the entrance of chloride
Also located in the basolateral membranes of the corneal endothelium is another membrane protein, the co-transporter. This acts to bring ions into the cell (hence co-transport). Each entry of Na ion is accompanied by the entry of one potassium ion and two chloride ions – Na/K/2Cl. The co-transporter redistributes energies between the ions and so the downhill crash of the Na ions into the cell results in the uphill accumulation of chloride ions, i.e., the chloride ions in the endothelium have a higher energy than the chloride ions in the corneal stroma. The chloride ions within the cell are bursting to get out (Figure 6.7).

Step 3: the exit of chloride and the entry of bicarbonate
Also located in the basolateral membranes of the corneal endothelium is another membrane protein, often called band III, because it is the third apparent membrane protein of red blood corpuscles, which acts to exchange the anions of chloride for bicarbonate. As chloride exits the cell (downhill) it drives bicarbonate uphill into the cell (Figure 6.8). Bicarbonate is, as a consequence, found in the corneal endothelium

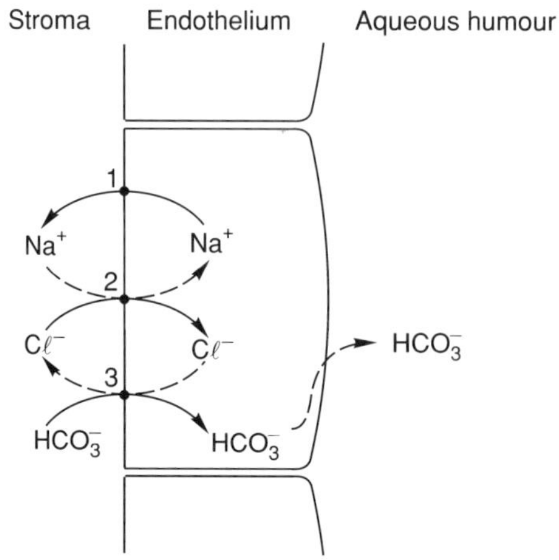

Figure 6.9 An abbreviated summary of the transendothelial bicarbonate flux. Solid arrows indicate the uphill flow of ions, dashed arrows indicate their downhill direction of flow. Membrane traffic proteins are 1: Na-K-ATPase, 2: co-transporter, 3: band III exchanger and 4: a putative HCO_3 channel. The mechanisms result in no net Na or Cl transendothelial transport but only in net HCO_3 transport

with a higher energy than the bicarbonate ions in the surrounding media, either in the stromal fluid perfusing through Descemet's membrane or in the aqueous humour.

Let us look briefly at a summary of steps 1, 2 and 3 before we close the story with a description of step 4.

If we look at the exit and entrance of Na (steps 1 and 2, Figures 6.5 and 6.6), it can be seen that there is no net translocation of Na across the endothelium between the stroma and aqueous humour. Na acts as a circulating current (into and out of the stroma, with no osmotic consequences for the stroma) whose role is to give energy to the chloride ion. If we look at the exit and entrance of Cl (steps 2 and 3, Figures 6.6 and 6.7) a behaviour similar to that for Na is observed. There is no net translocation of Cl across the endothelium between the stroma and the aqueous humour. Cl, too, acts as a circulating current (into and out of the stroma, with no osmotic consequences for the stroma) whose role is to pass some of the energy (given to it by the sodium ion) on to the bicarbonate ion.

Na gives energy to Cl; Cl then gives energy to bicarbonate and here, as we unravel the properties of the corneal endothelium, we are probably transecting an ancient evolutionary development. In the beginning, move Na and K, then, later, learn how to couple the energy to move Cl as well. Then as the organisms learn to oxidize matter and produce significant quantities of CO_2 and, consequently, bicarbonate, couple the energy to move bicarbonate as well.

Step 4: the exit of bicarbonate

Bicarbonate exits from the corneal endothelium via the opposite apical face. The membrane traffic protein responsible for the downhill exit of bicarbonate and whose presence can be proved directly and indirectly, is not yet characterized. The best evidence suggests that bicarbonate exits via a bicarbonate selective ion channel.

A composite of some of the ion flows of steps 1, 2, 3 and 4 is shown in Figure 6.9 and this is the main story of the mechanisms resulting in the bicarbonate pump of the corneal endothelium which regulates corneal stromal hydration. There are a number of complications to this relatively simple scheme which arise from the need to regulate the activity of the pump.

These concern the second major re-entry route of Na into the corneal endothelium (to generate a non-osmotic transendothelial ion flow), and the exit of K from the cell (not shown in steps 1, 2, 3 and 4 above) in order to regulate membrane potential and indirectly the activity of the co-transporter (step 2). Insufficient is yet known about the second above but the first process works this way.

Step 2b: Na entry, proton exit

Na re-enters the endothelium via a Na–H antiport located on the basolateral membranes of the corneal endothelium.

Step 2c

This is a non-membrane, non-enzymic event. A water molecule in the cytoplasm of the cell dissociates to provide a proton (to fuel step 2b) and a hydroxyl ion:

$$H_2O \rightarrow H^+ + OH^-$$

Step 3b

This is a non-membrane, cytoplasmic enzyme event. The hydroxyl ion combines with a CO_2 molecule via the soluble cellular enzyme carbonic anhydrase:

$$OH^- + CO_2 \rightarrow HCO_3^-$$

Step 4

The resulting HCO_3^- exits the cell via the same step 4 described in the osmotic pathway outlined earlier. The overall result of steps 2b, 2c, 3b and 4 are summarized in Figure 6.10.

This pathway has interesting aspects because, although it is electrogenic, the ions into the stroma coupled with the ions into the aqueous humour are equivalent electrically to either a negative current into the aqueous humour or a positive current into the stroma, either way the aqueous humour side shows a negative electrical potential with respect to the stromal side. Although it is electrogenic, it is not osmotic (one osmoticum into the stroma, a proton, exactly neutralizes one osmoticum into the aqueous humour, a bicarbonate ion).

This alternative pathway (non-osmotic) is potentially a way of de-tuning the sodium pump from coupling an osmotically effective bicarbonate pump. It may have, however, an alternative *raison d'être* as yet undiscovered.

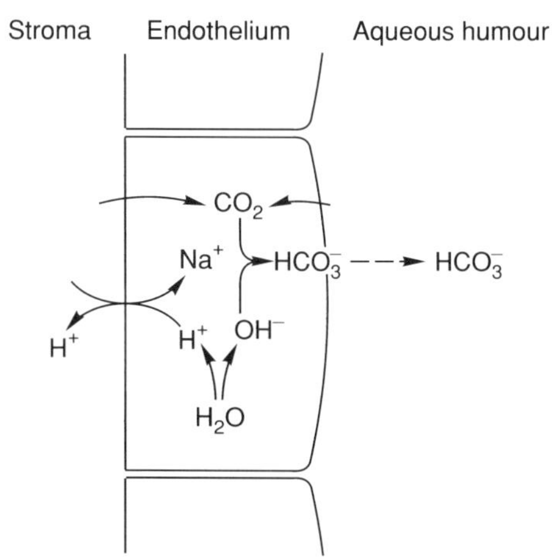

Figure 6.10 The regulatory (non-osmotic) pathway. Sodium re-entry across the basolateral membrane can also be associated with the ionization of a water molecule. The proton goes through the Na–H exchanger, the OH^- combines with CO_2 via the enzyme carbonic anhydrase to give HCO^-_3, which exists through the apical membrane. The pathway is electrogenic but is not seen to be osmotic

Gel pressure: the driving force behind corneal stromal swelling

Gel pressure results from the fixed negative charges on the very large molecules which make up the solid matrix of the corneal stroma. Gel pressure is related to the concentration of stromal fixed charges, Q, which has units of milliequivalents per litre of stromal fluid. As the cornea swells, so Q (the charge concentration) diminishes in consequence of its dilution by the increased stromal fluid and so the amount of fluid in the stroma is important in influencing the magnitude of Q. The state of hydration of the stroma is called H and is the fluid mass in the stroma divided by its dry mass. H is therefore a ratio and a dimensionless number and at physiological hydration $H = 3.2$ (i.e., 3.2 mg of fluid interpenetrates each milligram of dry stromal tissue). If the stroma swells, H increases and in consequence Q is diluted proportionately. The relationship is:

$$\mathrm{Q.H} = \text{constant} \tag{1}$$

$$\text{or } \mathrm{Q.H.} = \mathrm{Q_p\ H_p} \tag{2}$$

where subscript p denotes the physiological state. As already mentioned, $\mathrm{H_p} = 3.2$ and, incidentally, $\mathrm{Q_p} = 40\,\mathrm{mM}$. (Purists demur at these units of mM but it is a convention that works well enough.)

Gel pressure is very simple to visualize: it results from the mutually repulsive forces of the fixed matrix negative charges which collectively make up Q. Gel pressure is an electrostatic potential and because coulombic electrical repulsion is proportional to the square of electrical charge so gel pressure ($\Delta\gamma$) is proportional to Q^2 (very nearly, anyway), but the integration of all the charges in the stromal matrix is made tricky by the presence of mobile cations (mainly sodium, Na^+) and mobile anions (mainly chloride, Cl^-) also present in the corneal stroma. So, of the three ways of mathematically deriving the relationship between gel pressure ($\Delta\gamma$) and stromal charge density (Q), an easier (and more informative) way uses the principle of salt disparity.

To derive the relationship of salt disparity we will consider the simplest case of a biopsy of corneal stroma bathed in a salt solution of NaCl. Water molecules, sodium ions and chloride ions are all perfectly free to diffuse into and out of the stroma. (Life itself is a little trickier, there are more ions than just Na^+ and Cl^- in aqueous humour and tears but the arguments used here are reliable simplifications.) Three conditions occur:

1 There is an electrically neutral balance both in the bathing medium and also within the stromal fluid (where the presence of the fixed negative charge, Q, has to be included in the balance)
2 There is a salt chemical potential difference between the stromal fluid and the bathing medium
3 There is an osmotic potential difference between the stromal fluid and the bathing medium.

Let us designate all things in the bathing medium with a subscript 'o' and all things in the stromal fluid with a subscript 'i'. Let us also indicate a concentration (units: mM) with square brackets so $[Cl_i]$ represents the concentration of freely diffusible chloride ions in the stromal fluid. The difference of chemical potentials of the salt

(μ_S) and of osmotic potentials of the salt (π_s) is designated by Δ. So $\Delta\mu_s$ is the salt chemical potential excess within the stroma compared to the bathing medium and $\Delta\pi_s$ is the osmotic pressure excess within the stroma compared to the bathing medium. Finally, it is convenient to call the salt concentration in the bathing medium c_o because it keeps turning up in the relationships. Also for convenience I incorporate RT (molar gas constant times absolute temperature) into $\Delta\pi_s$ and $\Delta\mu_s$ so the term never appears in the following equations.

The first condition above gives two relationships:

$$[Na_o] = [Cl_o] = c_o \tag{3}$$

The salt in the bathing medium, c_o, just dissociates into equal amounts of sodium cation and chloride anion,

and

$$[Na_i] = [Cl_i] + Q \tag{4}$$

Q is the negative charge density of the fixed matrix anions which generate the gel pressure.

Equation (**4**) means that $[Na_i]$ must always be greater than $[Cl_i]$ by the magnitude of Q and this imbalance poses problems for the chemical and osmotic balances.

The chemical potential of a salt is proportional to the logarithm of the product of its two ions and so:

$$\Delta\mu_s = \ln\frac{[Na_i].[Cl_i]}{[Na_o].[Cl_o]} \tag{5}$$

Note (for those who have had thermodynamics represented to them previously): RT is incorporated into $\Delta\mu_s$ which becomes dimensionless.

The osmotic potential excess within the stroma is given by:

$$\Delta\pi_s = [Na_i] + [Cl_i] - [Na_o] - [Cl_o] \tag{6}$$

Note RT is incorporated into $\Delta\pi$. The macromolecules of the stromal matrix are so huge that they express no significant osmotic potential; their molar concentrations are minuscule and so the osmotic imbalance is found entirely within the ionic distributions. This makes corneal stromal swelling easier to understand.

If we substitute for $[Na_i]$ (**4**) and for $[Na_o]$ and $[Cl_o]$ (**3**) in the relationship for $\Delta\pi_s$ (**6**) we get:

$$\Delta\pi_s = 2\,[Cl_i] + Q - 2c_o \tag{7}$$

i.e.,

$$[Cl_i] = c_o + \frac{\Delta\pi_s - Q}{2} \tag{8}$$

and (**8**) into (**4**) gives:

$$[Na_i] = c_o + \frac{\Delta\pi_s + Q}{2} \tag{9}$$

We can finally eliminate [Na_i] and [Cl_i] from the relationship by substituting (**8**) and (**9**) (together with (**3**)) into (**5**) to give:

$$\Delta\pi_s = \ln \frac{\left(\frac{c_o + \Delta\pi_s + Q}{2}\right)\left(\frac{c_o + \Delta\pi_s - Q}{2}\right)}{c_o^2} \quad \textbf{(10)}$$

Multiplying out

$$\Delta\mu_s = \ln\left\{1 + \frac{\Delta\pi_\sigma}{c_o} - \frac{Q^2}{4c_o^{\,2}} + \frac{\Delta\pi_s^{\,2}}{4c_o^{\,2}}\right\} \quad \textbf{(11)}$$

This relationship can be simplified by expanding the logarithm into its series. Under physiological conditions, $c_o = 150\,\text{mM}$, $Q = 40\,\text{mM}$ and $\Delta\pi_s = 2.5\,\text{mM}$ and most terms are vanishingly small. The main terms of the expansion of the logarithm are given by:

$$\Delta\mu_s = \frac{\Delta\pi_s}{c_o} - \frac{Q^2}{4c_o^{\,2}} \quad \textbf{(12)}$$

and this relationship (ignoring the very small term $\Delta\pi_s^{\,2}/4c_o^{\,2}$ and other smaller terms) has an error of less than 1%. Good enough for practical use!

or

$$c_o\Delta\mu_s = \Delta\pi_\sigma - \frac{Q^2}{4c_o} \quad \textbf{(13)}$$

which is the relationship of salt disparity.

Gel pressure, $\Delta\gamma$, is the last term in the equation and this is what makes the cornea swell.

$$\Delta\gamma = \frac{Q^2}{4c_o} \quad \textbf{(14)}$$

Now as isotonic saline c_o is 154 mM and Q is 40 mM, $\Delta\gamma$ is calculated to be 2.6 mM (at physiological hydration of 3.2).

General considerations of gel pressure and the relationship of salt disparity

Equation (**13**) is central to the understanding of the water relations of all biological tissues and, in particular for our purposes, the fluid balances of the cornea. Equation (**13**) embodies the principle of salt disparity which states that, in the presence of fixed charges (i.e., Q greater than 0 and therefore $\Delta\gamma$, the gel pressure, is greater than zero), then it is *not* possible for salt to be distributed into a gel so that simultaneously it can be in osmotic balance ($\Delta\pi_s = 0$) and in chemical balance ($\Delta\mu_s = 0$). The presence of a gel pressure always means that the salt is in osmotic imbalance or in chemical imbalance (or a combination of the two imbalances) and in order to reach a balanced and stable system, other forces have to be brought into play. If other forces are not brought into play, the gel swells.

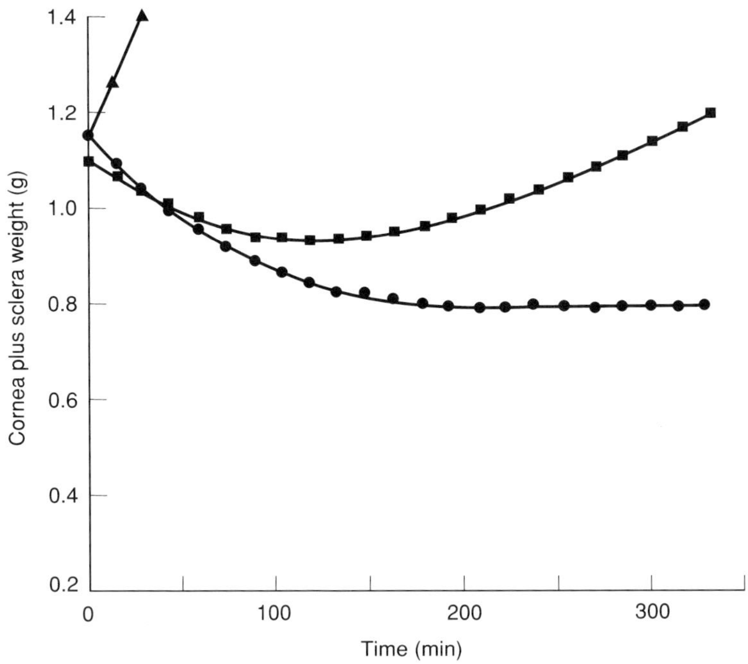

Figure 6.11 The measurement of corneal gel pressure. Whole cornea (plus scleral rim) equilibrates its weight after immersion in 8% polyethylene glycol (nominal molecular weight, 100 000 Da) in 154 mM NaCl (●). If either the epithelium (anterior surface) or Descemet's membrane (posterior surface) is removed from the preparation, equilibrium is not achieved (■). For illustration, the triangles show the well-documented rapid swelling of corneal stroma when immersed in saline alone

To take our particular example, the corneal stroma, the principle of salt disparity (**13**) predicts that if a corneal stroma is immersed in a salt solution it swells. This is just a manifestation of inability to achieve an equilibrium.

The measurement of gel pressure

We can measure stromal gel pressure by balancing it against an external osmoticum as follows: take a non-metabolising whole cornea (which will swell in a solution of NaCl) and add a non-penetrating solute to the bathing medium which generates an external osmotic pressure excess ($\Delta\pi_e$). Freshly manufactured polyethylene glycol of nominal molecular weight 10 000 Da is a suitable non-penetrating solute. The cornea will equilibrate (Figure 6.11). This is what has happened in Figure 6.11 according to the principle of salt disparity (**13**). At equilibrium, the salt, sodium chloride, is free to diffuse into and out of the corneal stroma and so $\Delta\mu_s = 0$. Consequently, the osmotic pressure excess within the stroma is according to (**13**) ($\Delta\mu_s = 0$) $\Delta\pi_s = \Delta\gamma$ and for the water also to be at equilibrium, $\Delta\pi_s$ (the internally generated stromal osmotic pressure) must be at equilibrium with the osmotic pressure excess generated by the external polyethylene glycol ($\Delta\pi_e$). The osmotic pressure of polyethylene glycol solutions can be measured by ordinary means. When the stroma is equilibrated at a particular hydration (H) we can estimate its corresponding gel pressure ($\Delta\gamma$). From $\Delta\gamma$ we can calculate Q (because $\Delta\gamma = Q^2/4c_o$).

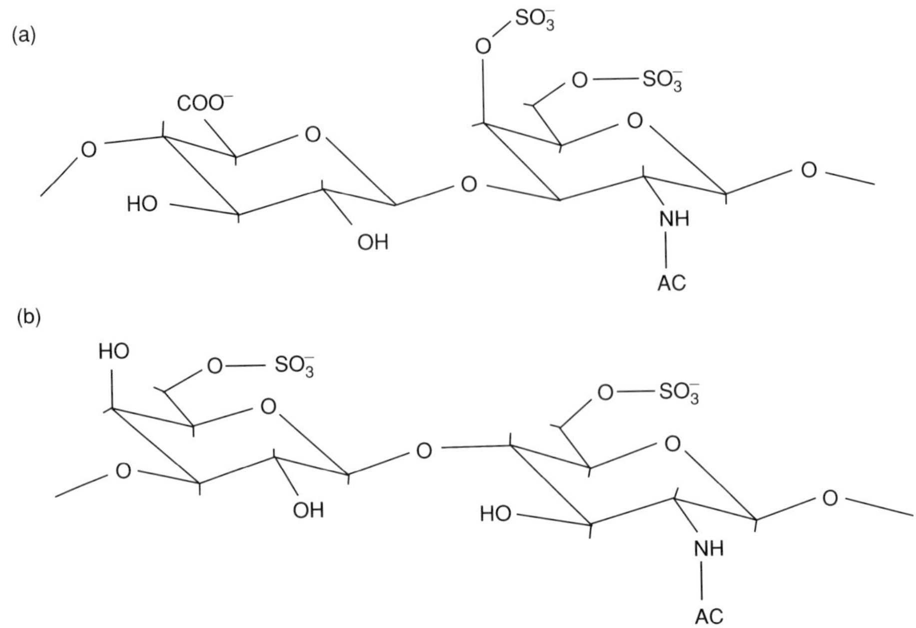

Figure 6.12 The structures of chondroitin sulphate and keratin sulphate. The degree of sulphation in the repeating disaccharide unit of both (*a*) chondroitin sulphate and (*b*) keratan sulphate can vary. Near maximal sulphation examples of the structure are given. The fixed negative charge of the polymers depends on the presence of both carboxylic and sulphonic acid groups

If the concentration of polyethylene glycol dissolved in the bathing medium is altered then the final equilibrium hydration of the cornea alters, but you would expect that. If $\Delta\pi_o$ goes up, $\Delta\pi_s$ goes up, $\Delta\gamma$ goes up and Q goes up, i.e., the corneal stroma thins itself down in order to concentrate its Q ((**13**) again). The equilibrium hydrations of the non-metabolizing corneas immersed in solutions containing polyethylene glycol give a figure for Q of 40 mM at the physiological hydration of 3.2 when the cornea is immersed in 150 mM (i.e., near physiological) NaCl. The gel pressure, under these conditions, can be calculated at ($\Delta\gamma = Q^2/4c_o$) 2.7 mM.

The chemical identification of *Q*

One very interesting result which has come out of the analysis of corneal swelling is in the identification of the molecules in the corneal stroma on which Q (the fixed negative charges) reside. Formerly, it was believed that stromal charge was generated entirely by the carboxylic and sulphonic acid groups of the glycosaminoglycans, chondroitin sulphate and keratan sulphate (Figure 6.12 and see Figure 6.1) but there is a slightly greater contribution to stromal fixed charge from elsewhere. It had been recognized for several years that corneal swelling rates were anomalous in differing salt solutions. If corneas were swelled in solutions of differing concentrations of NaCl, then they swelled 'too slowly' in low salt and 'too quickly' in high salt. (Gel pressure, which drives the swelling is equal to $Q^2/4c_o$. The argument was that swelling rate should be inversely proportional to c_o, the concentration of salt in the bathing medium, but it was not.) Elliott[1] first suggested that Q had two components, the acid groups of the glycosaminoglycans plus a contribution from a chloride binding ligand. Elliott's suggestions of a chloride binding ligand have been confirmed experimentally. The ligand (L) reversibly combines with free chloride in the corneal stroma (Cl_i^-) to make a complex LCl_i^-

$$L + Cl_i^- \rightleftarrows LCl_i^- \qquad \textbf{(15)}$$

The total concentration of ligand [L_T] is the sum of the concentrations of the free ligand [L] plus the ligand complexing a chloride ion [LCl_i^-]

$$[L_T] = [L] + [LCl_i^-] \qquad \textbf{(16)}$$

and [L_T] (at physiological hydration H of 3.2) is 75 mM of which (under physiological conditions) [LCl^- is about 20 mM and [L] is about 55 mM. As the concentration of chloride increases, so more of the ligand is complexed into the LCl_i^- form and it would require a bathing medium containing 300 mM chloride ions to achieve half occupancy of the ligand ([L] = [LCl_i^-) at $H = 3.2$). The net result is that the fixed charge Q increases with chloride (because one of its components, LCl_i^-, increases with increasing chloride). The experimental data are shown in Figure 6.12. The value of Q, as the concentration of chloride in the bathing medium is reduced to zero, and consequently [LCl_i^-] reduces to zero, arises from the contribution from the fixed negative charges of the glycosaminoglycans alone and is estimated at 18 mM. The rising values of Q, as [Cl_o] increases, reflects the action of the chloride binding ligand (**15**). Around physiological values, it is interesting to note that the magnitude of the stromal fixed charge has nearly equal contributions from the fixed charges (carboxylie and sulphonic in acid groups) of the glycosaminoglycans and from the bound chloride ions.

It seems clear that nature settled on this dual method of generating stromal fixed negative charge in order to help stabilize stromal gel pressure in varying salt concentrations (i.e., chloride ion binding is a device to help in the osmoregulation of the corneal stroma). The reasons are sketchcd out as follows.

Gel pressure ($\Delta\gamma$) results from two Components: Q, the fixed negative charge of the stroma, and c_o, the concentration of salt in the bathing medium:

$$\Delta\gamma = \frac{Q^2}{4c_o} \qquad \textbf{(14)}$$

Consequently, if c_o were to vary and Q were invariant, $\Delta\gamma$ would vary inversely with c_o. Let us call this gain in gel pressure $d\Delta\gamma/dc_o$, G′. Then it can be calculated that the change in gel pressure, under the same circumstances, with unit change of c_o, nominated G, will be six times smaller than G because of the tendency of Q to increase as c_o increases and vice versa. The attenuation of gel pressure change (G′/G) as a consequence of chloride binding increasing the stromal fixed negative charge would be six-fold. The practical consequences are considerable. If one immerses one's eyes in tap water for 2 minutes the corneal stroma swells by about 15 μm (from 520 to 535 μm) and as a consequence of this, haloes may be observed around point light sources. This effect would be nearly six times greater without the attenuation affect of the stromal chloride binding. If chloride binding did not exist, then the cornea would be sufficiently hydrated to impede vision, and our perception of water as a 'friendly' medium in which to immerse our face would be influenced adversely.

Backinq off stromal gel pressure *in vivo*

Although it is convenient to use experimentally non-penetrating solutes in order to balance the principle of salt disparity (**13**) and measure gel pressure, this is not the way the cornea works the trick *in vivo*. What the cornea does is to reduce its $\Delta\mu_s$ to negative values and let its osmotic potentials between the stroma and bathing media equilibrate ($\Delta\pi_s = 0$). It does this by actively pumping bicarbonate ions out of the corneal stroma to values below its equilibrium concentration and, by this action, reduces the osmotic pressure within the corneal stroma. We have already seen that this action (the pump-leak model) of the bicarbonate 'pump' resides virtually exclusively in the corneal endothelium, the monolayer of cells lining the posterior surface of the corneal stroma.

Combining the pump and the leak

The endothelial pump (J_p), which lowers the osmotic pressure by 'pumping' bicarbonate from the stroma to the aqueous humour can be combined with the gel pressure of the corneal stroma ($\Delta\gamma$) by including the third element in the equation, P_e, which is the permeability of the endothelium to bicarbonate ions. At equilibrium the relationship is:

$$J_p = P_e.\Delta\gamma \qquad \textbf{(17)}$$

(To digress a little: the full equation is $J_p = \dfrac{P_e.\Delta\gamma_s}{\sigma_e}$ **(18)**

where σ_e is the reflection coefficient of the endothelium to bicarbonate ions. Careful experiments indicate that $\sigma_e = 1$, i.e., corneal endothelium acts as a perfect semipermeable membrane and it is clear that the very high endothelial water permeability required for this experimental determination arises from the presence of CHIP 28 water channels in the corneal endothelial cell membranes described recently by Jorge Fischbarg[3] in an elegant series of experiments. As $\sigma_e = 1$, then (**18**) becomes identical with (**17**)). In (**17**), J_p is the pump and $P_e.\Delta\gamma_s$ collectively form the leak.

The third element in the dynamic 'pump-leak' balance which maintains corneal hydration is P_e, the endothelial permeability are two distinct routes for molecules/ions to pass across the endothelial monolayer and these are between the cells (the paracellular route) and through the cells (the transcellular route) in what is always a two step process: one step is getting into the cell, the other step is getting out of the other face of the cell. The barrier permeability properties of the paracellular route are surprisingly simple: the time of passage of any small molecule permeating through the paracellular route depends only upon its free diffusion coefficient and the physical dimensions of the paracellular route (to a very good approximation). The junctional complex at the apical end of the paracellular route offers no significant permeability barrier to ions or small molecules. (The junctional complex may filter larger proteinaceous molecules.) The paracellular route is the passive permeability route of all small molecules passing across the endothelium with the two important exceptions of water molecules, which passively permeate also (and at a much higher rate than the paracellular route) through the cells via the CHIP 28 water channels, i.e., through the transcellular route, and CO_2 molecules which pass freely through cell membranes. Nobody has yet discovered if they have special membrane channels, or whether they can move through the phospholipid bi-layers directly.

Measurement of the endothelial barrier function

Although it is usually simple to measure the barrier properties of any epithelial layer, such measurements are more complicated in corneal endothelium. The reason is that corneal endothelium is so permeable (it is classified as a 'leaky' epithelium) and fragile. It is not possible to isolate a preparation of endothelial membrane alone (although numerous heroic attempts have been reported) and when the endothelium is prepared together with a thickness of corneal stroma (whose presence provides the necessary mechanical support), the permeability of the stroma is about the same magnitude as the permeability of the endothelium and, consequently, the presence of the stroma interferes with the determination.

Reliable measures of permeability can be recorded by the following procedure. First, measure the permeability of the stroma and endothelium preparation (P_{e+s}) and then wipe off the endothelium and measure the permeability of the stroma alone (P_s). The permeability of the endothelium (P_e) can then be calculated from the equation:

$$\frac{1}{P_{e+s}} = \frac{1}{P_e} + \frac{1}{P_s} \qquad \textbf{(19)}$$

which can be re-jigged to

$$P_e = \frac{P_{e+s} . P_s}{P_s - P_{e+s}} \qquad \textbf{(20)}$$

It is a cumbersome procedure but when it is done it gives some interesting results, some of which have been sketched above. For example, these determinations of permeability show that it is the shape of the paracellular route (its length, width and frequency) alone which determines endothelial permeability and not the junctional complex at the apical end of the paracellular route. There are two adaptations which alter endothelial permeability. One concerns frequency. Frequency diminishes as cell numbers diminish (less cells mean less paracellular routes) and cell numbers diminish naturally with ageing. The well-documented decrease in corneal endothelial permeability with age in humans correlates well with cell loss and (consequently) paracellular route loss. The other adaptation is more immediate. As the cornea cools (walk about in the Arctic, for example) the endothelial pump, J_p, diminishes and the compensation (to maintain the balance in **(16)**, ($J_p = P_e \Delta\gamma$)) is interestingly enough caused by a suitable compensating decrease in P_e. The paracellular route simply narrows itself. How the endothelium works this trick is a great mystery, but it does, and in a matter of seconds.

Finally with respect to endothelial permeability, it can be noted that because it is such a simple non-selective phenomenon, the electrical resistance of the corneal endothelial is exactly what one would expect from knowledge of the permeabilities of all the ions in the aqueous humour. Measurement of endothelial electrical resistance (which takes only a second or two, at least in isolated corneas) gives us an immediate and reliable measurement of endothelial permeability.

The quantitative pump-leak model

Equation (**17**) describes the pump-leak model

$$J_p = P_e \, \Delta\gamma$$

When we measure the three components of the equation experimentally do they balance? The answer is yes, within experimental limits. The argument goes this way.

When we inhibit the pump re-entry route (Figure 6.7, step 2 of the model) with the loop diuretics bumetamide or furosemide at concentrations of less than 5×10^{-4} M (when the permeability of the endothelium is little affected) the transendothelial short circuit current is diminished by 16 μA/cm^2 which is equivalent to inhibiting a bicarbonate flux of 0.62 μmoles/cm^2 per hr. (Associated with this inhibition is a reduction of fluid flux of 40 μm/h which is also equivalent to an (isotonic) active flux of 0.6 μmoles/cm^2 per hr.)

$\Delta\gamma$ is about 2.6 mM (see above) which is 2.6 μmoles/cm^3 and the permeability of corneal endothelium to bicarbonate ions is estimated at 0.23 cm/hr. Consequently, the pump is estimated at 0.62 μmoles/cm^2 per hr and the leak ($P_e.\Delta\gamma$) is estimated at 0.60 μmoles/cm^2 per hr. The correspondence is within experimental error.

References

1 Elliot, G. F. (1980) *Biophysical Journal*, **32**, 95
2 Farrell, R. A. and Hart, R. (1969) *Bulletin of Mathematical Biophysics*, **31**, 727
3 Fischbarg, J. and Lim, J. J. (1974) *Journal of Physiology*, **241**, 647
4 Maurice, D. M. (1957) *Journal of Physiology*, **136**, 263

Chapter 7

Contact lens wear and the epithelium

Introduction

The corneal epithelium is adversely affected by most forms of contact lens wear. It is probably only in haptic lens wear, where the entire cornea is bridged by the lens, that negligible epithelial trauma occurs[9].

Changes to the integrity of the epithelium can best be examined with the aid of a slit lamp biomicroscope and vital stains. The stains have specific modes of action and differing stains can reveal differing features of epithelial disturbance. The use of vital stains often reveals characteristic patterns of epithelial response, which may be related to deficiencies in the lens or manner of blinking. However, much corneal staining fails to conform to any particular pattern, and histological examination of affected epithelial areas reveal a variety of complex changes to have occurred in the epithelium.

A loss of epithelial integrity is not the only adverse effect on this tissue. Both infiltrates and microcysts occur in differing forms of contact lens wear. The pathogenesis of these differing conditions is complex and by no means understood, although some useful clinical guidelines are available to aid detection and assist prevention.

Loss of corneal epithelial integrity

The corneal epithelium has been held to be the 'primary barrier against infection in the eye'. Yet from the inception of contact lens wear it was suggested that disruption of this barrier occurred[13]. The advent of modern forms of slit lamp biomicroscopes and particularly the use of vital stains has allowed the loss of integrity resulting from contact lens wear to be examined in some detail. However, before describing these effects it is well to consider the question of vital stains, as the appearance of the effects of corneal trauma are strongly influenced by the differing types of stain used.

Vital stains

Fluorescein

Undoubtedly the most widely used stain in contact lens work is sodium fluorescein. Fluorescein is a weak dibasic acid with a molecular weight of 330. It was first

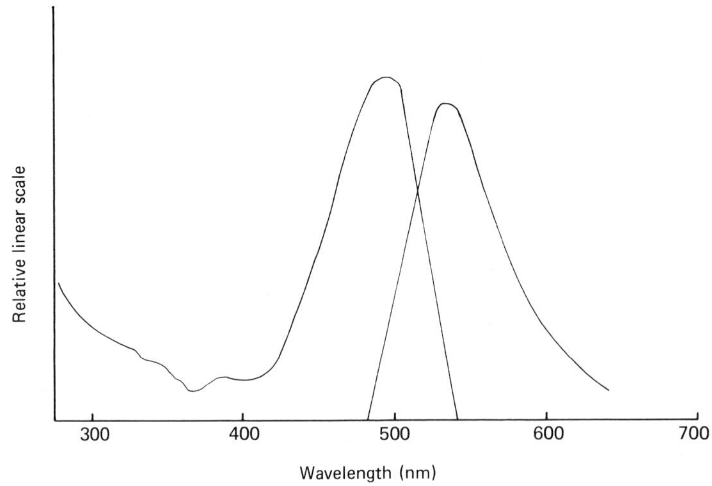

Figure 7.1 The absorption and emission spectra of sodium fluorescein (reproduced by permission of Maurice, *Investigative Ophthalmology*, 1967[39])

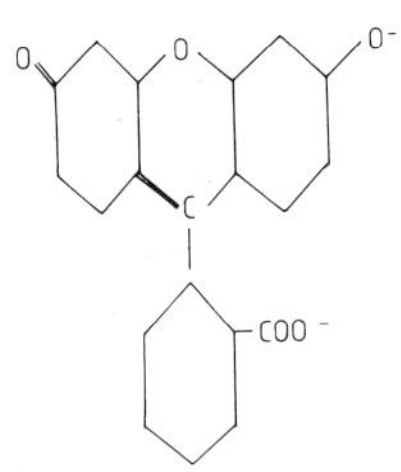

Figure 7.2 The molecular structure of the fluorescein ion (reproduced by permission of Maurice, *Investigative Ophthalmology*, 1967[39])

synthesized by Baeyer in 1871[39] from resorcinol and phthalic anhydride. Fluorescein is not particularly soluble in water and it is usually used as its sodium salt which dissolves in an equal weight of water. The absorption spectrum of sodium fluorescein lies in the blue region with a maximum at 490 nm while the emission spectrum lies principally in the green with a maximum at 520 nm (Figure 7.1). Fluorescein absorbs almost all the light incident upon it, and is remarkable in that the emission spectrum is maintained even in very dilute solutions, as low as 10^{-9} g/ml[39]. The structure of fluorescein is shown in Figure 7.2.

Although widely used as a stain in both research and practice, fluorescein does not form firm chemical bonds with cellular components[12], but rather diffuses through tissues which permit its passage. Since the intact corneal epithelium is essentially impervious to water soluble substances, fluorescein does not penetrate an intact epithelial layer. However, should surface disturbance occur fluorescein will penetrate the damaged areas[29], and this together with its role as an aid to fitting, is its principal use in contact lens practice. Sodium fluorescein is widely available in a variety of single dose disposable preparations in strengths of 1% and 2%, and possibly due to its reluctance to form strong chemical bonds has a very low toxicity.

Rose bengal

Another vital stain which has achieved wide usage in contact lens practice is rose

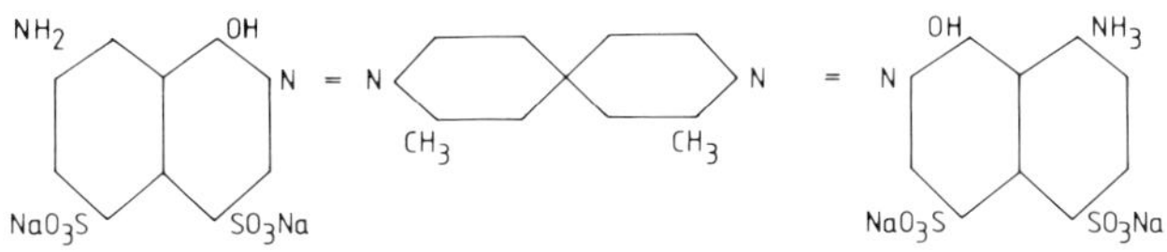

Figure 7.3 The structure of trypan blue (reproduced by permission of M. S. Norn, *Acta Ophthalmologica*, 1967[30])

bengal, which is an iodine derivative of fluorescein. It was probably first used as an ophthalmic stain by Kleefeld in 1919[38], who used rose bengal to stain a corneal ulcer. Rose bengal is a true stain in that it binds strongly and selectively to cellular components. Its essential role in cellular tissues has been carefully and exhaustively examined by Norn[28,32,34]. Norn has shown that rose bengal stains degenerate cells. Dead cells are stained a uniform intense red colour, while cells that are viable but degenerating are stained a weaker colour with the nucleus stained more strongly than the cytoplasm. Ocular mucus is also stained red by rose bengal which occasionally gives rise to confusion, although double staining with rose bengal and alcian blue can remove this difficulty. There is little doubt that rose bengal is most appropriately used as a 1% solution[35].

Even when used in as low a strength as 1% rose bengal is irritating to the eye. Patients typically complain of a 'gritty' sensation which can occasionally be severe. Because of the discomfort associated with the use of rose bengal it is rarely used as a matter of routine by contact lens practitioners. Its use is confined to the further examination of defects revealed by white light or fluorescein examination. Rose bengal remains particularly appropriate for the examination of corneal ulcers which, in their early stages, can sometimes be confused with pre-existing corneal nebulae.

Fluorexon

Fluorexon is a high molecular weight (710) fluorescein derivative initially suggested for use with soft lenses[42]. Fluorexon is BIS (*N*, *N*-BIS carboxymethyl-aminoethyl)-fluorescein tetrasodium. It is not readily absorbed by low water content soft lenses. Fluorexon has a number of the features of both fluorescein and rose bengal in that it may diffuse into tissues and also become associated with degenerated cells. However, it exhibits both properties to a lesser extent than the stains to which it is chemically related and as a consequence has not achieved wide usage.

Trypan blue

Trypan blue is a blue diazo compound having the structural formula shown in Figure 7.3. The dye possesses acidic groups and becomes associated with alkaline cellular components. The stain may act in two ways: it may become associated with degenerated cells in a similar manner to rose bengal, and it may also be ingested by a kind of phagocytosis and become visible as course grains in the cytoplasm. However, the latter property is limited to cells in the reticuloendothelial system[30]. Staining with trypan blue is reliable but not as pronounced as with rose bengal and for this reason it has not become widely used.

Methylene blue

Methylene blue is a complex blue compound (N N dimethylamino-3H-isophenthiazinylidendimethyl ammonium imdroxide). It was probably first used on the eye in

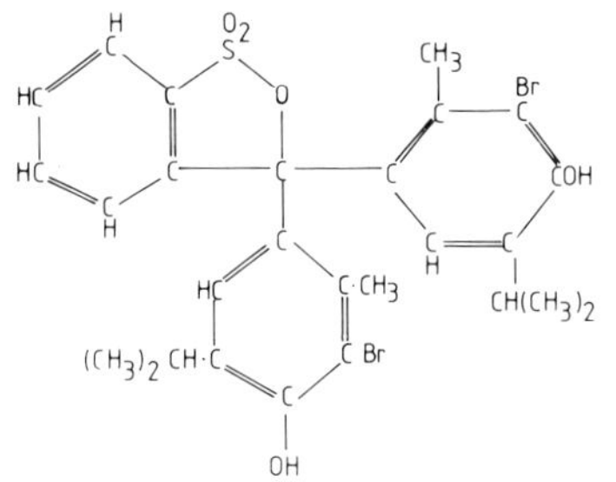

Figure 7.4 The structure of bromothymol blue (reproduced by permission of M. S. Norn, *Acta Ophthalmologica*, 1968[31])

1911[43] and has recently been re-evaluated by Norn[30]. Norn's study demonstrated that methylene blue is taken up by dead cells but not by degenerate cells.

The stain is unreliable for use in the eye as it may readily be precipitated from solution in granular form.

Bromothymol blue

Bromothymol blue has the structural formula shown in Figure 7.4. When used in a 1% solution iodonitrotetrazolium only stains epithelial cells with enzymatic activity, although it is probable that these cells are in some way degenerated to permit the absorption of the stain. Hence, the staining produced by iodonitrotetrazolium is similar in nature to that produced by rose bengal. The duration of stain is considerably longer than rose bengal and may on occasion give rise to permanent tattooing of very disturbed tissues[31].

Preferred stains for contact lens practice

In addition to the stains so far described a variety of other stains has been examined: scarlet red, merbromine, lissamine green and alcian blue (which is particularly useful for staining mucus but which does not stain the cornea)[32]. However, for a variety of reasons, which often include toxicity and permanence of stain, only sodium fluorescein and rose bengal have achieved wide usage. In his exhaustive studies of vital stains, Norn has frequently compared the clinical results obtained with various stains with either sodium fluorescein or rose bengal and on occasion with a mixture of 1% of each of these stains[37].

Vital staining of the non-lens wearing (normal) eye

Before describing disturbance to the corneal epithelium resulting from contact lens wear it is of clinical interest to note that vital staining also occurs in the non-lens wearing eye.

In the rabbit cornea, staining patterns are almost invariably revealed with the instillation of sodium fluorescein[24]. The suggestion has been made that these staining patterns are a normal feature of epithelial desquamation[24], although this seems rather unlikely.

In man, the author[26] has observed sporadic punctate stain among non-lens wearing control subjects who participated in various clinical experiments.

The degree of corneal stain observed in man is effected by the ageing process[33]. Patients in the sixth and subsequent decades of life are frequently observed to exhibit extensive but superficial areas of stain. These disturbances are effervescent in character, being present on one occasion and not on another and also changing location.

Instillation of fluroescein into the human eye can also be used to reveal the natural 'mosaic' which is thought to arise from the structure of Bowman's layer[1,15,50].

Vital staining: classification and incidence

Vital staining as the result of contact lens wear has been widely reported[25], although there is a scarcity of controlled comparative information.

Until the event of hard corneal contact lenses, corneal epithelial disturbances were only occasionally observed, although 'dimpling' (small regular depressions of the corneal surface) was occasionally encountered in poorly fitting haptic lenses. However, as corneal lenses became more widely accepted, disruptions to the integrity of the epithelium became widely recognized. One of the earliest attempts to classify epithelial disturbances in a systematic manner was probably that of Cochet and Bonnet[5] who described epithelial disruptions arising from contact lens wear as:

1 Small 'dots' resulting from pressure
2 Lines formed as the result of insufficient aspiration.

A rather wider classification has been produced by Schulman[48] who divided vital staining into seven categories:

1 Arcuate abrasions
2 Punctate abrasions
3 Superficial abrasions
4 Deep epithelial abrasions
5 Linear abrasions
6 Limbal abrasions
7 Superficial conjunctival abrasions.

The author has also attempted to classify staining patterns according to type, severity and area[26].

Type was categorized as:

1 Punctate stain (small localized areas of stain giving distinct margins and found singly or in groups)
2 Diffuse stain (an area of stain having an undifferentiated appearance with ill-defined margins)
3 Line stain (typically the 'tracking mark' made by a foreign body)
4 Dimple stain (strictly not a form of staining, but rather a series of regular indentations in the corneal surface.

Severity of stain was ranked at three levels:

1 Superficial stain confined to the outermost layers of the epithelium
2 Moderate stain involving the epithelium down to Bowman's layer
3 Deep stain which involved the entire epithelium with penetration of fluorescein into the corneal stroma.

Area of stain was assessed with the aid of a squared graticule introduced into one eye piece of the slit lamp biomicroscope where each square represented 0.75% of the total area of a cornea.

Although these and other classifications of vital stain have been proposed, none has achieved wide usage, and one of the difficulties of interpreting the available literature remains the variety of terminology used to describe essentially similar phenomena.

The incidence of differing types of vital staining in contact lens wear is not particularly well documented in the literature, although the majority of contact lens practitioners have a clear concept of the phenomena and a judgement as to what constitutes an acceptable degree of staining.

The author[26] found a fourfold increase in the incidence of punctate stain in patients who commenced corneal lens wear. The incidence of diffuse stain also increased from 10% to approximately 20%, while 10% of the patients examined presented with dimple 'stain' which had not been observed in any patient prior to contact lens wear. An increase in the incidence of punctate stain was also observed among soft lens wearers; the occurrence rising from 25% prior to fitting to approximately 50% after fitting. No increase was observed in the incidence of diffuse stain among soft lens wearers and no instance of dimple 'stain' was observed.

Mechanisms of vital staining

Epithelial disturbance as shown by vital stains often has a characteristic appearance. Perhaps the most well documented is '3 and 9 o'clock stain' arising from reduced or incomplete blinking habits (see Chapter 1). Various other patterns of vital stain have also been widely recognized. An arcuate appearance is often considered to arise from a poorly polished intermediate lens zone or edge, while the 'dimpling' pattern already referred to has been associated with a 'tight fitting' area particularly in a haptic lens[46]. However, many areas of vital stain have an ill-defined appearance, and may simply be referred to as 'mechanical' or 'chemical' type staining.

Little experimental work has been reported on the mechanisms of epithelial disturbance, but that which has been done is interesting. Animal eyes histologically examined after various periods of hard lens wear show a number of changes in the appearance of epithelium[16]. In the contact lens bearing area, the thickness of the epithelium has been found to be reduced to two thirds of the equivalent areas of control corneas. In these areas a layer of wing cells was observed to be absent and the basal cells were compressed in both height and width. Surprisingly, a substantial increase was observed in the rate of cell mitosis, the incidence rising from 1 per 100 cells in the control corneas to 1 per 10 in the 'bearing areas.'

The changes observed in this study suggest that the effects of contact lens wear on the integrity of the corneal epithelium are more subtle and complex than often supposed by the arbitrary classification of 'mechanical or chemical type' staining.

Epithelial erosions

Erosion of discrete areas of the corneal epithelium as a result of contact lens wear may occasionally be encountered. In rabbit studies, erosions are by no means uncommon[17]. However, among human subjects epithelial erosions have been only infrequently observed, and on the occasions when they are present they are often associated with patient abuse of the contact lens.

In a study of 2550 soft lens wearing patients, 57 were observed who wore their contact lenses for more than 20 hours, against professional advice. In 18 of these cases the patient presented with epithelium adhering to the posterior surface of the contact lens, which had sloughed off from the central epithelium[8]. These patients were also characterized by marked blepharospasm, injected conjunctivae and oedamatous corneas.

The eroded area of the cornea forms a discrete and usually circular 'hole' in the epithelium which is wholly devoid of cells. Specular reflection reveals a uniform bright area with light directly reflected from the basement membrane. Recovery from corneal erosions presents difficulties. Initially, the superficial epithelial cells surrounding the epithelium will slip and progressively extend across the denuded area. Once an intact single layer of cell is achieved cellular proliferation will occur under the outer protective layer, but it may be a matter of 2 weeks or more before a normally structured tissue is restored. During the period of tissue repair, growth factor is liberated into the extracellular spaces and this may result in the formation of synechiae during sleep. These adhesions formed between cells of the regenerating epithelium and cells of the tarsal conjunctiva will break when the eyes are opened upon waking resulting in recurrent erosion. There are a number of approaches to the treatment of recurrent erosion and rather surprisingly the use of a large 'bandage' soft lens during periods of sleep is often useful.

Epithelial infiltrates

Discrete infiltrates presenting as small (0.5 mm) intraepithelial lesions and larger (1.0–1.5 mm) subepithelial lesions have been observed in a variety of ocular conditions[19]. Although often associated with viral infections of the cornea, they may also occur in a variety of inflammatory processes. The infiltrates have been described as being 'composed of minute respersive granules that may be white, buff or grey. These vesicular granules may concentrate in the centre of the lesion and gradually decrease in density towards the periphery. They can effervescent presenting a different clinical picture from visit to visit[11,23]. The infiltrates may be composed of discrete collections of inflammatory cells of limbal origin[23].

Josephson and Caffery[23] have reported a careful and well-documented retrospective study of epithelial infiltrates in soft contact lens wear. Over a period of 18 months, 149 patients were examined who presented in private practice with infiltrates. The patients represented rather less than 4% of a fitted population sample. A careful examination was made of the patients' records and the severity of infiltrates was ranked on a scale of 1 to 5. In addition, the recovery time for the loss of infiltrates was recorded and comparison was made with a control group of subjects who had not worn contact lenses but who presented with infiltrates. Based on the patients' case histories eight groups of differing aetiologies were proposed:

1 Traumatic
2 Viral
3 Allergic
4 Preserved solutions
5 Lens fit

6 Coated lenses
7 Toxic vapours
8 Idiopathic.

The patients were assigned to the various groups and a statistical analysis of the incidence, severity and recovery from infiltrates was undertaken. The results of this analysis led to a number of conclusions:

1 Patients whose infiltrates were considered to be viral in origin had longer recovery times (mean 5.5 months) than the idiopathic group (mean 2.75 months). In addition there was:
   (a) a statistically higher incidence of subepithelial involvement
   (b) a lighter incidence of recurrence
   (c) a higher incidence of binocular involvement
   (d) a significantly larger incidence of previous contact lens wearing problems
2 Patients whose infiltrates were considered to be due to the use of preserved solutions, in conjunction with soft contact lens wear, had a higher incidence of subepithelial involvement, and took longer to recover from infiltrates than the idiopathic group, and there was also a higher incidence of female patients in this group
3 For all groups of subjects the contact lens wearers took longer to recover from infiltrates than non-lens wearers, however, this arose from the more severe forms of infiltrates observed among the contact lens wearers
4 Recovery time was related to severity for all of subjects and was also related to the severity of lens coating among the contact lens wearers.

In discussing their study, Josephson and Caffery speculated on their conclusions. They felt that the infiltrates attributed to viral origins formed a distinct clinical entity which seemed more likely to be stimulated by a contact lens related stimulus, which could be a virus other than an adenovirus or an adenovirus of low virulence. In addition, the infiltrates attributed to the use of preserved solutions had a greater incidence of subepithelial involvement. However, the wearing of hydrogen lenses resulted in an increased severity of keratitis with longer recovery times than non-lens wearers and thus it was felt that 'the wearing of hydrogen lenses causes exacerbation of infiltrative keratitis no matter what the etiology'. As a result of these and other considerations the writers 'proposed a mechanism of infiltrative keratitis specific to hydrogel lens wear'. The essence of this proposed mechanism is the migration of inflammatory cells from affected limbal blood vessels in response to a variety of stimuli caused, or exacerbated by hydrogel lens wear. The stimuli may consist of antiseptics or environmental toxins absorbed by the lens and leached onto the eye surface. The stimuli may also arise from contaminants on the lens surface, or from the accumulation of cellular debris and other metabolic by products trapped and held against the eye by a steeply fitted soft lens.

Although this proposed mechanism remains unverified, the application of the study to clinical practice has been suggested. Proper diagnosis and management of patients presenting with infiltrative keratitis should cover a number of features:

1 Symptoms should be discussed with the patients as the incidence of symptoms is known to be different (Table 7.1)

2 History questions should include time of onset, recent environmental exposure, general health (particularly the onset of recent sore throats or influenza)
3 Associated signs. In addition to a thorough slit lamp biomicroscope examination, the facial derma should be examined for the appearance of regional adenopathy. Further signs are included in Table 7.2
4 Lens observations. The degree of lens coating should be noted as well as any accompanying changes in wettability, colour and transparency. In addition, the fitting characteristics of the lens should be recorded.

Table 7.1 Symptoms associated with infiltrative keratitis (reproduced by permission of Josephson and Caffery, International Contact Lens Clinic, 1979[23])

Symptoms	*No lens* (%)	*Viral* (%)	*Preserved solutions* (%)	*Lens fit* (%)	*Coated lens* (%)	*Toxic vapours* (%)	*Idiopathic* (%)
Redress	3	15	65	50	50	13	31
Reduced vision or blur	–	–	40	20	31	50	6
Discomfort or irritation	–	8	45	20	31	37	31
Discharge	–	23	20	20	22	–	9
Burning	–	–	–	–	–	–	6
Itching	–	–	–	–	–	–	3
Light sensitivity	3	–	10	–	–	–	3
Dryness	–	–	–	–	–	–	6
None	94	46	5	20	22	13	33

Table 7.2 Signs of infiltrative keratitis (reproduced by permission of Josephson and Caffery, International Contact Lens Clinic, 1979[23])

Signs	*No lens* (%)	*Viral* (%)	*Preserved solutions* (%)	*Lens fit* (%)	*Coated lens* (%)	*Toxic vapours* (%)	*Idiopathic* (%)
Oedma	66	23	70	60	69	87	39
Follicles	41	75	15	20	12	12	18
Papules	22	–	15	–	12	–	6
Bulbar conjunctival hyperaemia	9	–	25	30	9	12	3
Perilimbal chemosis and hyperaemia	–	–	30	10	19	12	6
K change	–	–	–	–	–	75	3
Stain	–	–	–	–	–	12	–
Regional lymphadenopathy	–	20	–	–	–	–	–

Given the variety of possible causes proposed for infiltrative keratitis, prevention remains a difficult problem. As with contact lens associated giant papillary conjunctivitis (see Chapter 2), suitable and effective lens cleaning is of importance (see Chapter 3). Since the length of recovery is related to the severity of the condition, early diagnosis is essential and patients should be encouraged to seek advice with the onset of symptoms. A number of slit lamp photomicrographs showing instances of infiltrates are shown in Plate 32.

One form of infiltrative keratitis in contact lens wear has a well-established aetiology – so-called papain allergy. In the presence of mercury found in a number of contact lens solutions, papain will complex with protein residues left after enzymatic lens cleaning. The resulting residue is toxic to the ocular surface and infiltrates are rapidly formed by inflammatory material migrating from the limbal arcades. The infiltrates are invariably accompanied by a red eye which has led to the assertion of 'allergy to papain' for which there is no foundation. The treatment of affected patients consists of the supply of replacement lenses to be used in conjunction with solutions which are free from thimerosal and other organic mercury compounds. Resolution of the infiltrates and red eye is rapid and this form of infiltrative keratitis is by far the easiest to manage.

Epithelial cystic formations

Small cysts in the epithelium have been observed in a number of keratoconjunctival disorders (for a review of the clinical features of the various cystic disorders see Bron and Tripathi[2]). The cysts are a common feature of such conditions as Meesmann's dystrophy[40], Cogan's microcystic dystrophy[6], recurrent corneal erosions, and a number of other epithelial keratopathies. The pathogenesis of such disorders has been carefully examined by Bron and Tripathi[2]. In a histological and electron microscope study of epithelial biopsies obtained from a variety of patients Bron and Tripathi observed a number of common features:

1 The cysts which were observed clinically to have a globular profile and smooth outline preserved a similar appearance in the histological sections and were mostly located in the mid and superficial regions of the epithelium. The cysts were lined with a plasma membrane of adjacent epithelial cells which was usually occupied by degenerate epithelial cells as well as general cellular debris.
2 Pale cells: the majority of cells in the sections were of normal appearance and responded normally to histological stains. However, a number of cells which were swollen in appearance responded poorly to the histological stains, and were therefore pale in appearance. The nuclei of the pale cells were weakly basophilic while the cytoplasm showed small vacuoles and weak eosinophilia. Electron microscopy showed the cell membranes to be poorly demarcated with ill-defined desmosomal attachments. The cells were relatively depleted of glycogen and the cytoplasmic matrix and tonofilaments were of low electron density, giving rise to a pale appearance. A number of degenerative changes such as swollen mitochondria, dilated endoplasmic reticulum, nuclear blebs, and coarsely granular chromatin were observed and some cells showed clear evidence of cellular lysis.
3 Spongiosis: that is an increased width of the intracellular spaces between adjacent cells, was observed in most of the specimens examined. In most samples the intracellular junctions were intact although excessively widened and filled with a 'flocculent material probably proteinaceous elements of oedema fluids'.

The observation of cysts, pale cells and spongiosis led Bron and Tripathi to propose a hypothesis for the pathogenesis of cystic disorders of the epithelium. The observation of both pale cells (suggesting intracellular oedema) and spongiosis (suggesting extracellular oedema) supports the contention that epithelial cysts were

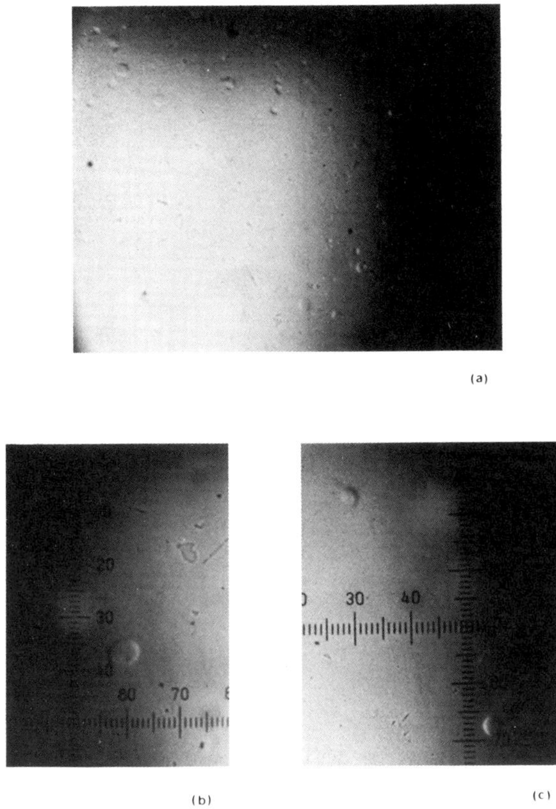

Figure 7.5 Microepithelial cysts provoked by extended contact lens wear. Photographed with a Holden/Zantos attachment on a Nikon Photo Slit Lamp Biomicroscope. Ten scale divisions = 140 μm

intimately related to both these oedematous processes. It was felt that pale cells were the precursors of cysts arising from intracellular oedema, which as cellular lysis took place, led to the accumulation of cellular debris in a cyst occupying an intracellular space. The initial event in the formation of an intraepithelial cyst was felt to be the accumulation of fluid in the intracellular spaces. Thus, a cyst may form from fluid accumulation around one cell, or a group of cells, leading to the complete lysis of these cells, with the resultant cellular debris being incorporated in a cyst. The fate of a cyst depends very much on its site of origin. Smaller cysts containing cellular debris would gradually migrate forward and eventually erupt on the epithelial surface. Larger cysts would either burst at a localized point forming a sinus to the surface, or crupt causing a partial loss of epithelium.

The observation of microepithelial cysts in hard contact lens wear was probably first reported by Frederick Burnett Hodd in 1964[18]. Microepithelial cysts have also been observed in both daily and extended soft lens wear[3,18,20,22,45]. In a study carried out in the author's laboratory by Judith Humphrys[21], microepithelial cysts were observed to occur in all patients participating in a controlled group comparative study, originally designed to examine the incidence and severity of neovasculariza-

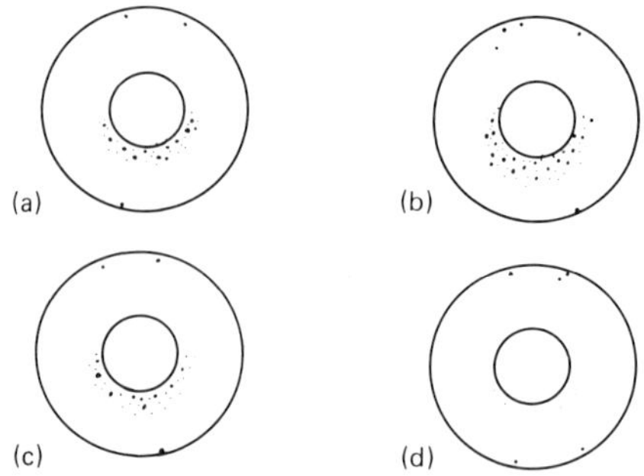

Figure 7.6 The rate of recovery from microcysts: (*a*) upon cessation of lens wear microepithelial cysts were observed to conform to an accurate pattern roughly coincident with the projected lower pupillary margin; (*b*) one week after ceasing lens wear the affected area was observed to be larger, more densely packed with cysts to show cysts which were grey or opaque and to exhibit grey infiltrates; (*c*) after a further 3 weeks grey infiltrates were no longer present and the density of the cysts had reduced; (*d*) 5 weeks later the central corneal area was almost devoid of cysts, although occasional cysts could be observed in the corneal periphery (reproduced by permission of Humphrys, 1982[21])

tion in extended soft lens wear. At the eighteenth week of the study a patient presented with a superficial epithelial erosion secondary to a damaged lens. Slit lamp biomicroscopic examination revealed the presence of microepithelial cysts. Subsequent examination of the 43 other participating subjects revealed 42 to have cysts while the remaining patient developed cysts 2 weeks after the termination of lens wear. The severity, intensity, and area occupied by the cysts was recorded and ranked at five levels and the rate of recovery monitored. The appearance of the cysts was also photographed and examples are shown in Figure 7.5.

The cysts were observed to conform to an arcuate pattern, roughly coincident with the projected lower pupillary margin. One week after ceasing lens wear the affected area was observed to be larger, more densely packed with cysts, to show cysts which were grey or opaque, and to exhibit grey infiltrates.

After a further 3 weeks the grey infiltrates were no longer present and the density of the cysts had reduced. Five weeks later the central area of the epithelium was almost devoid of cysts, although occasional cysts could be observed in the periphery of the cornea. The recovery from the cysts is illustrated in Figure 7.6. In considering our work we concluded that the cysts provoked by extended contact lens wear most nearly resembled those reported to occur in Meesman's dystrophy in both size (10–15 mm), and appearance (smooth globular structures which were clear in retro-illumination). Following the work of Tripathi and Bron we attempted to provoke cysts in rabbit corneas by the use of extended wear lenses. After sacrifice we observed pale cells and spongiosis, but not the cysts themselves. In addition we also observed fine changes beneath the epithelium, an observation also reported in man by Montague Ruben[44]. The cysts may not of themselves be particularly serious, and because of their small size they are difficult to observe and photograph. However, in view of the proposed pathogenesis they may indicate serious dysfunction of the basal cells of the epithelium with cellular degeneration and lysis.

A distinction between microepithelial cysts, and vacuoles and bullae has been made by Steven Zantos[51]. Epithelial vacuoles appear as discrete round transparent structures enclosed within the epithelium, while bullae are clear oval-shaped structures with a tendency to coalesce. Bullae would appear to be associated with excessive corneal oedema and discontinued lens wear is often indicated by their presence. Vacuoles, on the other hand, may be innocuous and an intermittent feature of various types of lens wear. As with microepithelial cysts, the pathogenesis of these conditions is unknown. It may be that they are all clinical manifestations of differing degrees of the same underlying epithelial dysfunction, or it is possible that they represent different clinical entities. As with so much of contact lens wear, the mechanisms responsible for these conditions has yet to be determined.

Sattler's veil

The subjective impression of 'haloes from light' is a well known complication provoked by various forms of lens wear. The condition was probably first described by Sattler[47] and has been attributed to epithelial oedema[7]. The epithelium, when viewed in retroillumination by slit lamp biomicroscopy appears bedewed with a grey epithelial haze. Oxygen deprivation has long been held to be the cause of the disorder[49]. Initial measurements[14] showed the half arc of the halo seen by contact lens wearers could have been produced by cells approximately 10 mm in diameter. A more plausible suggestion for the origin of Sattler's veil has been the proposal of a circular diffraction grating formed by the basal epithelial cells and the extracellular spaces[41]. Confirmation of the feasibility of this idea has been provided by an ingenious experiment described by Lambert and Klyce[27]. Using an excised rabbit cornea perfused with hypoxia (7 mm HgO_2) ringer's solution, the epithelial surface of the cornea was examined by specular microscopy and photographed. The hypoxia solution resulted in a polygonal mesh of scattered light which outlined the basal and intermediate wing cells of the epithelium. The resulting negatives were projected and the image outlined with india ink on an acetate background. The india ink pattern was then re-photographed and an optical transform or diffraction pattern was made with a laser diffractometer. The resulting negative showed a central maximum with a surrounding halo, with a half arc which corresponded to the calculated value of a first order maximum for a plane diffraction grating. Measurements from the specular microscope showed no consistent change in epithelial thickness, although stromal swelling was observed after 15–60 minutes. The stromal swelling was found to be reversible if under 10%, and to produce stromal back scatter of light at values greater than this. The absence of a consistent change in epithelial thickness suggests that any increase in cell volumes could only have occurred in a radial direction. The polygonal light pattern and subsequent diffraction pattern gives strong support to the contention that Sattler's veil is a circular diffraction pattern, the origin of which is the back scatter of light from the intracellular space.

References

1 Bron, A. J. and Tripathi, R. C. (1969). *British Journal of Ophthalmology*, **53**, 760
2 Bron, A. J. and Tripathi, R. C. (1973). *British Journal of Ophthalmology*, **57**, 361

3 Brown, N. A. and Lobascher, D. (1975). *Proceedings of the Royal Society of Medicine*, **68**, 2
4 Buschke, W., Friendenwald, J. S. and Fleischmann, W. (1943). *Bulletin of the Johns Hopkins Hospital*, **73**, 143
5 Cochet, P. and Bonnet, R. (1959). *Bulletin de la Société d'Ophthalmologie de France*, **1**, 20
6 Cogan, D. G., Donaldson, D. D., Kuwabara, T. and Marshall, D. (1978). *Transactions of the American Ophthalmological Society*, **62**, 143
7 Dallos, J. (1946). *British Journal of Ophthalmology*, **30**, 607
8 De Rothe, A. (1954). *Archives of Ophthalmology*, **68**, 139
9 Doggart, J. H. (1950). *Ocular Signs in Slit Lamp Microscopy*. 2nd edn. London: H. Kinson. p. 24
10 Duke Elder, S. (1965). *System of Ophthalmology*. London: Kimpton
11 Duke Elder, S. Cited by Josephson, J. E. and Caffery, B. E. (1979). *International Contact Lens Clinic*, **6**, 47
12 Ehrlich, P. (1878). In: *The Collected Papers of Paul Ehrlich*, Vol. 1 (1956). London: Pergamon
13 Fick, A. E. (1888). Translation by C. H. May (1906) *Archives of Ophthalmology*, **19**, 215
14 Finkelstein, I. S. (1952). *Archives of the American Academy of Optometry*, **29**, 231
15 Fisher, F. P. (1930). *Archiv für Augenheilkunde*, **102**, 146
16 Greenburg, M. A. and Hill, R. M. (1973). *American Journal of Optometry*, **50**, 699
17 Hirano, J. (1972). *Japanese Journal of Clinical Ophthalmology*, **16**, 1403
18 Hodd, F. A. B. (1965). *Contacto*, **2**, 18
19 Hogan, M. J. and Zimmerman, L. E. (1962). *Ophthalmic Pathology*. Philadelphia: W.B. Saunders
20 Holden, B. A. and Zantos, S. G. (1979). *The Optician*, **177**, 52
21 Humphrys, J. A. (1982). *Doctoral thesis*. University of Aston, Birmingham
22 Josephson, J. E. (1979). *International Contact Lens Clinic*, **6**, 40
23 Josephson, J. E. and Caffery B. E. (1979). *International Contact Lens Clinic*, **6**, 47
24 Kikkawa, Y. (1972) *Experimental Eye Research*, **14**, 13
25 Koverman, J. J. and Hoefle, F. B. (1971). *Proceedings of the Vth Ohio State Contact Lens Seminar*, Ohio State
26 Larke, J. R. (1969). *Doctoral thesis*. University of Aston, Birmingham
27 Lambert, S. R. and Klyce, S. D. (1981). *American Journal of Ophthalmology*, **95**, 51
28 Norn, M. S. (1964). *Acta Ophthalmologica*, **40**, 389
29 Norn, M. S. (1964). *Acta Ophthalmologica*, **42**, 1038
30 Norn, M. S. (1967). *Acta Ophthalmologica*, **45**, 380
31 Norn, M. S. (1968). *Acta Ophthalmologica*, **46**, 231
32 Norn, M. S. (1969). *Acta Ophthalmologica*, **47**, 1102
33 Norn, M. S. (1970). *Acta Ophthalmologica*, **48**, 108
34 Norn, M. S. (1970). *Acta Ophthalmologica*, **48**, 132
35 Norn, M. S. (1970). *Acta Ophthalmologica*, **48**, 546
36 Norn, M. S. (1971). *Eye, Ear, Nose and Throat Monthly*, **50**, 28
37 Norn, M. S. (1972). *Acta Ophthalmologica*, **50**, 286
38 Cited by Marx, E. (1924). *Grafes Archiv für Ophthalmologie*, **114**, 465
39 Maurice, D. M. (1967). *Investigative Ophthalmology*, **6**, 464
40 Meesman, A. and Wilke, F. (1939). *Klinische Monatsblätter für Augenheilkunde*, **103**, 361
41 Miller, D. and Benedek, G. (1973). *Intraocular Light Scattering*. Springfield Illinois: Charles C. Thomas. p. 82
42 Refojo, M. J., Miller, D. and Fiore, A. S. (1972). *Archives of Ophthalmology*, **87**, 275
43 Reuss, A. (1911). *Grafes Archiv für Ophthalmologie*, **78**, 297
44 Ruben, M. (1979). Personal communication
45 Ruben, M., Brown, N., Lobascher, D., Chaston, J. and Morris, J. (1976). *British Journal of Ophthalmology*, **60**, 529
46 Sabell, A. G. (1982). Personal communication
47 Sattler, G. H. (1931). *Deutsche Medizinalgeitung*, **52**, 312
48 Schulman, S. N. (1974). *Journal of American Optometric Association*, **46**, 242
49 Smelser, G. K. and Chen, D. K. (1955). *Archives of Ophthalmology*, **53**, 677
50 Tripathi, R. C. and Bron, A. J. (1972). *British Journal of Ophthalmology*, **56**, 713
51 Zantos, S. (1983) *International Contact Lens Clinic*, **10**, 128

Chapter 8

Corneal touch thresholds

Introduction

The surface of the human cornea is exquisitely sensitive to touch. This low threshold of sensation forms part of the eye's defence mechanism against mechanical trauma and allows lid closure to be provoked by the mildest of stimuli.

The sensitivity of the cornea is adversely affected by all forms of contact lens wear. Sensory loss is probably the commonest response that the eye makes to the presence of a contact lens. The rate of sensory loss is different for differing lens types. Hard lens wear results in a dramatic rise in touch threshold with a two-fold increase being observed in a single day's wear. The rate of reduction in sensation is slower with soft lenses. Some forms of high water content hydrogel lens require 12 weeks of extended wear before a loss equivalent to a day's hard lens wear is observed.

The loss of corneal touch sensation is progressive after the initial years of lens wear, and there is no current evidence of a revised stabilized threshold. Even among long-term hard lens wearers who may have worn their lenses for more than 2 decades, the threshold of sensation is still observed to decline, although at a very slow rate.

The rate of recovery of sensation upon cessation of contact lens wear depends upon the period of wear and hence the extent of sensory loss.

The essential mechanism responsible for sensory loss has not been clearly illustrated at the time of writing. However, it has been shown that a reduction in sensation may be provoked by anoxia exceeding 4–5 hours' duration. It is possible that the effect of oxygen deprivation on neurological tissue is to reduce substantially the availability of high phosphate energy, and hence embarrass transport function. Since the propagation of nerve impulses depends upon a high and continuing utilization of transport function, any reduction in the oxygen environment of the cell may directly impede its ability to transmit a wave impulse.

Sensory loss in contact lens wear may be regarded from at least two viewpoints:

1 The dramatic loss of lid sensation allows lens wear to become comfortable and the patient to be essentially unaware of the presence of the lens
2 The loss of corneal sensation may allow small unfelt particles to become trapped beneath the contact lens and abrade the cornea, thus opening the route for infection.

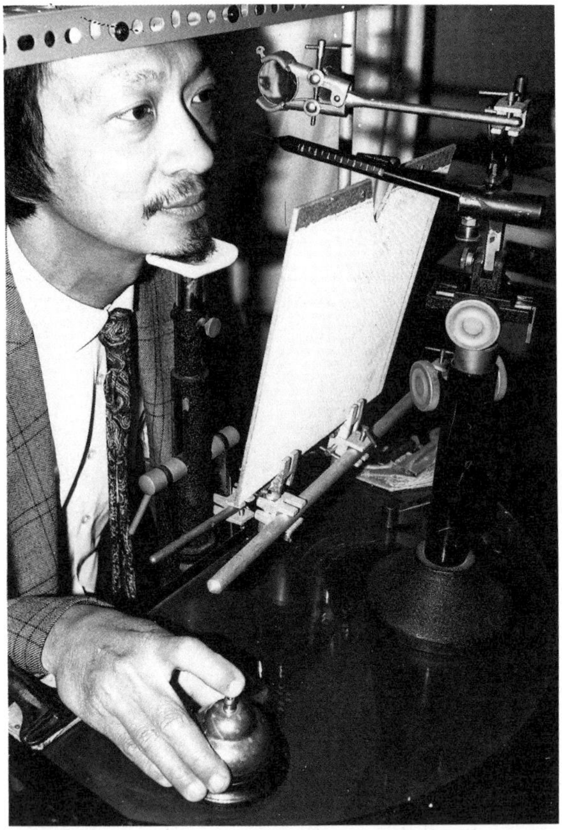

Figure 8.1 A suitably mounted arrangement of the Cochet-Bonnet aesthiometer (Reproduced by permission of Millodot, 1978)

The measurement of corneal sensation

The earliest attempt to measure corneal sensation has been attributed to Von Frey[4] who used a series of different length hairs pushed against the cornea to provoke a sensation.

Boberg-Ans[3] has described an instrument in which the length of a nylon filament may be altered by a simple rachet mechanism and the tip of the nylon held against the cornea. A commercial form of this instrument, the Cochet-Bonnet aesthiometer[6], has become widely available and will be familiar to most contact lens practitioners. Various improvements have been suggested since the introduction of the Cochet-Bonnet instrument in 1960. Some novel forms of instrument have been advocated with plastic discs held against the cornea[8], and springs utilized to apply a force to the surface of the eye[5]. Perhaps the most useful improvements have been suggested in an instrument described by Larson[14]. In this modification, the nylon filament was replaced by a longer length of platinum wire, thus avoiding the influence of humidity on nylon and increasing the range of measurement. As it touched the cornea the wire displaced a lever which in turn broke a light beam incident upon a photoelectric cell, causing the wire to retract. The instrument could be finely set; the force with which the wire touched the cornea being increased by a spring mechanism. The instrument had the further advantage of linear calibration which overcame the non-linear characteristics of the Cochet-Bonnet aesthiometer, which is least sensitive to changes in the length of the nylon thread, when it is close to full extension. The instrument known as the Larson Millodot aesthiometer was used successfully to measure the topographic distribution of touch threshold for the human cornea[27], but has not been made commercially available although a dissimilar device has been constructed by at least one group other worker in this area[7].

In the absence of the Larson Millodot aesthiometer the Cochet-Bonnet instrument remains the best known apparatus and a suitably mounted arrangement is shown in Figure 8.1. The essential feature of this system is the use of a moveable frame which allows displacement of the instrument in the x, y and z meridians, thus eliminating the imprecision of hand-held devices.

Mode and precision of measurement

In the measurement of corneal touch threshold it is important that a minimum of stimulation is used and measurements are made starting with a low pressure until threshold is reached. Random stimulation may lead to an elevation of the corneal touch threshold and give rise to a sensation of afterglow making further measurement difficult[29]. The correlation between subjective and objective measurement is good in the corneal periphery, and objective methods may be used in clinical and animal research[18].

The precision of measurement is high; repeated sequential measurement on the same subject gave a repeatability of ±4% for the Cochet-Bonnet aesthiometer[10]. However, this value is misleading as the instrument gives a stepwise non-linear reading. The progressive reading and linear characteristics of the Larson Millodot instrument would be likely to improve upon this level of measurement precision considerably. One surprising feature of the measurement of the corneal sensation is that the measured threshold is above the level at which damage to the cells of the epithelium occurs[29]. It has been suggested that the threshold to pain is determined by the threshold to tissue damage[32]. However, this is not the case for the corneal epithelium where damage precedes sensation and *a fortiori* pain.

Corneal touch thresholds and the influence of environmental variables

The surface of the human cornea is not uniformly sensitive to touch[27]. The most sensitive region of the cornea is the central zone where the touch threshold has been measured as 10.5 mg/mm^2 to 13.8 mg/mm^2[2,27]. The least sensitive region of the cornea is the superior zone which is frequently covered by the upper lid. In this region, touch thresholds as low as 35–45 mg/mm^2 have been recorded. The threshold for the nasal, temporal and inferior regions of the cornea are intermediate between those of the central and superior zones. A diagram illustrating mean touch thresholds of the human cornea is shown in Figure 8.2. The topographic distribution of corneal touch threshold is similar to the relative corneal distribution of acetylcholine[30].

In addition to a topographic distribution, corneal sensation has been shown to be subject to both a circadian[17] and menstrually[26] related variation. In man, the cornea is least sensitive in the early morning and the touch threshold declines throughout

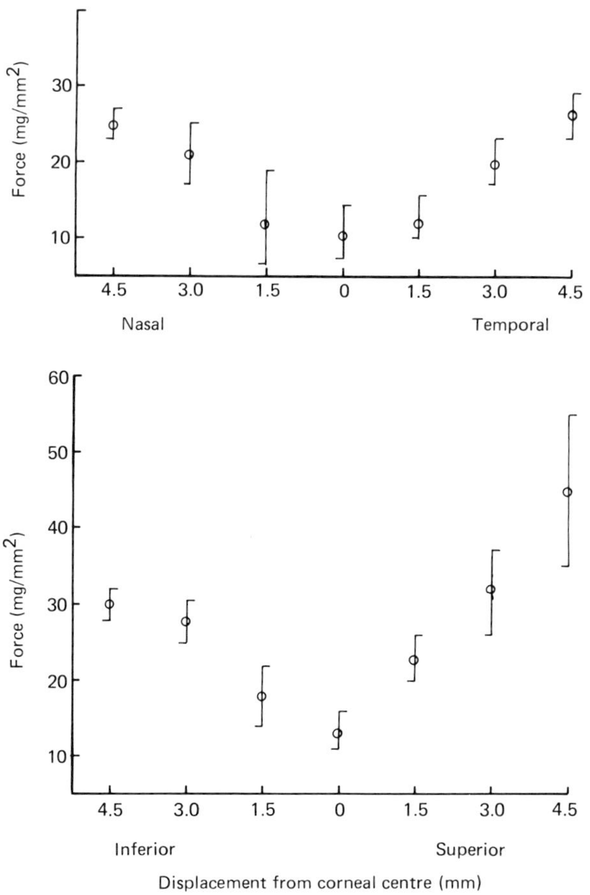

Figure 8.2 The topographic distribution of the touch threshold of the human cornea (reproduced by permission of Millodot and Larson, *American Journal of Optometry*, 1969[27])

the day until the late evening. During periods of sleep some sensory loss occurs until the eyes are opened on the following day when sensation again increases[15]. A graph illustrating circadian patterns in corneal touch sensation is shown Figure 8.3.

The menstrual cycle has been shown to affect corneal sensation with the cornea becoming markedly less sensitive during the premenstruum and during the time of menstruation. Corneal sensation is not noticeably affected during the remainder of the menstrual cycle and depressed levels of sensation have not been observed when oral contraceptives have been used. The depressed level of sensation has been attributed to the oedema associated with the onset and duration of menstruation and a graph illustrating menstrually related changes in corneal touch threshold is shown in Figure 8.4.

Both age and iris pigmentation have been shown to be related to corneal sensation. Corneal touch thresholds decline uniformly and progressively with age[23] and a graph illustrating age related corneal sensory loss is shown in Figure 8.5. Surprisingly, iris pigmentation shows a strong correlation with corneal touch threshold[21], with

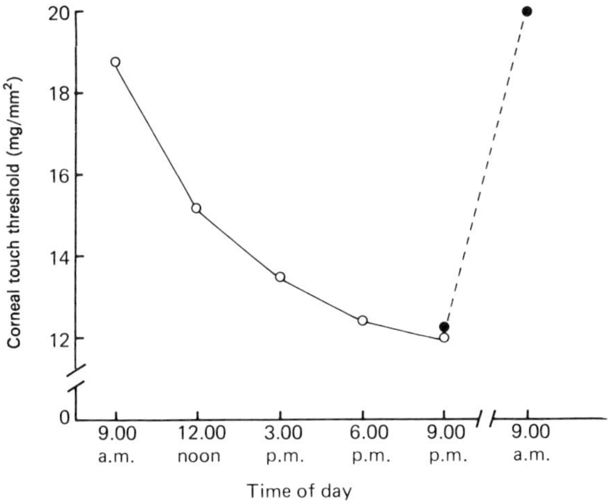

Figure 8.3 Circadian patterns in corneal touch thresholds (reproduced by permission of Millodot, *British Journal of Ophthalmology*, 1972[17])

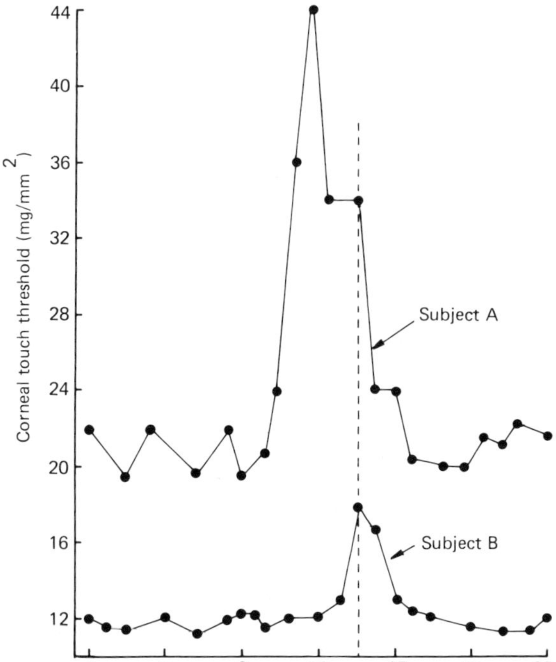

Figure 8.4 Menstrually related changes in corneal touch threshold (reproduced by permission of Millodot and Lamont, *British Journal of Ophthalmology*, 1974[26])

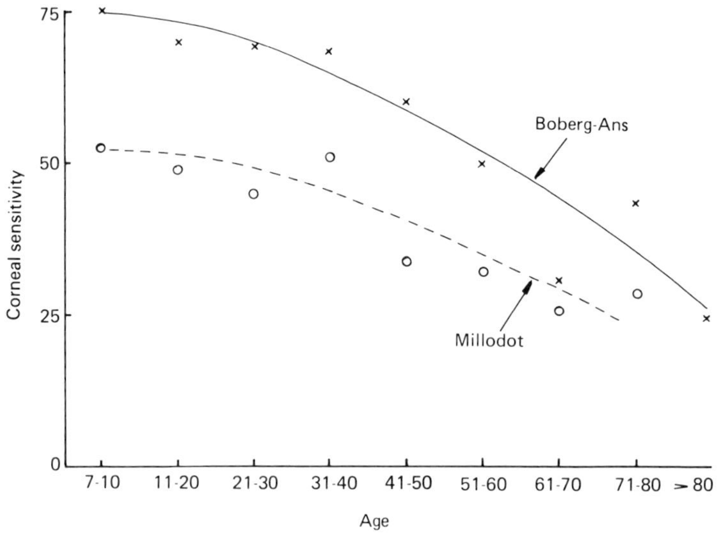

Figure 8.5 Corneal touch thresholds and age (reproduced by permission of Millodot, *Investigative Ophthalmology*, 1977[23])

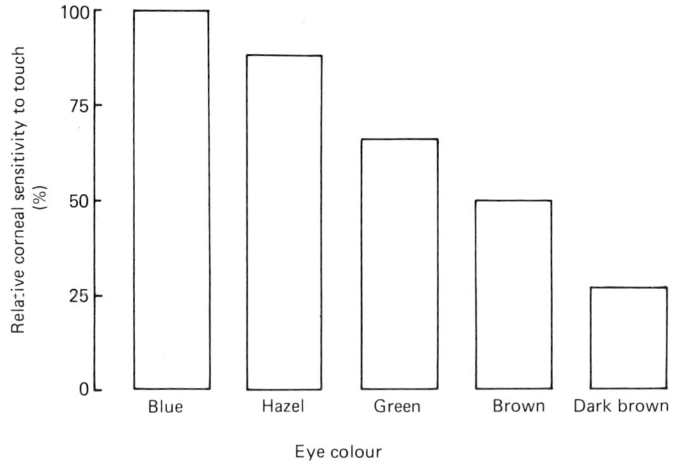

Figure 8.6 Corneal touch thresholds and iris pigmentation (reproduced by permission of Millodot, *Nature*, 1975[21])

subjects having blue, essentially unpigmented irides, being the most sensitive to touch while those with heavily pigmented brown irides exhibit the highest touch threshold (Figure 8.6).

Corneal temperature has also been shown to influence corneal sensation[12]. A change from an ambient temperature of 22°C to −14°C produces a nine-fold reduction in corneal sensation as measured by a Cochet-Bonnet aesthiometer. This dramatic loss of sensation has been proposed as the mechanism of improved contact lens comfort levels reported by Scandinavian cross-country skiers.

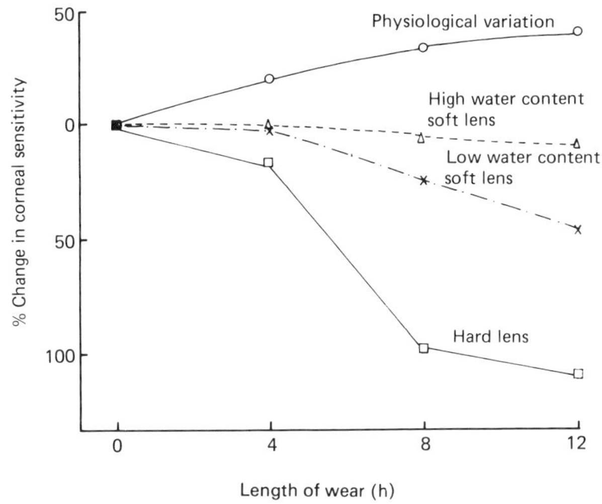

Figure 8.7 Comparative rates of sensory loss during 12 hours of different types of contact lens wear (prepared from data in Millodot, 1974, 1975, 1976, 1978[19,20,22,25] and Larke and Hirji, 1979[13])

Corneal touch thresholds and contact lens wear

It has long been known that the wearing of contact lenses reduces corneal touch sensation[3,5,9,31]. Boberg-Ans in his early thesis on corneal sensation[2], observed corneal touch sensation to be reduced by short periods of contact lens wear, and further observed the extent of sensory loss to be influenced by the fit of the contact lens. Michel Millodot in his definitive studies of corneal sensation in contact lens wear has carefully documented the degree of sensory loss provoked by differing periods and differing types of lens wear, and has monitored the rate of recovery when lens wear is discontinued[19,20,22,24,25].

The greatest degree of sensory loss to date reported is among wearers of hard contact lenses where a single 12-hour period of wear results in a two-fold increase in the touch threshold. The extent of loss among wearers of low water content soft lenses is less, with a single day's wear resulting in a 50% increase in the touch threshold. Among wearers of high water content extended wear lenses, a barely detectable 10% increase in touch thresholds has been observed[13]. A graph illustrating comparative rates of sensory loss during 12 hours of differing types of lens wear is shown in Figure 8.7.

Although the extent of sensory loss is considerable among wearers of hard lenses, recovery is rapid, often being substantially complete after one hour of non-lens wear. Following a period of sleep, the touch threshold is invariably restored to pre-fitting levels. However, the restoration of normal corneal sensory levels occurs only in the first few years of lens wear. After approximately 5–7 years, sensory loss becomes cumulative with time and progressively decreases over, at least, the next 2 decades. This cumulative rate of loss has been shown to be linear if a log of corneal sensitivity is plotted against years of wear[24], (Figure 8.8). At the time of writing it is not known if a similar cumulative loss is occurring in long-term soft lens wearers. Among wearers of extended wear contact lenses, sensory loss is cumulative, although at a

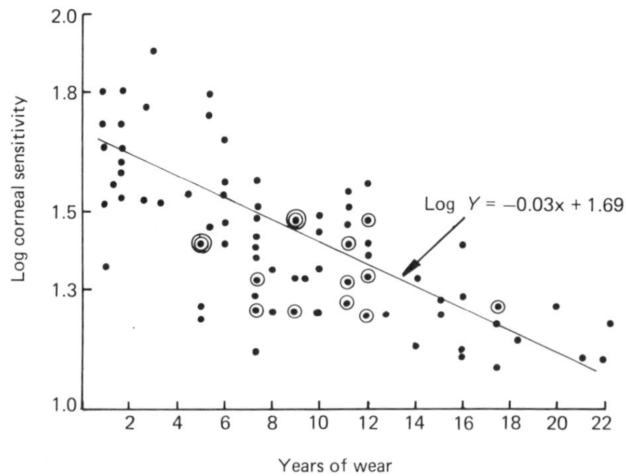

Figure 8.8 Cumulative rate of sensory loss in long-term hard lens wearers (reproduced by permission of Millodot, *Contacto*, 1978[24])

very slow rate, at least in the short term. The extent of sensory loss after 12 weeks of extended wear is approximately equal to one day's wear of a hard lens[10].

Rate of recovery of sensory loss

The rate of recovery of sensory loss following the cessation of lens wear depends upon the extent of loss resulting from lens wear which, in turn, depends upon the nature and duration of wear. Although an hour's non-lens wear may be sufficient to restore sensation following a single day's wear of a hard lens during initial wearing periods, considerably longer is required after many years of contact lens wear. After 16–20 years of hard lens wear, 4 or 5 months of non-lens wear may pass before the restoration of a normal level of corneal sensation. This observation has clinical implications. In the early years of hard lens wear sensation is rapidly restored upon lens removal. Hence, although the patient may be at some risk from unfelt foreign bodies trapped between the contact lens and the cornea, their presence will usually become apparent shortly after ceasing lens wear. In a long-term hard lens wearer this will not be the case and it may be wise to fit such patients with thin gas permeable lenses in an attempt to restore some level of corneal sensation.

Mechanisms of corneal sensory loss

The underlying mechanism of sensory loss provoked by contact lens wear is not known at the time of writing. As the topographic distribution of corneal touch threshold is similar to the relative corneal distribution of acetylcholine[30], it is tempting to speculate on a causal relationship between corneal touch thresholds and acetylcholine concentrations. However, there are a number of reasons against so doing. The majority of the acetylcholine present in the cornea is located in the intracellular spaces where its presence would not appear to be associated with neural transmission[11]. Until recently, no classical acetylcholine receptors (muscarinic or nicotinic) could be found in the epithelium using specific radioactive ligand binding techniques[30]. Hence, the role of much corneal epithelium acetylcholine is not understood, although it would not appear to be associated with its classical function as a neurotransmitter. However, it has been observed that the concentration of corneal epithelial choline acetyltransferase, the enzyme responsible for the synthesis of acetylcholine, is suppressed by prolonged lid closure[16], as is corneal sensation. In addition, careful corneal sensory denervation by radiofrequency thermocoagulation of the appropriate ganglia, has been shown significantly to decrease wound healing ability, epithelial permeability and cell proliferation, suggesting a trophic function for the ciliary nerves in the maintenance of epithelial properties[1].

Although the initial experiments concerned with sensory loss and short-term anoxia were unproductive[33], when the period of anoxia was extended to beyond 4–5 hours, sensory loss occurred in a manner reminiscent of hard contact lens wear[28]. The possibility of sensory loss as a direct effect of depressed oxygen levels would seem a rational speculation. The efficiency of neural transmission is known to be decreased by reduced oxygen environments, probably as a direct result of low cellular energy states adversely affecting transport function. However, in contact lens wear, the lens is an ever present mechanical stimulus and some traumatic effects are also possible. A correlation between epithelial fragility and corneal touch thresholds has been demonstrated[29] and the corneas of contact lens wearers may be more prone to damage than normal. The length of recovery of sensory loss in long-term hard lens wearers suggests some neural damage may occur after the first few years of wear which may take some months to recover when lens wear terminates.

References

1 Beuerman, R. W. and Schimmelpfenning, B. (1980). *Experimental Neurology*, **69**, 196
2 Boberg-Ans, J. (1952). Thesis. *Om Corneasensibilitete Med Soerlig Henblik Pa Kliniske Under-Sogelsesmetoder*. Copenhagen, Denmark
3 Boberg-Ans, J. (1955). *British Journal of Ophthalmology*, **39**, 705
4 Cited by Boberg-Ans, J. (1955). *British Journal of Ophthalmology*, **39**, 705
5 Byron, H. and Wesley, A. (1961). *American Journal of Ophthalmology*. **51**, 675
6 Cochet, P. and Bonnet, R. (1960). *Clinical Ophthalmology*, **4**, 12
7 Draeger, J., Heid, W. and Luders, M. (1980). *Contactologia*, **2**, 83
8 Gotz, R. (1972). *Klinische Monatsblätter für Augenheilkunde*, **161**, 469
9 Hamamo, H. (1960). *Contacto*, **4**, 41
10 Hirji, N. K. (1978). *Doctoral Thesis*. University of Aston in Birmingham
11 Howard, R. O., Wilson, W. S. and Dunn, B. J. (1973). *Investigative Ophthalmology*, **12**, 418
12 Kolstrad, A. (1970). *Acta Ophthalmologica*, **48**, 789
13 Larke, J. R. and Hirji, N. K. (1979). *British Journal of Ophthalmology*, **63**, 475
14 Larson, W. L. (1970). *British journal of Ophthalmology*, **54**, 342
15 Mindel, J. S. and Mittag, T. W. (1977). *Experimental Eye Research*, **24**, 25
16 Mindel, J. S. and Mittag, T. W. (1978). *Experimental Eye Research*, **27**, 359
17 Millodot, M. (1972). *British Journal of Ophthalmology*, **56**, 844
18 Millodot, M. (1973). *Acta Ophthalmologica*, **51**, 325
19 Millodot, M. (1974). *Acta Ophthalmologica*, **52**, 603
20 Millodot, M. (1975). *Acta Ophthalmologica*, **53**, 5736
21 Millodot, M. (1975). *Nature*, **255**, 151
22 Millodot, M. (1976). *Acta Ophthalmologica*, **54**, 721
23 Millodot, M. (1977). *Investigative Ophthalmology*, **16**, 240
24 Millodot, M. (1978). *Contacto*, **22**, 7
25 Millodot, M. (1978) *Acta Ophthalmologica*, **56**, 1225

26 Millodot, M. and Lamont, A. (1974). *British Journal of Ophthalmology*, **58**, 752
27 Millodot, M. and Larson, W. (1969). *American Journal of Optometry*, **46**, 261
28 Millodot, M. and O'Leary, D. J. (1980). *Acta Ophthalmologica*, **58**, 434
29 Millodot, M. and O'Leary, D. J. (1980). *Acta Ophthalmologica*, **59**, 820
30 Mittag, I. W. and Mindel, J. S. (1980). *Proceedings of the International Societies for Eye Research*, **1**, 80
31 Morganroth, J. and Richman, L. (1969). *Journal of Pediatric Ophthalmology*, **6**, 207
32 Perl, E. R. (1971). *Journal of Psychiatry*, **8**, 273
33 Polse, K. A. (1978). *Investigative Ophthalmology*, **17**, 1202

Chapter 9

Corneal swelling and its clinical sequelae

Introduction

Contact lens wear invariably reduces the oxygen tension at the corneal surface, and as a result the cornea swells. The amount of anoxia-induced stromal swelling can be wholly accounted for by changes in stromal lactate concentration.

However, a lowered oxygen tension is not the only stimulus to provoke swelling, which may also be induced by changes in the oscularity of the tear film. The degree and extent of swelling depend upon the material and design of lens used. A hard lens will provoke swelling in that area of the cornea which is always covered by the contact lens, while a soft lens which covers the entire cornea, will induce swelling throughout the tissue. A consequence of the different extent of swelling is a difference in induced changes in the refractive state and topography of the cornea. In hard lens wear, where the swelling is localized, the centre of the cornea will become 'steeper' with respect to the periphery. The even swelling characteristics of soft lens wear will have little detectable effect on corneal topography or power.

The swelling provoked by contact lens wear is not constant. The initial phase of contact lens wear is almost always accompanied by excess lacrimation and as more normal tear flows are achieved, swelling attributable to tear osmolarity changes subsides. In the slightly longer term, anoxic swelling provoked in the first few weeks and months of lens wear may also partially subside, although the reasons for this are currently unknown.

Although much of the swelling associated with the early period of lens wear may decline, induced changes in corneal topography and refractive state do not. The reasons for this are unknown, but it may be that the oedematous cornea is more easily deformed by the presence of a contact lens which, during blinking, may be exerting considerable intermittent forces on the surface of the eye. A long-term consequence is a loss of regularity in the corneal surface which leads to a loss of resolving power and visual function. These changes can be quite marked and, if allowed to persist over many years, may become irreversible in a small proportion of badly affected patients.

Although corneal swelling and its clinical sequelae have been an invariable feature of hard lens wear, there is now no clinical reason why they should be accepted.

The development of thin, soft and gas permeable lenses enables practitioners to avoid provoking corneal swelling, although the use of both of these differing types of lenses may provoke other types of adverse response in the contact lens wearing eye.

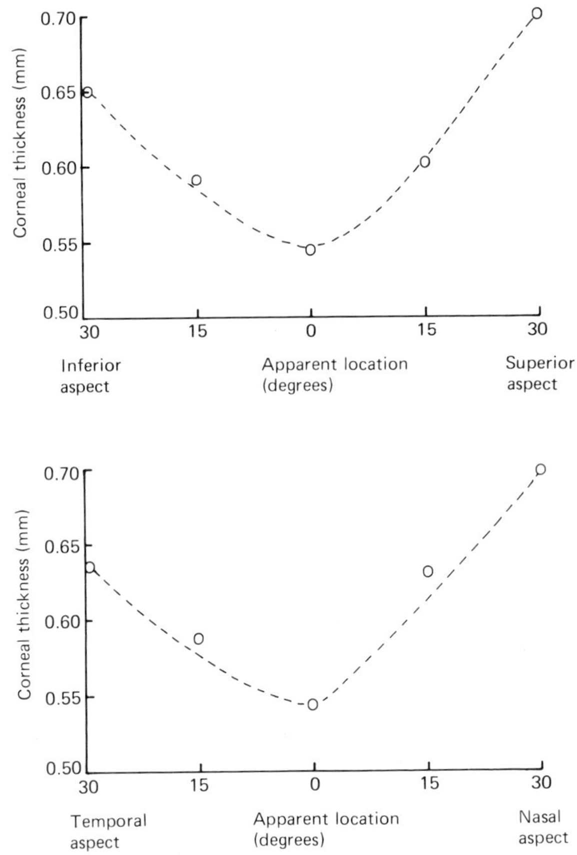

Figure 9.1 Cross-sectional thickness of the human cornea (from Larke and Hirji, *The Optician*, 1976)

The thickness of the cornea

The cornea is not uniformly thick, being thinnest at the centre and thickest in the periphery. Differing peripheral regions are also of varying dimensions. The cross-sectional form of the horizontal and vertical meridians are shown in Figure 9.1.

The cornea changes in thickness throughout the day. Initially when the eyes are opened, following sleep, a rapid thinning of approximately 4% takes place. This reduction in thickness is thought to be an osmotic stromal response to the change in tear toxicity levels brought about by evaporation of the tears after lid opening[31]. After this initial rapid thinning of the cornea, further but slower decreases have been observed, although the mechanism responsible for these changes is currently unknown[29]. Waking hours changes in corneal thickness are shown in Figure 9.2.

The relative thickness of the cornea may be measured with conventional pachometry. A number of expensive self-recording pachometers are commercially available. Satisfactory self-assembled instruments can be constructed from readily available components. The addition of a potentiometer above the upper plate of a

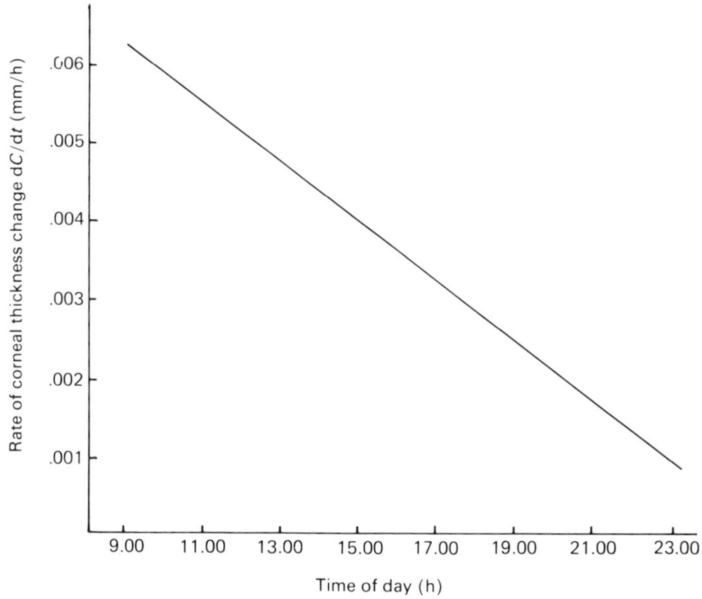

Figure 9.2 Change in corneal thickness during waking hours, expressed as dC/dt mm/h where C = corneal thickness and t = time (redrawn from Hirji and Larke, *American Journal of Optometry*, 1978[17])

Haag Streit pachometer enables a displacement dependent signal to be generated, while a mechanical device to move the rotatable prism will aid precision. A suitable arrangement which may be input into a microcomputer is shown in Plate 33.

The precision of pachometry is dependent upon the experience of the operator. A naive user will have difficulty in taking measurements to within ±10%, while experienced personnel may measure to less than ±2%[18]. The addition of 2% sodium fluorescein into the tear film will often aid measurement, particularly for the inexperienced users[10].

Micropachometry

While conventional pachometers are capable of measuring the thickness of the whole cornea to a precision of ±2%, micropachometry can achieve a precision of ± 5 μm, and can measure the thickness of the corneal epithelium and, by subtraction, the thickness of the stroma. The development of micropachometry is attributable to Dan O'Leary who described the first successful micropachometer in his doctoral thesis (Figure 9.3). In principle, a micropachometer is a high resolution conventional pachometer with a more intense light source and sophisticated optics on the illumination side and a high resolution monocular viewing system. Utilizing his micropachometer O'Leary successfully measured the thickness of human corneal epithelium *in vivo* and demonstrated that it was subject to oedema in anoxia. Indeed the thickness of the epithelium thins 2–3 μm when transferred from an ambient oxygen environment to anoxia.

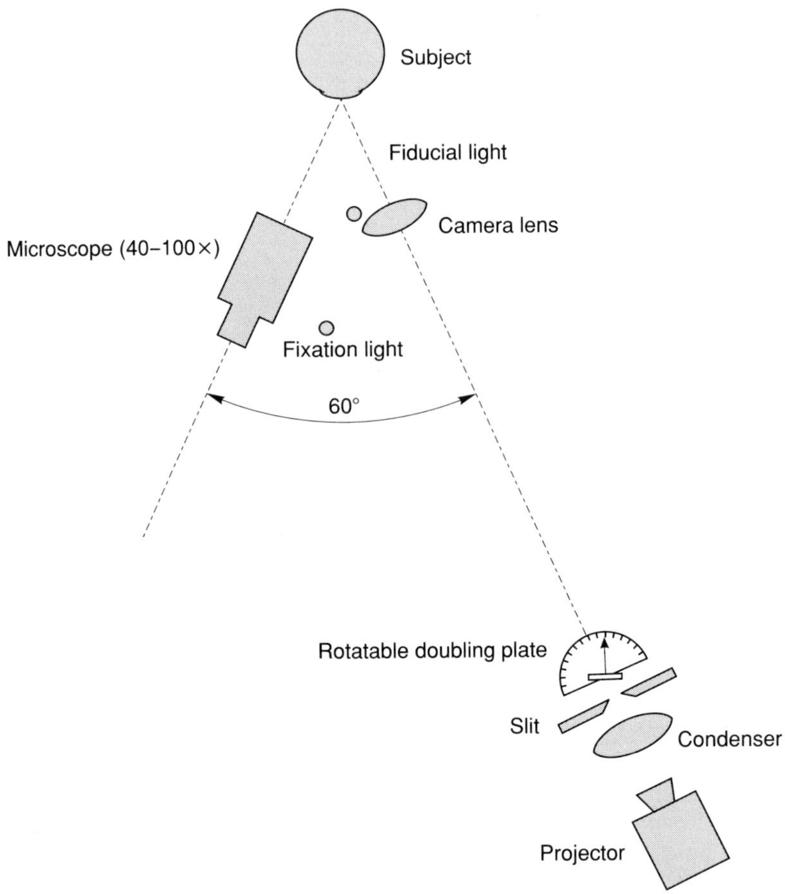

Figure 9.3 A schemia of the first micropachometer designed and constructed by Dan O'Leary (Doctoral thesis, 1974, University of Wales, Cardiff)

Corneal swelling provoked by contact lens wear

Corneal swelling in contact lens wear may be provoked by:

1 Changes in tear osmolarity (see Chapter 3)
2 Changes in corneal oxygen tension.

It has been held for some time among contact lens practitioners that the reason the cornea swells in contact lens wear is because the reduced oxygen tension provoked by contact lens wear gives rise to raised structural lactate levels which results in raised stromal water content and hence stromal swelling.

In 1984, Klyce published a set of complex yet elegant serial equations which established a mathematical model of anoxic provoked stromal swelling. The model proposed a causal relationship for lactate in stromal swelling[25]. Klyce was further able to show that changes in lactate concentration could account for all of the

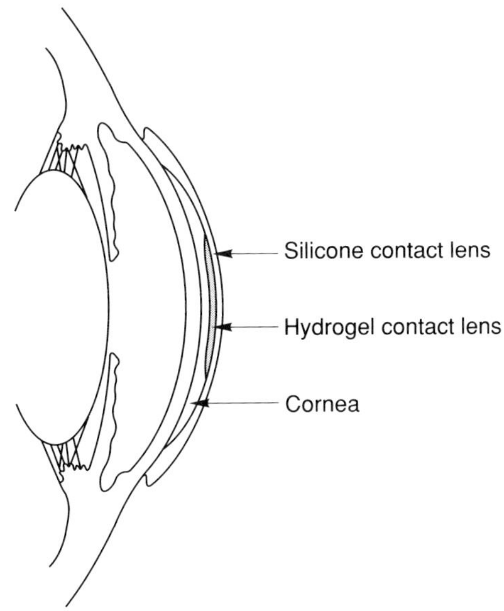

Figure 9.4 A method for the collection of corneal derived lactate

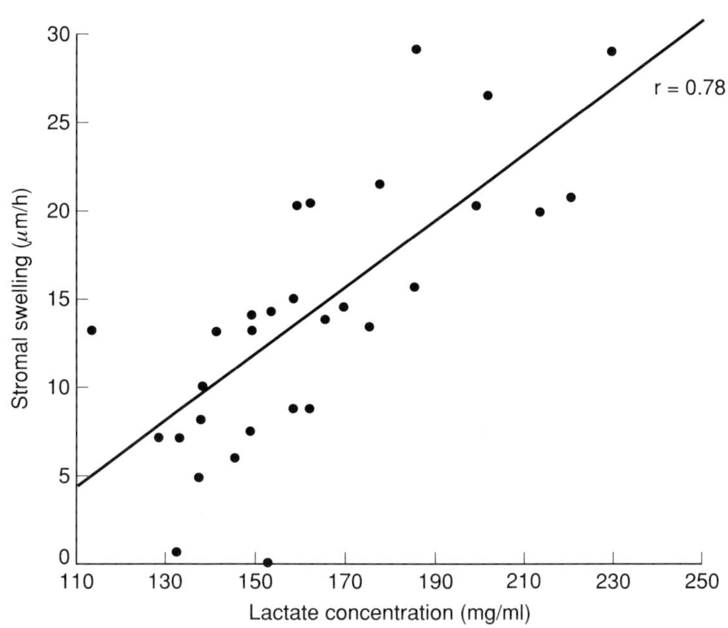

Figure 9.5 Stromal swelling collected corneal lactate

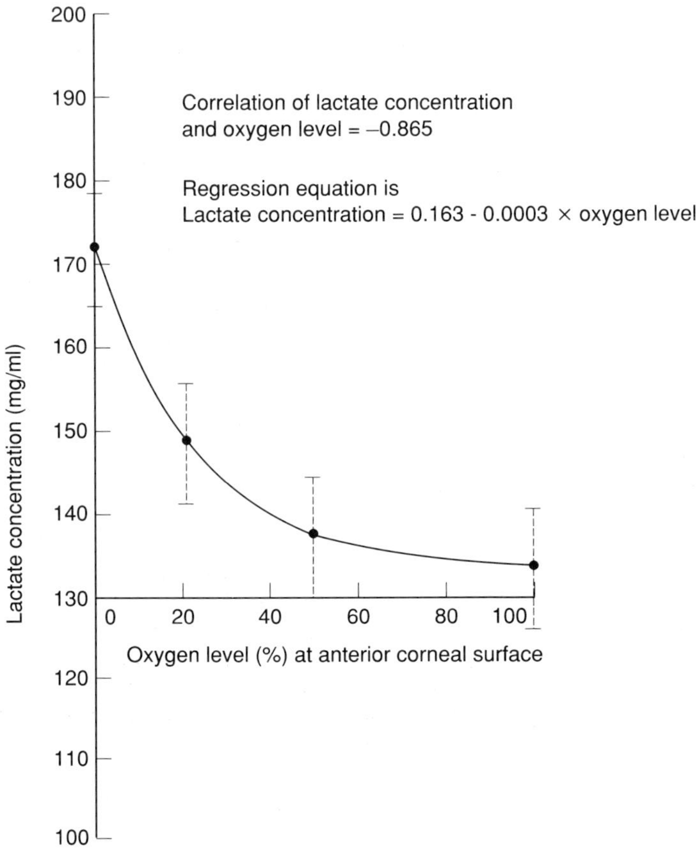

Figure 9.6 The relationship between corneal derived lactate and oxygen tension and the anterior corneal surface

changes in stromal thickness, that had been measured by various workers and that it was unnecessary to invoke the influence of a second variable to account for the phenomenon

Experimental evidence to support Klyce's model was provided by the author and Stella Briggs-Dokubo[6].

Our technique used a high water soft lens as a collecting medium, sealed against the surface of the cornea by a lactate intermediate silicone elastomer lens (Figure 9.4). The efficiency of the silicone membrane seal which excluded lactate derived from other ocular tissues was established with prolonged fluorescein irrigation, while the influence of cellular damage was examined in a series of traumatic experiments using the author's left cornea! This established the corneal origin of the collected lactate which had leaked between the cells of the tight epithelium of the cornea. It is of course true that this represents a small but constant fraction of all the lactate produced by the epithelium. The drainage route for the large majority of epithelial lactate is across the corneal stroma and into the aqueous humour.

The usefulness of this experimental approach was demonstrated when we examined the nature of the relationship between stromal swelling and collected lactate from 30 experimental subjects (Figure 9.5). It is readily apparent from Figure

9.5 that a correlation exists between stromal swelling and collected lactate. In addition, the correlation coefficient (0.78) indicated a particularly good agreement between these two sets of data (the precision of the stromal thickness measurement was ±1.4% while the precision of the lactate measurement was ±4.8%).

This experiment gives strong and convincing support to Klyce's mathematical model. Not only is stromal swelling directly related to collected lactate levels but the agreement is so good that it is unlikely that a further metabolic variable has a substantial effect on stromal swelling.

Having provided support for Klyce's model of stromal swelling we then looked at the relationship between corneal oxygen availability and collected lactate levels, in an attempt to describe the relationship and to answer such clinical questions as, 'how much oxygen does the cornea require in contact lens wear?' and 'what is the minimum oxygen tension necessary for satisfactory lens wear?'. These questions have been with us for some time!

The nature of the relationship between oxygen and lactate is illustrated in Figure 9.6.

It is apparent from inspection of Figure 9.6 that the relationship between stromal thickness and collected lactate is not linear. It is also apparent that there are no thresholds. The effect of decreasing oxygen environments is simply to provoke an ever increasing lactate level. The answer to the question, 'what is the minimum oxygen tension necessary for satisfactory contact lens wear?', is a clinical one; it is that level of oxygen, above which unacceptable clinical phenomena are not provoked. This level is somewhat arbitrary; all clinical judgements are, but 10–12 mmHg, (2–3% oxygen), a figure proposed for a long time, is probably as good a judgement as can be made. As to the question, 'how much oxygen does the cornea require in contact lens wear?', it is apparent that increasing oxygen levels produce a diminishing return in terms of reduced lactate levels. Certainly, above 100 mmHg (14% oxygen) very little reduction in lactate is gained by increasing oxygen availability.

It is also the author's view that the traditional approach to anoxia-provoked swelling is conceptually wrong. It is a better description to say that the cornea moves from one steady state thickness dependent upon one steady state lactate concentration, provoked by one particular oxygen tension. Swelling, although not necessarily deswelling, is simply the movement of the corneal stroma between two steady states.

Recently, the view of lactate as the principal determinant of anoxia-provoked change in corneal thickness has been challenged by various workers citing the work of McNamara *et al.*[28], who have provoked the cornea with differing mixtures of carbon dioxide, nitrogen and air. Interestingly, while the open-eye steady state thickness was not significantly affected by changes in CO_2 (at least up to 7%), the rate of return to air steady state thickness was reduced. The authors ascribed these observations to changes in stromal pH which they had measured independently, citing 'acidosis' (*sic*) provoked changes in the rate of lactate metabolism or 'altered endothelial hydraulic conductivity' as possible mechanisms. Certainly both are plausible, particularly endothelial mechanisms. The posterior endothelial surface is richly endowed with carbonic anhydrase which catalyses CO_2 to bicarbonate ion which is in turn utilized by the endothelium in the maintenance of corneal hydration via the bicarbonate dependent sodium ion pump. Why these observations and others should be held to influence the notion that anoxia-provoked changes in corneal thickness is a CO_2 dependent effect is not readily apparent to the author.

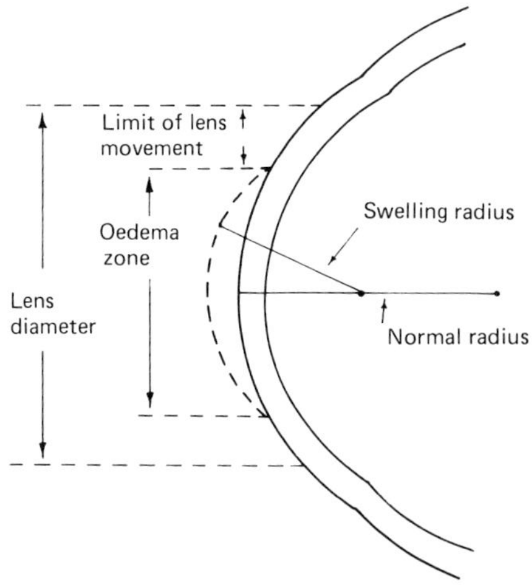

Figure 9.7 An illustration of corneal swelling provoked by hard lens wear

The manner in which corneal derived lactate influences corneal thickness can be summarized thus: when the oxygen tension of the anterior eye is altered this provokes a change in epithelial cellular lactate production rate. The principal drainage route for lactate is across the stroma via the endothelium into the aqueous humour. Lactate is a well dissociated acid, hence is principally present in the stroma as its sodium salt. The presence of stromal sodium lactate has an osmotic effect in a system which acts as a well nigh perfect osmometer (the epithelium is a 'perfect' semipermeable membrane). Hence, changes in lactate provoke osmotically-driven changes in stromal water content which in turn determine the thickness of the stroma (assuming endothelial homeostasis). The amount of stromal thickness changes observed in anoxia can be wholly accounted for theoretically by changes in lactate levels. The experimental correlation between corneal derived lactate levels and oxygen levels is remarkably good and is within the precision of the experimental techniques used.

Hard (PMMA) contact lens wear

Swelling in hard contact lens wear is confined to that region of the cornea which is always covered by the contact lens. Hence a lens 8.5 mm in diameter, which moves 1 mm in all directions on the cornea, will leave a central zone 6.5 mm in diameter in which stromal swelling will occur (Figure 9.7). The extent of swelling in this zone will depend upon the lens design and mode of fit.

The degree of corneal swelling provoked by hard contact lens wear has been characterized into three levels of response[32]: R1, R2 and R3 (Figure 9.8).

In response R1, a maximum stromal swelling of 2–4% is apparent during the first day of wear. After 2 weeks of wear the stroma no longer swells. R1-type patients may be considered to exhibit adequate levels of tear exchange and corneal oxygenation, and suffer only from changes in tear osmolarity.

Response R2 is characterized by a maximum swelling of 5–8% during the first day's wear, which decreases to a lower level after 2 weeks of wear. Such patients may have some problems in wearing their lenses but are usually able to continue with lens wear. Unfortunately, if a further problem is superimposed on the first, lens wear often becomes intolerable.

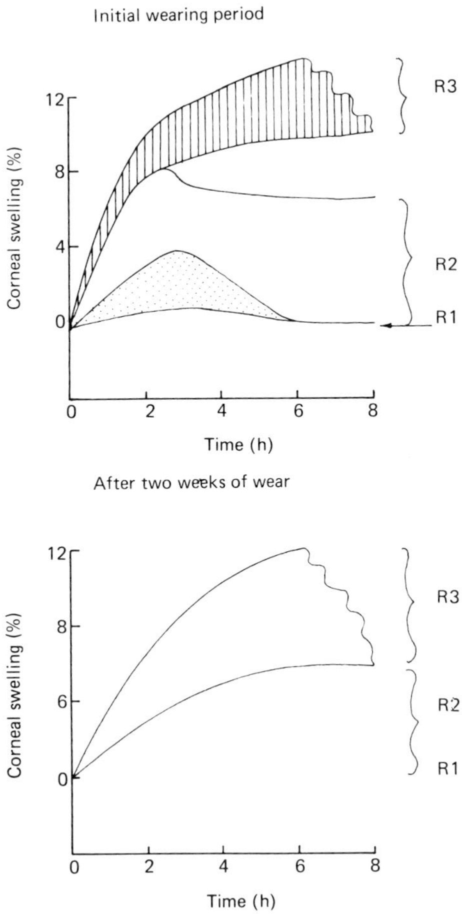

Figure 9.8 Categorized swelling response to hard lens wear (reproduced by permission of Mandell and Polse, *American Journal of Optometry*, 1969[32])

Patients exhibiting an R3-level of response to an initial day's lens wear have greater than 8% stromal swelling. Such patients are invariably unable to wear their lenses beyond 6 hours on the first day. Clearly corneal oxygenation is wholly inadequate and this level of response is usually provoked by a grossly tight fit.

If lens wear continues it may be possible slowly to 'adapt' such patients to their lenses, and after 2 weeks the extent of swelling may have declined. However, wearing times are invariably restricted and further problems are very common in this group of patients. Since there is always a risk of an overwear syndrome, patients should be advised against further lens wear.

The use of corneal swelling data and subsequent categorization into groups of responses is very appropriate to clinical hard lens practice. The careful measurement of corneal thickness at aftercare, 2 weeks after lens supply, will indicate those patients who are likely to be predisposed towards difficulties and who require refitting.

Soft contact lens wear

Unlike hard lenses, soft lenses cover the entire cornea and provoke swelling

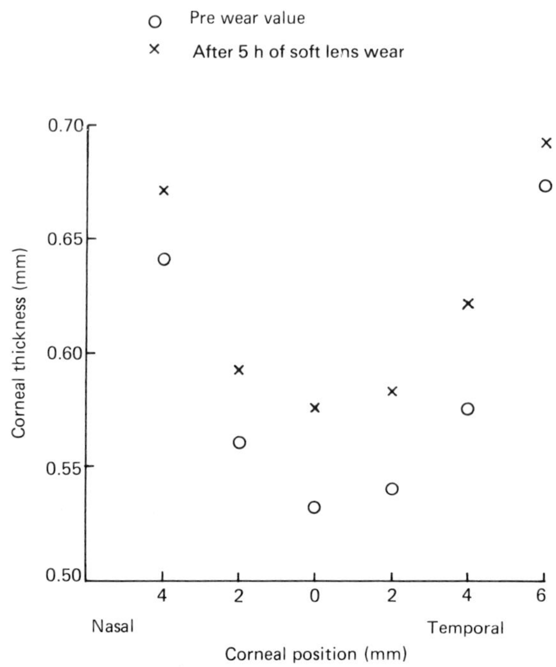

Figure 9.9 Corneal swelling provoked by 5 hours of soft lens wear (reproduced by pemission of Mandell, *Contacto*, 1976[29])

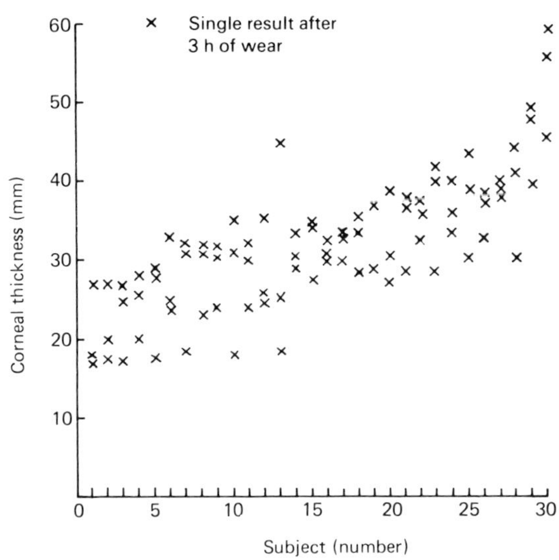

Figure 9.10 Corneal swelling response of 30 subjects to an identical experimental lens work on three separate occasions (reproduced by permission of Sarver, Polse and Baggett, *American Journal of Optometry*, 1983[43])

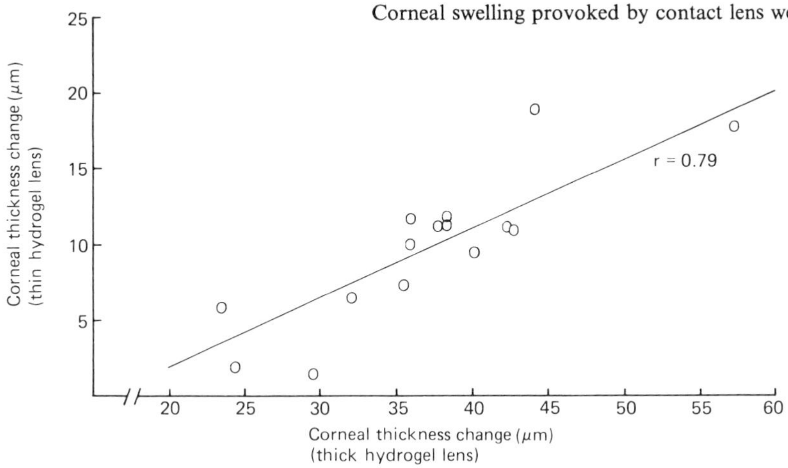

Figure 9.11 Correlation in corneal swelling response between wearing thick (0.4 mm) and thin (0.07 mm) HEMA lenses (reproduced by permission of Sarver, Polse and Bagget, *American Journal of Optometry*, 1983[43])

throughout the tissue[29] (Figure 9.9). This regularity of oedema may make detection difficult. The characteristic central epithelial haze so often observed by retro-illumination in hard lens wearers is usually absent in soft lens wear. Micropachometry remains the technique of choice in monitoring soft lens patients.

The extent of swelling occurring in soft lens wear is a function of the gaseous transmission characteristics of the lens material. Hence, lens thickness and water content are important criteria in soft lens wear. Even among aphakic patients, where there is evidence for a reduced swelling response to anoxia[19], low water content lenses provoke more corneal swelling than lenses of high water content[36].

In addition to lens characteristics, patient response also varies considerably. This arises from a high intra-subject variability to hypoxia which appears to be inversely related to corneal thickness[43]. The response of 30 consecutive patients to the same experimental lens worn on three separate occasions is shown in Figure 9.10.

Given this large variability among individuals in their swelling response to hypoxia and hence contact lens wear, it is difficult to give meaningful data on patients' response to differing lens types. However, some generalizations can be made:

1 As would be expected, thick hydrogen lenses provoke more stromal swelling than thin lenses (Figure 9.11)
2 The extent of swelling (whether induced by thick or thin lenses) declines with time[8,21] (Figures 9.12 and 9.13)
3 The extent of swelling rarely exceeds the maximum amount that can be provoked by anoxia alone (8%). In cases where this is not the case, the posterior stroma shows evidence of gross change in the form of 'striae' and folds in Descemet's layers
4 The use of thin (0.1 mm lenses) provokes, on average, less than 1% stromal swelling.

The clinical usefulness of pachometric data in monitoring soft lens wearers is limited. The widespread usage of thin soft lenses largely avoids the problems of stromal swelling, and it is only when unusually thick soft lenses are used that swelling data again become important.

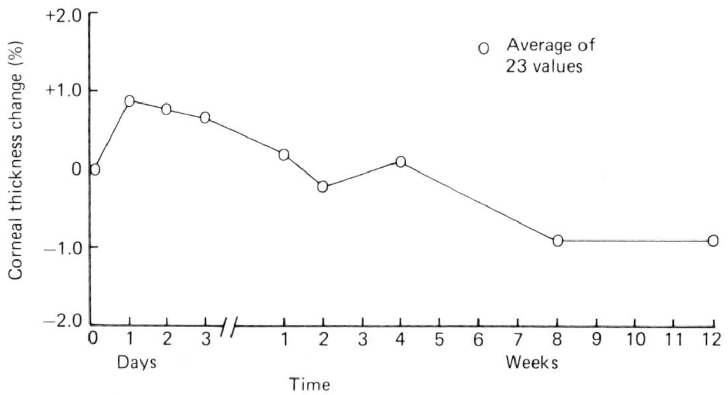

Figure 9.12 Corneal thickness with time for 23 eyes wearing a HEMA lens of 0.07 mm centre thickness (reproduced by permission of Callender, *Canadian Journal of Optometry*, 1979[8])

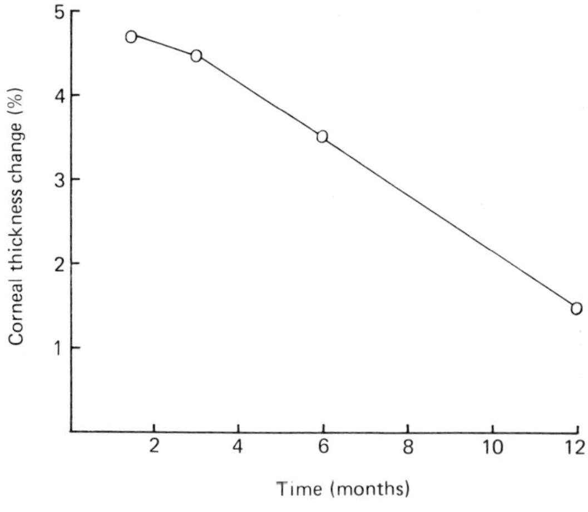

Figure 9.13 Corneal thickness with time for 35 subjects wearing HEMA lenses of average centre thickness of 0.1 mm (based on data in Høvding, *Acta Ophthalmologica*, 1982[21])

Although pachometric readings are of limited value in day wear soft lenses, stromal swelling is of much greater significance in extended soft lens wear, where increased levels of corneal thickness can be anticipated during periods of sleep.

The response to initial periods of extended lens wear shows the cornea to swell by 10–15% during eyelid closure in patients who, prior to lens wear, averaged no more than 3–4% overnight swelling[20] (Figure 9.14). However, as with day wear of soft lenses the degree of provoked swelling declines with time[44] (Figure 9.15). If hydrogel water content is increased to the maximum that is currently commercially available and soft lens thickness very carefully controlled, it is possible to provide lens wear that, during the day at least, will give rise to 'normal' corneal thickness. There is also some evidence to suggest that after many weeks of lens wear, the pattern of day time

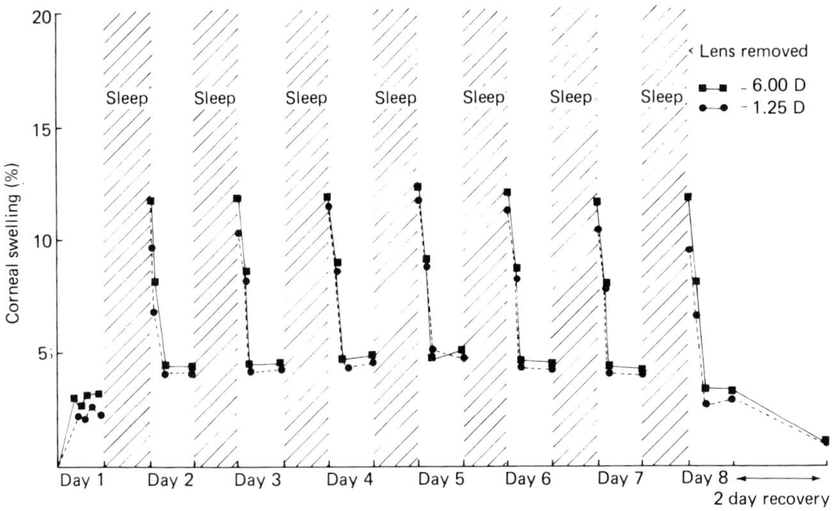

Figure 9.14 Corneal swelling with time for 5 unadapted patients wearing a high water content soft lens for one week (reproduced by permission of Holden, Mertz and McNally, *Investigative Ophthalmology*, 1983[20])

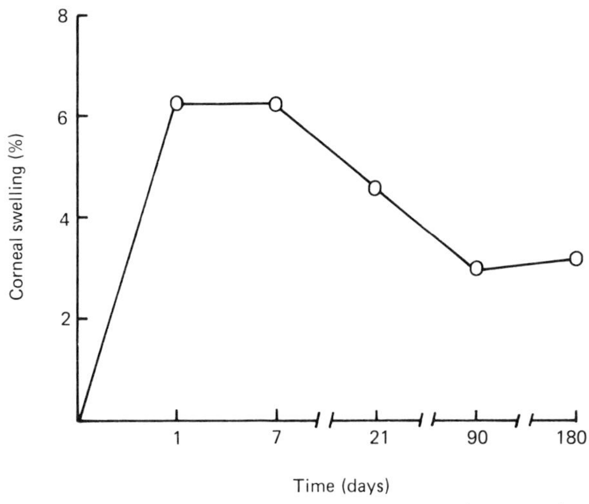

Figure 9.15 Corneal swelling with time for 38 patients wearing a high water content soft lens continuously for 180 days (reproduced by permission of Sorenson and Corydon, *Contacto*, 1979[44])

thinning of the cornea is also reduced, possibly as a result of 'adaptation' to contact lens wear[18].

Gas permeable lens wear

Conventional thickness (0.12 mm)

The advent of gas permeable lenses with Dk values in excess of 30 has resulted in levels of central corneal swelling that cannot be detected with conventional pachometry. As Dk is increased to 90–100 it becomes difficult to detect the increased thickness with micropachometry. So far as conventional thickness is concerned, the problem of oxygen availability and, hence induced increases in stromal thickness, has essentially been solved, at least for day wear gas permeable lenses. The pursuit of materials with Dk values in excess of 90–100 is illusionary. There is no detectable clinical gain in such material and since other polymer properties (dimensional stability, wettability, etc.) may have to be sacrificed to achieve such high Dk values, the clinical desirability of such materials may be less than those with lower Dk values. At the time of writing (September 1994) research expenditure and effort is still being made in the pursuit of ever high Dks. In this author's view this effort and expenditure is being wasted. The 'Dk problem' is solved for gas permeable lenses and there are other areas of polymer materials research which require attention and which will give real clinical benefit to practitioners and patients alike.

Clinical sequelae

Corneal shape change

The causal relationship between corneal swelling and corneal shape change would appear to be unknown. Clearly in hard lens wear, central swelling of the cornea will cause a steepening of this region with respect to the rest of the unaffected cornea. However, corneal shape change is usually a long-term phenomenon often being at its greatest after much early corneal swelling has partially subsided. Probably, the forces of the lid acting through a contact lens play a role, as may longer-term changes in a chronically hypoxic cornea.

Detecting changes in corneal topography requires a suitable measurement system. The majority of keratometers have mire image sizes of 2–4 mm and thus provide an average measurement over a considerable corneal area. Small mire instruments having image sizes of 0.2–0.3 mm are more suitable for precise topographic measurement but are extremely laborious in use. Photokeratoscopes, on the other hand, are very rapid but only suitable for detecting gross corneal distortion. Perhaps the most satisfactory solution to the problem of detecting changes in the shape of the cornea would be the use of small mire keratometers in conjunction with photokeratoscopes. However, the author is not aware of any work carried out in this way.

The majority of reported studies have used large mire keratometers and their value is limited for this reason. However, a number of observations have been made which are valid at least in qualitative terms. Initially, there is little doubt that the central cornea steepens in hard lens wear by 0.1–0.3 mm[7,9,16,41]. This steepening is most apparent towards the end of a wearing period and is considerably in excess of any circadian changes that may be anticipated[27]. During periods of sleep, after hard contact lens wear, the cornea flattens, although generally speaking base line curvature is not achieved before the next period of lens wear[39].

Over the first year of hard lens wear the induced corneal steepening gradually decreases and the cornea may eventually become flatter than its refitting value. In addition to the notion that the cornea 'steepens' and 'flattens' in hard contact lens wear, it is apparent that curvature changes are more apparent in the horizontal than

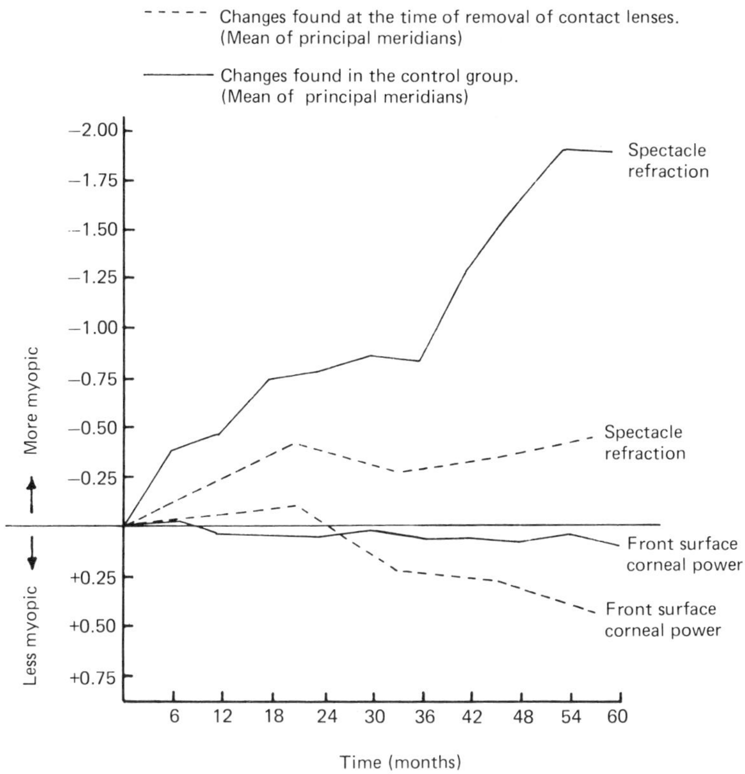

Figure 9.16 Progression of myopia in spectacle and contact lens wearers monitored over a period of 5 years (reproduced by permission of Janet Stone, *British Journal of Physiological Optics*, 1976[45])

in the vertical meridian[40]. These changes frequently present as induced irregular astigmatism[22]. The term 'corneal warpage' has been used to describe this effect[12].

In addition to gross changes in corneal topography, hard lenses have been observed to induce fine irregularities in surface contour[26]. Such irregularities can best be described as corneal corrugation with adjacent corneal zones alternately steepening and flattening. The corrugation is not static with time but moves rather in the manner of fine undulations on a sandy beach. The effect of this loss of surface regularity is to reduce corneal resolving power even in the absence of gross corneal change.

The effect of soft lens wear on corneal topography is far less marked than hard lenses. A slight corneal flattening may be observed in the first 2 or 3 weeks of lens wear, followed by a period of relative steepening[1]. However, the changes are of a very low order and do not seem adversely to affect visual function.

Refractive state

Changes in refractive state in hard lens wear are very common. The extent of refractive error can frequently exceed ± 0.50 D and there is frequently an increase in

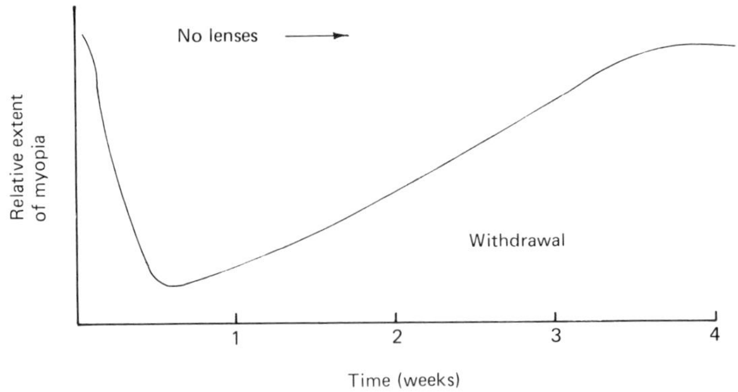

Figure 9.17 The nature of refractive change upon cessation of contact lens wear in long-term wearers (reproduced by permission of Rengstorff, *International Ophthalmology Clinic*, 1980[42])

astigmatism. The fit and design of hard lenses influences the degree of response. Generally, poorly fitted large lenses (9 mm diameter) will provoke more change than well fitted smaller lenses. The duration of the power change increases with both the period of wear and the extent of the change. Changes in refractive state, which will subside during a single period of sleep during initial periods of lens wear, may persist for days or even weeks after some years of lens wear. In rare instances, changes in refractive state may be essentially irreversible[39] and these cases correspond to permanently disturbed corneas (see preceding section). However, in general terms, the correlation between changes in corneal topography and refractive state is not particularly good. One possible reason has already been referred to in the discussion of a satisfactory measurement system for corneal topography.

The advent of gas permeable lenses with satisfactory Dk values has resolved the problem of the clinical sequelae to corneal swelling in hard lens wear, and the author is not aware of reported case histories of problems arising in gas permeable lenses wear. For this reason, if for no other, the continued fitting of hard (PMMA) lenses by a small minority of practitioners has become indefinable and ethically unsustainable.

The observation of changes in refractive state has led a minority of contact lens practitioners to propose utilizing this unwanted effect deliberately to alter refraction, and the doubtful practice of orthokeratology has developed.

The published literature on orthokeratology runs to many dozens of papers. Unfortunately the majority are of little value as the experimental work described is so poorly designed and executed. Indeed, many consist of little more than anecdotal information used to support a previously held viewpoint. Some of the proponents of orthokeratology apparently claim that the extent of refractive change may be predicted from the mode of contact lens fit[35,46]. However, it would seem common practice successively to refit the lens as refractive state alters and some regimens include the use of lenses worn through periods of sleep. The conclusion that most 'orthokeratologists' work on a trial-and-error basis seems inescapable.

The success of orthokeratology is difficult to assess[24], and is clearly a contentious issue. The extent of refractive change is variable, although many articles indicate a marked trend towards the development of increased amounts of astigmatism. A definitive study by Brand *et al.*[5] at the University of Birmingham has clearly demonstrated the unsatisfactory nature of orthokeratology and demolished its claimed theoretical basis.

A more appropriate use of contact lens induced refractive change has been the attempt by a number of practitioners to arrest the progression of myopia, particularly in the young. Of the many studies reported in the literature[2,3,4,9,11,23,34,35], that carried out by Janet Stone[45] of the Institute of Optometry (formerly The London Refraction Hospital) stands out both in terms of its duration and meticulous nature. In a controlled group comparative study, the progression of myopia in spectacle and contact lens wearers was followed in a study which took a decade to complete. The collected data were carefully analysed with appropriate statistical techniques and the essential tenet of the virtual arrest of myopia among contact lens wearers has been established (Figure 9.17).

The study also stands out in contrast to much of the clinical literature as a cautiously interpreted piece of work based on a sound experimental basis.

The use of contact lenses for myopia arrest in the young presents a number of problems for practitioners. It may be considered wise that only those patients showing accelerated rates of refractive change are fitted, as very prolonged periods of lens wear are being contemplated. It is particularly important that corneal health is carefully monitored. In addition to normal after-care procedures, such features as endothelial cell density and appearance should be considered. An essential feature of contact lens wear in young children is that the eye should remain as nearly 'normal' in its development as would otherwise be the case with non-lens wear. This is difficult to achieve and is demanding, particularly in terms of time. However, the benefit to the patient is often considerable, and this area can be one of the most worthwhile forms of contact lens practice.

Visual function

It is not unusual for contact lens patients to experience a reduction in their visual performance, particularly following the removal of their contact lenses and their return to spectacle lens wearing. This is in part attributable to changes in corneal topography induced by the contact lens. However, just as there is no strong correlation between corneal topography and refractive cornea changes, visual acuity losses cannot always be shown to be related to keratometric changes. Where regular changes in corneal topography occur, appropriate over-refraction will result in good spectacle acuity. However, where small-scale surface irregularities are found, the best obtainable visual acuity with spectacles will be less than that possible before contact lens wear – this is true spectacle blur.

As well as causing corneal shape changes, the wearing of contact lenses can cause corneal swelling. Indeed, this corneal swelling can be partly responsible for the corneal shape changes when it is unevenly distributed across the cornea. Such corneal swelling can result in transparency losses and so affect visual function. Although visual acuity is not usually affected by mild corneal swelling, the use of more sensitive measures of visual function can demonstrate reduced visual performance. For example, glare sensitivity can be shown to be changed[34]. Perhaps more importantly, changes in contrast sensitivity can be detected. The clinical assessment of vision is routinely carried out by the assessment of the limit of resolution, or visual acuity. This provides no information on how well the patient sees objects within the resolution limit. Such an assessment is provided by the contrast threshold function, which relates threshold visibility to object size. Such measurements can be used to confirm the subjective observation that vision is reduced even when letter acuity is normal. Thus, when corneal swelling occurs without corneal distortion, there is an elevation of threshold visibility at all spatial frequencies[15]. Although the change at high spatial frequencies may be small and not detectable by normal clinical assessment of vision, the fact that there is a loss at low spatial frequencies as well is of significance. Attenuation of low spatial frequencies has a marked influence on visual performance and routine assessment of visual acuity loss may not in these cases be a reliable guide to the patient's disability. Indeed, this confirms the frequent clinical observation that such patients experience reduced visual performance despite normal visual acuity.

Corneal distortion, on the other hand, produces a different type of visual response. When corneal distortion occurs without corneal swelling, there is an elevation of threshold visibility mainly at the high and medium spatial frequencies[14]. In this instance, the loss of visual performance is very similar to that caused by dioptric defocus, and can be more reliably assessed by routine letter acuity assessment than in the case of corneal swelling.

Consequently, the nature of any corneal changes following contact lens wear will influence the visual function resulting on removal of the lenses. Patient complaints of poor visual function despite the finding of normal visual acuity can perhaps be better understood from these findings.

Corneal recovery from contact lens wear

Few contact lens problems are more irritating than the provision of spectacles for a patient who has been wearing hard (PMMA) contact lenses for some time. The reasons for this have been discussed in the preceding sections. The cornea of a long-term hard lens wearer is different in shape and refractive state than prior to wear. When contact lenses are removed, recovery takes place at a rate which varies considerably between different individuals.

The general effect of the removal of hard lenses is to induce a transient decrease in the state of myopia[38] and an increase of astigmatism[13]. The extent of these changes can be dramatic; refractive changes of as much as 7.50 D in myopia and 6.0 D in astigmatism have on occasion been observed. Perhaps the rigidity of the cornea is adversely affected by the prolonged hypoxia and the mechanical stress of contact lens wearer[42]. The contact lens may become a partial support for the softened corneal tissue which, upon removal of this restraint, becomes abnormally deformed. Whatever the reasons, the changes in refractive state are short lived and normally after 3–4 weeks the cornea has returned to its lens wearing values (Figure 9.17).

The provision of spectacles for established contact lens wearers is dependent upon the needs of the patient.

Supplementary wear

The spectacle prescription for the patient who requires reasonable vision after contact lens removal in the evening should be measured immediately after 8 hours of lens wear[42]. Spectacles made up to this prescription would also be useful for night time and prior to lens wear in the early morning.

Cessation of contact lens wear

Sudden cessation of contact lens wear presents the optometrist with an insoluble visual problem, and may be potentially harmful to the patient's vision. A long-term hard lens wearer should be 'de-adapted' to contact lens wear in the reverse of the manner in which they were 'adapted' to wear in the first instance. Spectacles provided in a similar manner to supplementary wear will provide good vision during increasing periods of non-contact lens wear. Usually a period of declining lens wear over 4–6 weeks will result in a stable and relatively unchanged refraction.

However, in the veteran wearer a further 4 weeks may be necessary before a wholly stabilized refraction can be established.

References

1 Bailey, I. A. and Carney, L. G. (1973). *American Journal of Optometry*, **50**, 299

2 Baldwin, W. R., West, D., Jolly, J. and Reid, W. (1969). *American Journal of Optometry*, **46**, 903

3 Benjamin, W. R., Armitage, B. S., Woldschak, M. J. and Hill, R. M. (1983). *Journal of the American Optometric Association*, **54**, 243

4 Bier, N. (1960). *The Optician*, **135**, 427

5 Brand, R. J., Polse, K. A. and Schwalbe, J. (1983). *American Journal of Optometry*, **60**, 175

6 Briggs-Dokubo, S. (1986). *Doctoral Thesis*. University of Wales, Cardiff

7 Brungardt, T. F. and Potter, C. E. (1972). *American Journal of Optometry*, **49**, 41

8 Callender, M. (1979). *Canadian Journal of Optometry*, **41**, 79

9 Carney, L. G. and Bailey, I. L. (1972). *Journal of the American Optometric Association*, **43**, 669

10 Crook, T. G. (1979). *American Journal of Optometry*, **56**, 124

11 Graz, H. V. (1976). *Contact Lens Journal*, **4**, 4

12 Hartstein, J. (1965). *American Journal of Ophthalmology*, **60**, 1103

13 Hartstein, J. (1967). *Current Concepts in Ophthalmology*, edited by Becker and Drew. St Louis: Mosby. p. 207

14 Hess, R. F. and Carney, L. G. (1979). *Investigative Ophthalmology*, **18**, 476

15 Hess, R. F. and Garner, L. F. (1977). *Investigative Ophthalmology*, **16**, 5

16 Hill, J. F. (1974). *Journal of the American Optometric Association*, **46**, 290

17 Hirji, N. K. and Larke, J. R. (1978). *American Journal of Optometry*, **55**, 97

18 Hirji, N. K. and Larke, J. R. (1979). *British Journal of Ophthalmology*, **63**, 274

19 Holden, B. A., Mertz, G. W. and Guillon, M. (1980). *Investigative Ophthalmology*, **19**, 1394

20 Holden, B. A., Mertz, G. W. and McNally, J. J. (1983). *Investigative Ophthalmology*, **24**, 218

21 Høvding, G. (1982). *Acta Ophthalmologica*, **60**, 57

22 Ing, M. R. (1976). *Annals of Ophthalmology*. **8**, 309

23 Kemmetmuller, H. (1972). *Contact Lens Journal*, **1**, 9

24 Kerns, R. L. (1975). *Journal of the American Optometric Association*, **47**, 1047, 1275, 1505; **48**, 345, 1134; **49**, 227, 308

25 Klyce, S. (1984). *Journal of Physiology*, **251**, 348

26 Larke, J. R. (1969). *Doctoral Thesis*. University of Aston in Birmingham

27 McLean, W. E. and Rengstorff, R. H. (1978). *Journal of the American Optometric Asssociation*, **49**, 305

28 McNamara, N. A., Polse, K. A. and Bouaund, J. A. (1994). *Investigative Ophthalmology and Visual Science*, **35**, 846

29 Mandell, R. B. (1976). *Contacto*, **1**, 8

30 Mandell, R. B. and Farrell, R. (1980). *Investigative Ophthalmology*, **19**, 697

31 Mandell, R. B. and Fatt, I. (1965). *Nature*, **208**, 292

32 Mandell, R. B. and Polse, K. A. (1969). *American Journal of Optometry*, **46**, 479

33 May, C. H. and Grant, S. (1971). *Journal of the American Optometric Association*, **42**, 1277

34 Miller, D., Wolf, E., Geer, S. and Vassallo, V. (1967). *Archives of Ophthalmology*, **78**, 448

35 Morrison, R. J. (1958). *Contacto*, **2**, 20

36 Nilsson, S. E. and Morris, J. A. (1983). *British Journal of Ophthalmology*, **67**, 317
37 Rengstorff, R. H. (1965). *American Journal of Optometry*, **42**, 156
38 Rengstorff, R. H. (1967). *American Journal of Optometry*, **44**, 149
39 Rengstorff, R. H. (1971). *American Journal of Optometry*, **48**, 239
40 Rengstorff, R. H. (1971). *American Journal of Optometry*, **48**, 810
41 Rengstorff, R. H. (1973). *American Journal of Optometry*, **44**, 291
42 Rengstorff, R. H. (1980). *International Ophthalmology Clinic,* **21**, 85
43 Sarver, M. D., Polse, K. A. and Baggett, D. A. (1983). *American Journal of Optometry*, **69**, 128
44 Sorenson, T. and Corydon, L. (1979). *Contacto*, **23**, 28
45 Stone, J. (1976). *British Journal of Physiological Optics*, **31**, 89
46 Ziff, S. L. (1970). *Contacto*, **14**, 44

Chapter 10

Contact lens associated infections and related conditions

J. Dart and F. Stapleton

Introduction

Infections in contact lens users differ in their differential diagnosis, epidemiology and pathogenesis compared to infections in other groups[24]. These differences demand their separate consideration from other causes of ocular infection and understanding them is fundamental to the recognition, management and prevention of infections in contact lens users. This chapter examines the relationship of contact lens wear to ocular infections in users of contact lenses for the correction of low refractive errors. The problem of distinguishing infection from the other causes of conjunctival and corneal inflammation in contact lens users is discussed together with strategies for prevention based on our current understanding of the epidemiology and pathogenesis.

Conjunctivitis

Microbial conjunctivitis in contact lens users may be caused by bacteria, chlamydia

Table 10.1 Clinical characteristics of the principal causes of conjunctivitis in contact lens users

	Contact lens associated papillary conjunctivitis	*Thiomersal keratoconjunctivitis*	*Microbial conjunctivitis*
Symptoms	Subacute onset. Symptoms relieved by refitting with new lenses for 1–2 weeks, or by a period without lens wear, before recurring. Mucous discharge, with minimal inflammation, greasing of lenses, itching on lens removal, increased mobility of soft lenses with blinking. Itching after lens removal in early stages, moderate to severe irritation or severe discomfort during lens wear in the later stages with variable loss of tolerance. Acuity unaffected	Irritation and severe hyperaemia with discomfort and epiphora building up over 1–2 weeks. Rapid relief of symptoms, following lens removal, in early disease. Symptoms recur within hours of lens reinsertion or exposure to thiomersal. In chronic disease vision is blurred with contact lenses and deteriorates further with spectacles	Acute onset in hours. Mucopurulent discharge. Diffuse hyperaemia from outset. Vision affected by pus in tear film in bacterial conjunctivitis and by keratopathy in some viral infections. Systemic symptoms usual in viral and chlamydial infections
Conjunctival signs	Upper tarsal conjunctiva only affected. Rarely bulbar conjunctival hyperaemia. In mild cases conjunctival infiltrate only. Moderate cases show micropapillae and advanced cases giant papillae (>1 mm) with apical fibrosis. Clear mucous discharge	Intense hyperaemia soon after exposure to lens or to thiomersal in solution. Few conjunctival signs except some follicles after hyperaemia has resolved	Diffuse conjunctival hyperaemia and infiltrate with formation of micropapillae, and a mucopurulent discharge, within hours of onset of bacterial infection. Viral and chlamydial infection similar but with early follicle formation, often on the bulbar conjunctiva in chlamydial disease
Corneal signs	None	Superior limbal hyperaemia, oedema, and neovascularization of superior cornea. Keratopathy affecting superior cornea and extending down to include visual axis in advanced cases. Corneal changes include epithelial infiltrate, microcysts and anterior stromal opacity	Keratopathy uncommon in bacterial disease. Punctate corneal infiltrates common in viral and chlamydial disease. Coarse anterior stromal infiltrates develop several days after onset of adenoviral infection. Pseudomembrane formation common with adenovirus
Contact lens related associations	All lens types. Commoner with extended wear. Associated with spoiled lenses, poor lens hygiene and a history of allergy	Strongly associated with the use of thiomersal in soft lens care solutions. May develop after years of uneventful use of the same solutions. Very rare in rigid lens users	No established association with any lens type

or viruses and must be differentiated from other causes of conjunctival inflammation. Contact lens associated papillary conjunctivitis and thiomersal keratoconjunctivitis are the principal conditions that may be confused with conjunctival infection[129]. Table 10.1 outlines the major features of these diseases which can be distinguished from microbial conjunctivitis by the differences in their onset, symptoms and signs. These conditions are illustrated in Plates 34–38. Conjunctival culture is seldom necessary and may be misleading as a light growth of organisms from the conjunctival sac is a normal finding.

Bacterial conjunctivitis

It is not clear whether this is an intercurrent event unrelated to the use of lenses or whether it may be precipitated by lens wear. The well-established contamination of contact lens storage cases by bacteria might be expected to result in an excess of conjunctivitis in contact lens users, but it is also possible that the ocular surface defences against infection largely neutralize this potential. There have been several studies on the conjunctival microbial flora of contact lens wearers. A common finding has been a decreased frequency of positive cultures from contact lens wearers compared with controls. This flora has usually been reported as qualitatively unchanged from the findings in normal eyes or in eyes before lens wear[53,71,101,110,121]. However, an increase in Gram-negative organisms has been shown in two studies, one in a hard lens wearing group[53] and in one in a group with hydrogel lenses[85]. It is possible that the source of contamination was the lens care materials in the daily wear subjects but this was only confirmed in one study[85]. The decreased frequency of positive cultures reported in many contact lens wearers has been ascribed to increased hygiene in those lens users during the study period and the effect of antimicrobial lens solutions, introduced by the contact lenses, on the resident flora in the conjunctival sac.

This evidence suggests that, at least in the short term, there is rarely any qualitative change in the conjunctival flora towards a more pathogenic spectrum of organisms, although contaminated contact lenses may introduce Gram-negative bacteria from the lens case. The numbers of bacteria in the conjunctival sac of contact lens users may be reduced.

Viral and chlamydial keratoconjunctivitis

Viruses and chlamydia are common causes of a mixed follicular and papillary conjunctivitis with an associated keratitis. Contact lens wear has not been recognized as a cause of these infections, although potentially they may be transmitted by inadequately disinfected trial lenses. Chlamydial infection by non-endemic strains (inclusion conjunctivitis) is often sexually transmitted and is a common cause of chronic follicular conjunctivitis in sexually active contact lens users. Its diagnosis demands treatment in a sexually transmitted disease clinic to exclude and manage asymptomatic genital infection. Adenovirus, one of the numerous viral causes of keratoconjunctivitis, is highly infectious and may be transmitted by hand to eye contact, upper respiratory droplet infection or contaminated solutions. Contact lens fitting carries a risk of transmitting these viral and chlamydial infections as well as bacterial infections[19]. There is also a theoretical risk of transmitting human immunodeficiency virus type 1 (HIV-1) which has been isolated from both the tears and ocular surface cells of AIDS patients[1]. However, most lens care regimens are probably effective against HIV-1[3] although not necessarily against adenoviruses[95]. For these reasons, both hard and soft trial lenses should be disinfected in hydrogen peroxide 3%, or by heat if appropriate, to prevent transmission in the clinic setting[122].

Suppurative keratitis

Suppurative keratitis describes a wide spectrum of disease ranging from small, generally non-infected, usually peripheral, corneal infiltrates and ulcers, to large ulcers associated with uveitis. Differentiating non-infected from infected keratitis lesions in contact lens users has been the cause of both controversy and confusion.

The terminology surrounding suppurative keratitis in contact lens users is unclear. This has arisen because of the difficulty of differentiating, either clinically or with laboratory investigations, between corneal ulcers due to replicating organisms (microbial keratitis) and corneal ulcers resulting from hypersensitivity responses to a variety of stimuli (sterile or aseptic keratitis). This has led to the use of the terms 'ulcerative keratitis'[104] and 'presumed microbial keratitis'[28] to describe keratitis probably due to replicating organisms, but in which laboratory investigations may have been negative. The terms 'peripheral sterile ulcers'[45] 'peripheral corneal infiltrates'[14] and 'sterile corneal infiltrates'[9,117] have been used to describe keratitis resulting from hypersensitivity reactions in which there is no evidence of replicating organisms and for which analogies have been drawn with 'marginal keratitis', an entity often associated with staphylococcal blepharitis[4]. Here, the terms *microbial keratitis* will be used to describe suppurative keratitis resulting from invasion by replicating microorganisms and *aseptic keratitis* for keratitis due to these other causes.

Differentiating between aseptic and microbial keratitis

Current laboratory techniques cannot be used to differentiate microbial from aseptic causes of suppurative keratitis with reliability. Aseptic keratitis is a diagnosis of exclusion because there are no laboratory investigations to substantiate the different causes and microbiological investigation in contact lens associated keratitis has a low sensitivity. It is well established that a negative corneal culture cannot be used to eliminate a microbial cause or, conversely, to validate an aseptic cause; large series of microbial keratitis cases have documented a culture positive rate of 50% in inpatient populations comprising the more severe cases[22], whereas a high proportion of contact lens related keratitis cases are small lesions which may be expected to be culture positive less often. Negative culture resulting from microbial lesions may occur for several reasons: small volumes of necrotic material available for culture; viable organisms present in deep tissues less available to corneal sampling methods; and pretreatment with antibiotics reducing the viability of invading organisms.

For these reasons, clinical criteria have to be used for diagnosis of individual patients and in studies designed to investigate these disorders. The size and position of the lesion are not diagnostic although these criteria alone have often been used to attempt to differentiate the lesions. The use of clinical criteria incorporating the severity of the symptoms and signs of clinical inflammation, in addition to the size and position of the lesion, has been recommended[113]. Clinical criteria used to differentiate these lesions are summarized in Table 10.2[9,117]. That these definitions

Table 10.2 Definition of presumed microbial and aseptic keratitis with distinguishing clinical characteristics

	Presumed microbial	*Presumed aseptic*
Definition	There is a high probability that replicating bacteria are the principal factor in the pathogenesis. Therefore microbiological investigations are appropriate, although they may not be positive	There is a high probability that replicating bacteria are *not* involved in the pathogenesis. Consequently, microbiological investigations will be irrelevant to the management. No laboratory investigations are available to confirm the diagnosis
Clinical criteria	Central lesions	Peripheral lesions, occasionally central, often multiple
	Lesions >1mm in diameter	Lesions usually <1 mm, may be >1 mm, sometimes arcuate in the limbal zone
	Epithelial defect	Intact epithelium in early lesions with ulceration in late lesions
	Pain, progressively deteriorates and may be severe	Mild pain, non-progressive
	Diffuse and/or severe progressive corneal suppuration	Mild non-progressive corneal suppuration
	Uveitis	Minimal anterior chamber reaction

distinguish between distinct disease processes is supported by epidemiological data[113]. Examples of aseptic, indeterminate and proven bacterial keratitis cases are shown in Plate 39.

Aseptic keratitis

Symptoms and signs

Mild non-progressive pain develops, with localized redness in the quadrant of conjunctiva adjacent to involved cornea. Corneal infiltration is present, usually in the peripheral cornea, although identical, single or multiple, culture negative infiltrates may occur in the central corneal zones (see Plate 39*c*). The epithelium overlying the infiltrates is often intact in early disease (see Plate 39*a*) but will ulcerate if the inflammation is severe (see Plate 39*b*). Adjacent ciliary hyperaemia is present and there is no, or limited, anterior chamber response[117].

Pathogenesis

In non-contact lens wearers, sterile peripheral infiltrates, 'marginal keratitis', are seen in association with staphylococcal blepharitis[120]. Clinical[18,120] and animal studies[80,81] have shown that infiltrates may result from hypersensitivity to staphylococcal antigens. In contact lens users blepharitis may or may not be present and similar mechanisms have been invoked with the lens acting as a source of antigens[57] and toxins[96] from bacteria derived both from the lids and from lens case contaminants. These observations are supported by the demonstration that poor lens hygiene and bacterial contamination of the lens storage case have been shown to be associated with sterile infiltrates[9]. In addition, the lens may act as a vehicle for presenting antigen to the cornea which may be more susceptible as a result of the effects of lens wear on epithelial integrity. Other potential causes in lens users include delayed hypersensitivity to thiomersal in lens care materials[79,130] and a response to tight fitting lenses[130]. Other factors may be those associated with the acute red eye (ARE) reaction. This is associated with peripheral sterile infiltrates in extended wear hydrogel[76] and less commonly in rigid lens use[105]. It frequently occurs upon awakening, and has been attributed to the build up of cellular and metabolic debris under the lens. Epidemiological studies have confirmed that the highest relative risk of sterile keratitis occurs in extended wear hydrogel use, at 2.43 times greater than with RGP lens use[112]. The incidence of sterile keratitis in extended wear users has been estimated at 1% per year, with a greater risk for wearers with a previous history of infiltrates[44]. No association has been found between increased lens age and sterile infiltrates[113], which implies that a similar level of risk may be present for frequent replacement/disposable lenses as for conventional lenses.

Management

Progressive lesions should be treated as microbial keratitis. Typical lesions may be managed by discontinuing lens wear until the corneal signs have resolved, particularly in the case of infiltrates without ulceration when symptoms are minimal. In the presence of ulceration, prophylactic levels of topical antibiotics with activity against both staphylococci and Gram-negative organisms, including *Pseudomonas*, a quinolone or aminoglycoside, may be used to limit the risk of superinfection in the contaminated environment of contact lens wear. Topical steroids may also be used, when symptoms are more severe, to reduce inflammation and shorten the disease course, but their use demands specialist medical management.

Measures should be taken to reduce the risk of further attacks. These are based on what is known about the pathogenesis and include attention to lens and lens storage case hygiene, the elimination of thiomersal-based disinfection systems, changing from extended to daily wear hydrogel lenses, ensuring that the lens is a loose fit and, in recurring cases, changing from hydrogel to RGP lenses.

Microbial keratitis

Pathogenic organisms in contact lens wear

Bacteria and free-living amoebae are the principal causes of keratitis in contact lens users. Polymicrobial infections may also occur in contact lens users and can be mixed Gram-positive, Gram-negative and amoebic. A predisposition to pseudomonas and acanthamoeba keratitis is unique to contact lens wear. It has been an unfortunate accident of nature that *Pseudomonas* is one of the most virulent pathogens that can invade the cornea and *Acanthamoeba* among the most difficult to eliminate. Fungi, although contaminating the lens case and having the potential to invade soft lens materials have infrequently been implicated as a cause of microbial keratitis in lens users. Herpetic keratitis has not been associated with or modified by lens wear although it has often been misdiagnosed in contact lens users with amoebic keratitis resulting in sometimes long delays in reaching the correct diagnosis.

Bacteria

Gram-negative bacterial infections predominate in cosmetic contact lens wear. *Pseudomonas* is the predominant organism and *Serratia* has also been frequently isolated. Other Gram-negative enterobacteria including *Escherichia coli* and *Proteus* are occasionally isolated. Gram-positive infections with *Staphylococcus aureus* and *Staph epidermidis* are also common and more frequently reported than infection with *Serratia*[124].

Fungi

There have been few reports of fungal keratitis associated with contact lens wear and it is likely that contact lens use has a minimal effect on the predisposition to fungal infection. *Fusarium*, *Curvularia* and *Paecilomyces* have been reported[125,126].

Acanthamoeba

Acanthamoeba has recently become a frequent cause of keratitis in contact lens users. Concern about acanthamoeba keratitis has resulted not so much because of the numbers affected but because of the poor prognosis and the severe morbidity associated with the initial management techniques. The prognosis has now improved with early diagnosis and the availability of effective medical therapy, although the disease course is often prolonged and the outcome poor[7]. The disease was uncommon until the late 1980s. The number of cases in the USA had risen to about 200 by 1989 and it was proposed that this increase in cases partly resulted from the growth in popularity of contact lens wear[116], which is associated in about 85% of cases. In the UK, 72 cases (77 eyes) have recently been reported from the same centre over a 7.5-year period with a rapid increase in the number of cases occurring in 1991 and 1992, associated with disposable contact lens wear[8]. Although the number is still rising, the numbers of new patients at any one referral centre is usually small. The disease is possibly rarer, under-diagnosed or under-reported elsewhere.

Symptoms and signs

Progressive symptoms, after removal of the lens, are the hallmark of this disease. These include pain, redness and discharge with loss of vision in lesions that involve the visual axis. Lesions may be central, or less commonly peripheral[51,54]. Lesions are typically associated with an epithelial defect, although in the early stages of bacterial keratitis and acanthamoeba keratitis there may be epithelial infiltration only. Bacterial keratitis rapidly becomes severe and progressive with associated iritis, whereas in acanthamoeba keratitis the course is usually slowly progressive. Focal conjunctival hyperaemia adjacent to the affected quadrant of cornea gives way to generalized conjunctival and ciliary hyperaemia as the condition develops. The discharge may be watery or purulent.

Although the clinical features of keratitis resulting from these organisms differ, there is too large an overlap in these to allow clinical diagnosis with certainty and microbiological diagnosis is mandatory. Plates 39*d* and 39*e* demonstrate the similarity between early pseudomonas and staphylococcal keratitis and the difficulty of differentiating these from the aseptic or culture negative cases in Plates 39*a–c*. *Pseudomonas* rapidly causes a fulminating purulent keratitis associated with intense inflammation of the cornea surrounding the ulcer (Plate 39*f*) over which there is a mucopurulent exudate. Stromal thinning may be rapid leading to perforation within hours in some cases. Other bacterial causes generally result in a less intense keratitis. Although intense pain may be a feature of early acanthamoeba keratitis, a corneal ulcer usually takes days or weeks to develop with punctate keratopathy, pseudo-dendrites, focal and diffuse epithelial and subepithelial infiltrates (Plate 40*a*) and radial keratoneuritis (Plate 40*b*) being among the signs of early disease[7,51,69,84]. These features may be mistaken for those of herpetic keratitis, resulting in delayed diagnosis and treatment with a worse prognosis[7]. A ring infiltrate and corneal ulceration are usually late signs of disease[119]. *Acanthamoeba* must be considered in the differential diagnosis of contact lens users with an atypical keratitis in whom the diagnosis of herpes keratitis should be treated with scepticism.

Epidemiology

Until the results of the recent well-designed epidemiological studies of keratitis in lens wear became available, it was unclear whether there were real differences in the incidence and risks of keratitis for different lens types. Microbial keratitis was too rare to be identified as a problem in unpooled clinical trial data and it was case reports and case series that first identified the probability that there was an increased risk of keratitis associated with some lens types. In these, the number of extended wear soft contact lens users affected was higher than might be expected[2,42,90] as it has been in the accumulated literature of case reports[124]. These reports could not be used to give an estimate of the incidence or the risks for different lens types because the size of the populations at risk are unknown[25].

Incidence of keratitis in reusable contact lens wear

When the problem of lens related keratitis became apparent, efforts were made to establish incidence data. Analysis of the pooled results of 48 consecutive premarket approval studies (clinical trials) on 22 739 contact lens users for the US Food and Drug Administration provided annual incidence rates for keratitis of 6.8 : 10 000 ($n = 3907$) in gas-permeable daily contact lens wear, 5.2 : 10 000 ($n = 3591$) for daily wear soft contact lens wear and 18.2 : 10 000 ($n = 1276$) for reusable extended wear soft contact lens wear[72]. These studies were carefully carried out but were not comparative. They were also conducted on carefully monitored volunteer users giving informed consent and individuals failing to adhere to the follow-up schedules were often excluded. For these reasons, such trials may not be representative of the population of contact lens users in the real post-marketing situation.

The problems associated with the interpretation of the data on keratitis in contact lens wear from these descriptive studies and clinical trials, have been successfully addressed for estimating the incidence of ulcerative keratitis associated with reusable contact lens wear in New England. This study estimated an annual incidence for ulcerative keratitis in the USA of 20.9 (95% CI 15.1–26.7) : 10 000 for extended wear soft contact lens use compared with 4.1 (95% CI 2.9–5.2) : 10 000 for daily wear soft contact lenses[98]. This study did not have the power to identify differences between rigid and soft lens types.

Risks of keratitis in contact lens wear

Case control studies have recently been used to provide quantitative data on differences in risk for a wider range of different lens types. The influence of factors associated with these lenses which might contribute to these risks has been assessed by multivariable analysis, giving some insight into the pathogenesis of keratitis in contact lens wear.

Reusable cosmetic contact lenses

The principal findings of the recent case control[28,104] and incidence studies[98] for daily wear and extended wear reusable cosmetic lenses can be reasonably extrapolated to all countries where contact lenses are widely used. The UK study has shown that contact lenses are now the major associated cause of microbial keratitis in London, with a risk that is significantly higher than that for corneal trauma[28]. The relative risk (RR) with 95% confidence limits of keratitis associated with these causes, compared to cases without an identifiable predisposing factor (the referent with a baseline risk of 1.0) was 80 times (38–166) higher for contact lens wear and 14 times (6–32) for trauma. Contact lens wear, principally of soft contact lenses, was also shown to be responsible for 65% of all new microbial keratitis cases at this centre where no serious cases attributable to this cause had been reported a decade earlier. This trend for increased risk associated with contact lens wear persisted for all severities of microbial keratitis[29]. This study also showed that, compared to hard contact lenses, the risk for extended wear soft contact lenses was 21 times (7–60) and daily wear soft contact lenses 3.6 times (1–14) greater. Continuous periods of extended wear of more than 6 days were associated with a further increase in the risk of keratitis. The findings of the independent multicentre case control study in the USA, on the risks of keratitis associated with different types of soft contact lenses, were very similar. The risk of extended wear soft contact lenses use was 9–15 times higher than that for daily wear soft contact lenses and was incrementally related to the period of extended wear. The relative risks for hard contact lenses could not be assessed in this study[104].

Disposable cosmetic soft lenses

Disposable soft contact lenses have only become widely available since 1989 and the advantages and disadvantages of this lens disposal schedule are only now becoming established. Enthusiasm for this type of lens wear is based on the theoretical advantages due to the potential for elimination of problems relating to surface deposits, in particular contact lens associated papillary conjunctivitis, and problems associated with hygiene systems and compliance[35]. However, the effect of using a disposable lens wearing regimen on the risks of keratitis has been uncertain[55,64]. Soon after the introduction of disposable lenses, case series and reports described both bacterial keratitis due to *Pseudomonas*[43,59,93,100] and acanthamoeba keratitis with daily[37] and extended wear[41] use of these lenses. Clinical trials and retrospective cohort studies to date have not had the statistical power to establish whether there are differences in risk for microbial keratitis for disposable compared to reusable lenses[47,97]. However, a retrospective cohort study of hospitalized cases of microbial keratitis in Sweden has estimated a reduced risk associated with daily wear of disposable lenses compared with daily wear of re-usable lenses[89].

The uncertainty arising from these case reports and cohort studies of disposable lenses has been addressed by two case control studies. The results of one of these suggested that the risks for both sterile and microbial keratitis may be as great or greater than those for conventional soft lens wear[74] and that failure of compliance with recommended lens care and wear regimens may be one cause of this. The results of the other study suggested that the greater risk associated with disposable lens use compared to reusable lenses[15] can be attributed to their greater use for overnight wear[103].

The effect of lens related factors on keratitis risks

Multivariable analysis of case control studies has contributed to our understanding of the pathogenesis of keratitis in contact lens wear[28,104,113]. This is as a result of identifying additional factors that are associated with the use of different lens types and which contribute to the risk of keratitis. These studies have shown that the major risk factor for microbial keratitis is overnight wear of soft lenses and that this risk increases incrementally with the number of nights of continuous wear. This finding is not confounded by the misuse of lens materials or designs intended for daily wear use being worn overnight. Higher risks for keratitis are related to lower socioeconomic status, smoking and male sex; probably factors related to compliance with lens care advice. Although these studies had limited power to evaluate hygiene and compliance in the extended wear soft contact lens using population, neither the hygiene systems nor compliance with lens hygiene could be shown to have any effect on the risk of keratitis for extended wear.

Among daily wear soft lens users, poor hygiene itself was shown to have a small but significant effect on the risk of microbial keratitis and lens case cleaning was shown to have a small protective effect. However, levels of hygiene compliance were generally poor both in cases and controls[104]. For daily wear, soft contact lens use the effects of hygiene system and compliance have been further evaluated. For users with good compliance, the daily use of peroxide disinfectant systems minimized the risk of microbial keratitis, cold chemical systems had a slightly, but not significantly higher risk (2.4 times, with 95% confidence intervals 0.6–11.0), whereas the use of chlorine release and heat disinfection carried a significantly greater risk of keratitis at 5.6 times (1.02–31.0) and 5.74 (1.0–33.0) respectively. Poor compliance with any system increased the risk of keratitis by a factor of from 2 to 17 times, although this increase was only significant for poor compliance with chlorine release (16.38 times 1.2–226.0) and for those using no disinfection system at all (10.61 times, 2.2–52.0)[114].

Although both hygiene compliance and the disinfection system used increase the risk of keratitis for daily wear soft contact lens users, it has also been observed that a proportion of keratitis cases have good hygiene and uncontaminated lens care materials[22] suggesting that lens hygiene is not the only determinant of keratitis in this group[10]. This is not surprising when the high contamination rate of lens cases in asymptomatic lens users, associated with compliant use of current hygiene systems is considered[23].

For both daily and extended wear of reusable lenses, many other factors that had been anticipated to affect the risk of developing keratitis have not been shown to do so in these studies. These included factors that might be expected to have a relationship to decreased hygiene compliance; the age of the user, the number of years of lens wear and the period since the last follow-up visit.

In addition there was no effect of lens age on keratitis. This is at variance with what had been predicted from laboratory studies, described below, that show increased bacterial adherence to deposits on lenses. This could be expected to result in an increased risk of keratitis with lens age, whereas these epidemiological findings suggest that increased lens age does not affect the risks of keratitis and that other factors must be more important. For example, the overriding effect of extended wear as a risk factor for keratitis is probably related to increased susceptibility of the cornea to microbial invasion and lens bacterial interactions other than adherence.

These findings suggest that disposable lenses, when used for extended wear, cannot be expected to reduce the risk of keratitis. Also their use as frequent replacement daily wear lenses is unlikely to reduce the risk of keratitis because hygiene compliance failure is reintroduced. Although the disposable concept has potentially much to offer in terms of safety and convenience, these lenses should be treated with the same caution as other types of lens regarding the risks of keratitis for the present. However, true daily wear disposable lenses, where single-use lenses are worn daily and discarded, may be expected to reduce the risk of keratitis.

Risk factors for Acanthamoeba keratitis

In these case control studies of microbial keratitis the majority of cases were proven or presumptively bacterial with few *Acanthamoeba* cases. An early case control study of soft lens related amoebic keratitis had shown that these infections were associated with the use of home-made saline solution, as opposed to proprietary solutions, and with the habit of swimming in lenses[115]. Until recently no differences in risk had been identified in association with different types of lens[63,83,116]. However, a large case series of acanthamoeba keratitis from the UK, including all cases identified between 1984 and 1992, has shown that 28/64 consecutive contact lens users with acanthamoeba keratitis were disposable lens users[8]. Disposable lenses were not introduced into the UK until 1989 and this proportion is much higher than expected from the current penetrance of disposable lenses in the UK. The factors that may account for this apparent increased incidence of this disease in this group have not yet been investigated but are possibly associated with deficient lens hygiene[58].

Pathogenesis

These epidemiological studies have identified several factors that contribute to the pathogenesis of keratitis in contact lens users; overnight wear, soft lenses, disposable lenses, poor hygiene compliance and some types of hygiene systems. These studies, together with the clinical and laboratory investigations described here, have led to our current understanding of the pathogenesis of bacterial and acanthamoeba keratitis in contact lens users.

Until recently, theories of the pathogenesis of microbial keratitis in contact lens users were founded on two principal proposals. First, that contact lens wear, particularly the use of extended wear soft contact lenses, has extensive effects on the ocular surface[50] that might be expected to compromise its resistance to microbial invasion[17,70,82]. Second, that some of these eyes are exposed to large numbers of bacteria contaminating a high proportion of contact lens cases[65,75]. The combination of increased susceptibility to infection with increased exposure therefore resulted in the increased risk of infection.

Failure to review critically the evidence for the pathogenesis of infection in contact lens users and the mechanisms contributing to these two important proposals has contributed to both exacerbating and perpetuating the problem of microbial keratitis in contact lens wear. Examples are the introduction of extended wear, both reusable and disposable, as a means of reducing the exposure to contaminated contact lens solutions, and emphasis on improving contact lens hygiene compliance when there is doubt that the hygiene systems are adequately effective in use even when compliance is adequate. In addition, these proposals for the pathogenesis do not address why *Pseudomonas* and *Acanthamoeba* is more common in contact lens users with keratitis; why there is not a link between contact lens case contamination and keratitis in all patients with keratitis[22,40] and why rigid contact lens users are probably at a lower risk of keratitis than soft lens users.

The pathogenesis of bacterial keratitis

Any theory of the pathogenesis of keratitis in contact lens users must take into account the source of the organisms, the role of bacterial adherence and colonization of the lens and lens care materials, and the effect of lens wear on resistance to bacterial invasion.

The source of bacteria

The organisms that commonly cause keratitis in contact lens users may all be isolated from the ocular surface of normal individuals. These include *Staph. aureus*, *Ps. aeruginosa* and other coliform bacteria[54]. The studies on the conjunctival flora in

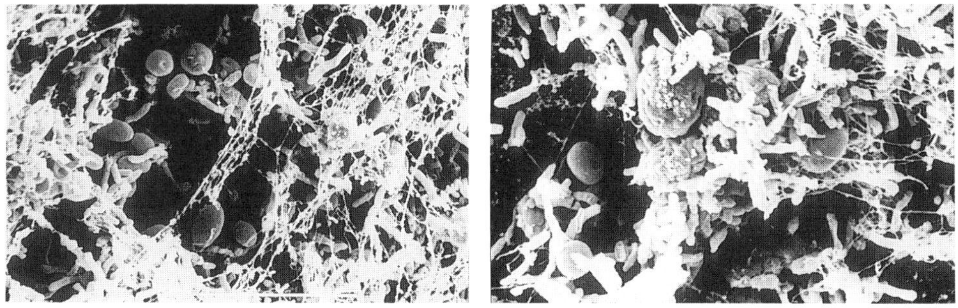

(a) (b)

Figure 10.1 (*a*) Scanning electron microscopy of the surface of the contact lens from a patient with pseudomonas keratitis. Bacterial rods and fungal spores are shown in a biofilm on the soft contact lens surface (stained with ruthenium red, ×3300); (*b*) the surface of the contact lens case from the same patient showing an identical flora (stained with ruthenium red, ×4500)

contact lens wear have been reviewed in the section on conjunctivitis. Although some of these have shown no qualitative change in the conjunctival flora towards a more pathogenic spectrum of organisms, others have shown that contact lenses may introduce Gram-negative bacteria from contaminated contact lens cases[85]. These have since been shown to be an important additional source of pathogens[31,33,128]. The importance of the contaminated contact lens case in the pathogenesis of bacterial keratitis in contact lens users has been identified for many years and the expected link between lens case contamination and keratitis has been confirmed for some subjects[75,127] although an association is not always present[22,127]. Lens case contamination probably results from a combination of poor hygiene and the failure of current disinfection systems in use.

The role of the contact lens case may be to amplify the concentration of these environmental bacteria contaminating contact lens care systems, thereby providing a large inoculum of bacteria to be presented to the eye by the contact lens. The discovery of the potential importance of the bacterial glycocalyx provides a theoretical mechanism whereby small numbers of bacteria from these environmental sources might be able to amplify in numbers both in the lens case and on the contact lens surface itself as demonstrated in Figure 10.1[23,128].

Bacterial adherence to the contact lens

Numerous studies have been carried out on bacterial adherence to contact lenses to explore the relationship of adherence to the lens as a source for bacteria in the pathogenesis of keratitis. Both *Ps. aeruginosa* and *Staph. aureus* adhere to new and worn soft and unworn polymethylmethacrylate (PMMA) lens surfaces with *Staph. aureus* having a much greater affinity for PMMA than *Pseudomonas* or for soft lenses[26]. Subsequent studies, principally on *Pseudomonas* have confirmed that *Pseudomonas* adheres in large numbers to both new[36] and worn lens surfaces, although greater numbers of bacteria adhere to worn surfaces[16] and to deposits on soft lenses to which *Pseudomonas* adheres more avidly than *Staph. aureus*[5].

Although the effect of ocular deposits in most studies has been seen to increase bacterial adherence[5,118] these experiments may represent an over-simplification of the situation *in vivo* and have masked interstrain differences and interhost variations in the effect of ocular deposits on adherence. It has been shown that interspecies and interstrain variations in bacterial adherence to lenses occur[62]. Surface deposits may or may not enhance the adherence of *Pseudomonas*[77,78]. Inhibition of *Pseudomonas* adherence in worn lenses has been shown in a rabbit model[67] and, in humans, to the predominantly lysozyme coating of Etafilcon A lenses[11]. Adherence to unworn lenses is likely to be mediated by non-specific surface interactions, such as ionicity and hydrophobicity. Interactions between bacteria and worn lenses are likely to be mediated by specific protein-to-protein interactions. The mechanisms of adherence to worn and unworn lenses are very different and are not directly comparable. Therefore, although bacterial adherence to the lens surface is probably an important factor in the pathogenesis of keratitis, the clinical relevance of *enhanced adherence* to lens surfaces, when this occurs, is not proven. The laboratory findings implying that enhanced adherence is due to surface deposits do not correlate with case control study findings which have failed to establish an association between lens ageing and keratitis[28].

Although these studies have all shown that the lens may act as a vector for the delivery of organisms to the eye from a contaminated lens case, the bacteria are also able to colonize (replicate in microcolonies on) the surface of the lens. This involves the elaboration of a glycocalyx by the bacteria and the maturing of this into a biofilm. As a strategy for bacterial survival on a surface, bacterial adherence is of importance in retaining viable bacteria long enough on the lens surface for a glycocalyx, and later a biofilm, to form[73]. The development of these structures results in conversion of reversibly adhering bacteria, that are simply passengers on the lens surface, into replicating bacteria colonizing the lens surface in strongly attached populations as shown in Figure 10.1*a*. Subsequent to this, adherence of individual bacteria to the surface is likely to be of little significance.

The role of bacterial colonization

In appropriate environmental conditions most bacteria will secrete a glycocalyx that serves to bind microcolonies of bacteria together. The glycocalyx is a polysaccharide-containing structure, produced by the bacteria, and lying outside the peptidoglycan and outer membrane of Gram-positive and Gram-negative organisms[21]. This structure is difficult to stabilize for visualization by electron microscopy and is lost when using routine fixation techniques with glutaraldehyde without using specific techniques for stabilization of the structure, such as the use of ruthenium red. Proliferation and organization of this bacterial glycocalyx leads to the development of a more complex biofilm that results in irreversible adhesion of the bacteria to the surface[73].

These biofilm enclosed organisms may become mobile, planktonic or ‘swarmer’ cells when they are free to invade surrounding tissues. In this latter state they do not have the protection afforded by the glycocalyx from phagocytosis, bacteriophages[21] and antibiotics. In addition these planktonic cells are genotypically identical but phenotypically different from the sessile cells and are particularly sensitive to antibiotics compared to the cells that remain within the biofilm[38,39]. This may result in eradication of the planktonic cells by biocides or antibiotics but persistence of viable bacteria within the biofilm from where further shedding can occur.

In vitro data show that the levels of antibiotic must be 20–1000 times greater to achieve adequate growth inhibition in a biofilm, compared to the same bacteria when they have been liberated into a planktonic state[46,86,87,99]. Similar data exist for biocides[101]. This resistance of biofilm to antibiotics and biocidal agents is complex and not completely understood.

It is probable that biofilm enclosed bacterial colonization of surfaces is the rule rather than the exception, and that the planktonic or free living mode of existence that has been studied in the laboratory test tube, is an artificial environment for most bacteria.

The kinetics of the development of glycocalyx suggest that this can occur rapidly enough for this to be the form in which bacteria are transported to the eye on a lens contaminated in the case. Therefore it is probable that, in different circumstances, the lens promotes keratitis both by acting as a vehicle for mature bacteria and as a surface for bacterial growth and replication. In addition, the lens may act as a reservoir for organisms introduced into the eye from environmental sources providing lower inocula than the contact lens case. Although in these circumstances adherence to the lens may result in a relative increase in the retention time of bacteria at the ocular surface from a few hours to several hours, as determined by the life of the bacteria, it will not result in an increase of their numbers, or more prolonged exposure, unless the adherence results in colonization of the lens surface. Recent interest has focused on the formation of lens surface biofilms which would allow this to occur[22,27,56,109,111]. This provides one explanation for the pathogenesis of the keratitis that occurs in subjects whose contact lens cases and solutions are not contaminated by bacteria, and in compliant disposable extended wear lens users. In such cases, bacteria arising in small numbers from the environmental sources could adhere to the lens, whereas in the normal eye they are cleared by the ocular surface defence mechanisms. If these adherent bacteria form a glycocalyx they will be able to colonize the lens surface and their numbers can then amplify on the lens itself. This has been demonstrated on lenses from patients who have developed lens related pseudomonas keratitis[52,113] as is shown in Figure 10.1*a*.

The role of the contact lens in reducing corneal resistance to bacterial invasion of the cornea

It has been postulated that the contact lens may reduce the resistance of the cornea to bacterial invasion by several mechanisms. However, none of these has yet been shown to result directly in bacterial keratitis. The profound effects on corneal oxygen supply resulting from all lens wear and extended wear soft contact lens wear in particular, the disturbance of the normal flow of tears over the cornea and interference with the normal lid/tear resurfacing mechanisms are among the mechanical and physiological stresses induced by lens wear. These may lead to a reduction in the clearance of bacteria contaminating the tear film and to breaches in the corneal epithelium common in contact lens users, and mandatory for the development of keratitis[10,17,48].

Contact lens wear may lead to the necessary epithelial injury in a number of ways. Trauma occurs during lens handling and disruption of the epithelium occurs in a number of other complications of lens wear, such as acute epithelial necrosis (overwear syndrome) and microcystic epitheliopathy. These are known to be more common in overnight wear of contact lenses. Soft contact lenses also reduce tear exchange under the lens and this is likely to prolong the retention of bacteria at the surface of the cornea. In experimental animal models of pseudomonas corneal infection, keratitis will not occur in the presence of a contaminated contact lens unless there is epithelial trauma[22,32]. However, suturing the lids together for a prolonged period will result in keratitis, in the absence of a mechanical defect in the epithelium, probably as a result of the effects of severe hypoxic stress on epithelial resistance to infection[5,66]. These findings correlate with the epidemiological findings of increased risk associated with overnight wear of soft lenses.

The pathogenesis of acanthamoeba keratitis

Acanthamoeba is found in air, soil, salt, fresh and chlorinated water and can be commonly isolated in nasopharyngeal cultures of human upper respiratory tract infections[6,10]. In the UK, *Acanthamoeba* can be isolated in association with limescale from domestic taps in hard water areas, particularly from tank stored water, common in the UK, rather than from the rising main[107]. The organism has been found in home-made saline solutions[33,116] and in the lens cases of lens users with acanthamoeba keratits[34]. They have also been isolated from the contact lens cases of 4–7% of asymptomatic lens users[31,65].

Acanthamoeba is almost always present in these environments as a co-contaminant with bacteria and/or fungi because these organisms are required as a food source for the organism[12]. Although heat disinfection is effective against *Acanthamoeba* cysts and trophozoite[69,70] it is not appropriate for use with all lens systems. Also acanthamoebae have been isolated from the cases of individuals using this method[31]. Cold contact lens disinfection systems are not yet required to be effective against *Acanthamoeba* by the licensing authorities in the UK or USA.

Evaluation of the effect of these disinfection systems on *Acanthamoeba* trophozoites and cysts has led to inconsistent results, possibly due to variations in the methodology, inoculum size and species or strain susceptibility[88]. Of the systems available, only hydrogen peroxide 3% with exposure times of from 2–4 hours[13,108] and chlorhexidine 0.004–0.005%, also with prolonged exposure times, have been shown to be effective *in vitro*[61]. None of the remaining systems has been shown to have a reliable effect in the concentrations available, including peroxide with short acting neutralization systems[68,70,108], chlorine release[30,94,106], polyquaternary ammonium, polyhexamethylene biguanide[20,94,106,108] or benzalkonium chloride 0.004%[94].

Successful disinfection of bacterial contaminants would reduce or eliminate the problem of *Acanthamoeba* contamination but this is currently not achieved in practice in 35–50% of asymptomatic users[31,34,65]. These individuals are likely to be at a higher risk of acanthamoeba keratitis if they are using a system that has no effect against the *Acanthamoeba* that may coexist in these cases.

Acanthamoeba cysts and trophozoites have also been shown to adhere to contact lenses[56] although they can be effectively removed by contact lens cleaners *in vitro*[60]. Of these cleaners, isopropyl alcohol has been shown to be very effective against both cysts and trophozoites[20,94].

Preventing contamination by *Acanthamoeba* is consequently of greater importance than for bacteria. Measures which may protect against this include avoiding the use of tap water for cleaning lens cases or lenses, avoiding home-made solutions, cleaning the contact lens with a surfactant cleaner, drying the contact lens case after use and the use of heat, chlorhexidine or peroxide with overnight soaking of the lenses. Specific adherence mechanisms have been shown for acanthamoebae to rabbit corneal epithelium[92] and it is probable that these are also important in the pathogenesis of keratitis in humans. However, unlike bacteria, amoebae may be able to invade the corneal epithelium in the absence of an epithelial defect as shown *in vitro* for human corneal epithelium[88] and in a pig model of acanthamoeba keratitis[49,91].

The rarity of acanthamoeba infection, and the frequency with which contact lens users may be exposed, implies that most strains of the organism are of low virulence in the cornea. However, for current contact lens users, the potential for acanthamoeba keratitis is continually present. Like bacteria, it is present in the contact lens users' ocular environment, it is resistant to current contact lens disinfection systems and it has mechanisms for invading the cornea.

Summary of theories of the pathogenesis of lens associated microbial keratitis

The presence of microbes on the lens results from a number of factors: the principal organisms causing keratitis are widespread in the contact lens users' environment; *Pseudomonas* and *Acanthamoeba* from contaminated water supplies and solutions. Contact lens users may also be exposed to *Pseudomonas* and other coliforms, such as *Serratia,* as a result of faecal contamination. Staphylococci colonize the lids, skin and upper respiratory tract. Microorganisms from these sources may be transferred to the lens and lens case directly during lens hygiene routines such as case washing and lens cleaning and insertion. Compliance failures with hand washing, lens and case cleaning and disinfection routines probably increase the load of microorganisms that are inevitably transferred to the lens and lens case. Organisms may contaminate the lens case as a result of both compliance failures and disinfectant system failures. It is probable that organisms may colonize the lens case in biofilms that increase their resistance to disinfection regimens. *Acanthamoeba* may require a case contaminated with bacteria to provide an intermediate food source.

Both bacteria and *Acanthamoeba* can adhere to the lens and bacteria have been shown to be capable of colonizing the lens surface as well as simply adhering to it. The lens material, degree of spoilation and hygiene compliance may all affect this step in the pathogenesis. The cornea may be exposed both to microorganisms adherent to the lens or derived from biofilm enclosed microcolonies on the lens surface.

Virulence factors may be important in determining the presence of organisms pathogenic for contact lens users, their ability to adhere to or colonize the lens, as well as their ability to invade the cornea.

Factors affecting the susceptibility of the cornea to keratitis include reduced resistance to infection as the result of the physiological effects of the lens on the cornea, and interference with physical factors important in resistance to infection, such as the tear flow over the ocular surface. The deleterious effect of the extended wear of soft lenses on these factors, together with the possibility of more prolonged exposure to microorganisms colonizing the lens, is likely to account for the increased risk associated with this lens type.

The development of keratitis in contact lens users is a multifactorial problem caused by numerous interrelated factors. The importance of these is likely to vary for different organisms and lens systems. It is hoped that a better understanding of the pathogenesis than is currently outlined here will lead to the development of safer contact lens systems.

Limiting morbidity in contact lens associated infection

When microbial keratitis does occur in contact lens users, the morbidity can be limited by prompt diagnosis and treatment. The preponderance of pseudomonas and acanthamoeba keratitis in contact lens users emphasizes the importance of considering these diagnoses in contact lens users presenting with keratitis, particularly because the penalties for misdiagnosis are serious.

In countries other than the USA, chloramphenicol eye drops are widely used for the prophylaxis and treatment of ocular infections. *Pseudomonas* is usually resistant to this antibiotic which remains a good choice for prophylaxis of ocular infection in non-contact lens users in whom *Pseudomonas* is rare. Although *Pseudomonas* infection of the cornea may result in an almost pathognomonic keratitis within 24–48 hours of the onset of symptoms, with ulceration surrounded by intense inflammatory cell infiltration and extensive corneal oedema peripheral to the abscess, an intense anterior uveitis and hypopyon, this picture is frequently not apparent in cases presenting early. At this stage, when appropriate treatment can limit severe morbidity, the ulcer may show no specific features. It is important that the choice of broad spectrum antibiotics for prophylaxis, or for the initial treatment of ocular infection before laboratory results are available, takes into account the epidemiology and the preponderance of *Pseudomonas*, *Serratia* and staphylococcal infections in cosmetic contact lens users. For this group of patients an aminoglycoside or quinolone antibiotic is currently the appropriate first line choice.

Acanthamoeba keratitis is now nearly as common as herpetic keratitis in some populations of contact lens users. It has been shown that misdiagnosis of acanthamoeba as herpes keratitis is common and the most frequent cause of delayed diagnosis[8]. This is significant because a critical factor determining the outcome of treatment of *Acanthamoeba* is the time to diagnosis and the institution of appropriate medical therapy[7]. Early signs of disease include mild inflammation, an irregular infiltrated epithelium with or without pseudodendrites and punctate keratopathy, coarse anterior stromal infiltrates and perineural infiltrates. Identification of these signs is facilitated if the index of suspicion for acanthamoeba keratitis in contact lens users is high. Patients with a presumptive diagnosis of herpes keratitis, who do not respond to treatment should have the diagnosis of *Acanthamoeba* considered.

Prevention of contact lens associated infection

The appearance of contact lens related disease as a new group of disorders over the last 30 years has proved challenging to diagnose, treat and to prevent. Microbial keratitis in contact lens users is proving to be a disease with a complex pathogenesis that is only now becoming understood. Microbial strategies for survival in the environment of the contact lens wearing eye and contact lens care system have too often been underestimated in the development of contact lens systems. It is probable that the development of hygiene systems against planktonic, rather than sessile, bacteria has led to an underestimation of the biocidal activity required by lens disinfectants to maintain a microbe free lens environment even in subjects having good compliance with lens care systems. The introduction of extended wear reusable and disposable lens systems to bypass the problems relating to solutions has resulted in increased risks for microbial keratitis that are still only partly understood. The reasons for the low risk of keratitis associated with hard lens use is not understood and investigation of this might be expected to provide some clues to the development of safer soft contact lens wear. Although daily disposable lens systems may be expected to reduce the risk of keratitis, the use of such a lens system will not necessarily overcome the problems of increased susceptibility of the lens-wearing cornea to infection, the possibility of microbial contamination and colonization of the lens in the eye or the likelihood of compliance failures for economic reasons leading to retention of lenses and overnight wear.

Our current understanding of the pathogenesis of lens-related keratitis suggests several practices that will reduce the risk of keratitis for contact lens users. The overnight wear of current soft lenses should be avoided unless patients are prepared to accept the substantially increased risk of keratitis. Acceptance of this risk places a substantial burden of unnecessary keratitis on the medical services by increasing the incidence approximately 20 times in this group. The use of rigid contact lenses is probably less often associated with keratitis compared to daily wear soft contact lenses, although the difference is probably small. Careful adherence to recommended lens hygiene regimens, and the choice of a system with a high margin of safety, does have a protective effect against keratitis. Use of non-sterile, non-preserved solutions for lens care, such as tap-water has been implicated in the development of acanthamoeba keratitis and should be avoided. Other measures, such as frequent lens case disposal, daily lens case cleaning and drying to control biofilm build up, have as yet no proven role in prevention but might be expected to be helpful on theoretical grounds and require evaluation in use. The contact lens user must also be educated about the risks of lens wear, and the importance of compliance with the appropriate hygiene and lens wear regimens, so that an informed choice can be made.

Contact lens wear has provided optical, occupational, sporting, and cosmetic advantages for millions of individuals. The risks of keratitis to the individual are small but, because of the large numbers of users at risk, the burden of unnecessary disease is substantial. In order to create a safer environment for contact lens users continued efforts are needed to understand the epidemiology and pathogenesis of lens related disease and to implement these findings in the development of improved contact lens systems.

References

1 Ablashi, D. V., Sturtzenegger, S., Hunter, E. A., Palestine, A. G., Fujikawa, L. S., Kim, M. K. *et al.* (1987). *Journal of Experimental Pathology*, **3**, 693–703

2 Alfonso, E., Mandelbaum, S., Fox, M. J. and Forster, R. K. (1986). *American Journal of Ophthalmology*, **101**, 429–433

3 Amin, R. M., Dean, M. T., Zaumetzer, L. E. and Poiesz, B. J. (1991). *AIDS Research on Human Retroviruses*, **7**, 403–408

4 Aquavella, J. V. and DePaolis, M. D. (1991). *International Ophthalmology Clinic*, **31**, 127–131

5 Aswad, M. I., John, T., Barza, M., Kenyon, K. and Baum, J. (1990). *Ophthalmology*, **97**, 296–302

6 Auran, J. D., Starr, M. B. and Jakobiec, F. A. (1987). *Cornea*, **6**, 2–26

7 Bacon, A. S., Dart, J. K. G., Ficker, L. A., Matheson, M. and Wright, P. (1993). *Ophthalmology*, **100**, 1238–1243

8 Bacon, A. S., Frazer, D. G., Dart, J. K. G., Matheson, M., Ficker, L. A. and Wright, P. (1993). *Eye*, **7**, 719–725

9 Bates, A. K., Morris, R. J., Stapleton, F., Minassian, D. C. and Dart, J. K. G. (1989). *Eye*, **3**, 803–810

10 Baum, J. L. and Boruchoff, S. A. (1986). *American Journal of Ophthalmology*, **101**, 372–373

11 Boles, S. F., Refojo, M. F. and Leong, F. L. (1992). *Cornea*, **11**, 47–52.

12 Bottone, E. J., Madayag, R. M. and Qureshi, M. N. (1992). *Journal of Clinical Microbiology*, **30**, 2447–2450

13 Brandt, F. H., Ware, D. A. and Vivesvara, G. S. (1989). *Applied Environmental Microbiology*, **56**, 1144–1146

14 Bruce, A. S. and Brennan, N. A. (1990). *Survey of Ophthalmology*, **35**, 25–58

15 Buehler, P. O., Schein, O. D., Stamler, J. F., Verdier, D. D. and Katz, J. (1992). *Archives of Ophthalmology*, **110**, 1555–1558

16 Butrus, S., Klotz, S. A. and Misra, R. P. (1987). *Ophthalmology*, **94**, 1311–1314

17 Chalupa, E., Swarbrick, H. A., Holden, B. A. and Sjostrand, J. (1987). *Ophthalmology*, **94**, 17–22

18 Chignell, A. H., Easty, D. L., Chesterton, J. R. and Thomsitt, J. (1970). *British Journal of Ophthalmology*, **54**, 433–441

19 Cohen, E. J. (1990). *Cornea*, **9**, (suppl. 1) S41–43

20 Connor, C. G., Hopkins, S. L. and Salisbury, R. D. (1991). *Optometry and Visual Science*, **68**, 138–141

21 Costerton, J. W., Irvin, R. T. and Cheng, K. J. (1981). *Annual Review of Microbiology*, **35**, 299–334

22 Dart, J. K. G. (1988). *British Journal of Ophthalmology*, **72**, 926–930

23 Dart, J. K. G. (1990). *British Journal of Ophthalmology*, **74**, 129–130

24 Dart, J. K. G. (1993). *British Journal of Ophthalmology*, **77**, 49–55

25 Dart, J. K. G. (1993). *CLAO J*, **19**, 241–246

26 Dart, J. K. G. and Badenoch, P. R. (1986). *Contact Lens Association of Ophthalmologists Journal*, **12**, 220–224

27 Dart, J. K. G., Peacock, L. J., Grierson, I. and Seal, D. V. (1988). *Transactions of the British Contact Lens Association Conference*, 95–97

28 Dart, J. K. G., Stapleton, F. and Minassian, D. (1991a). *Lancet*, **338**, 650–653

29 Dart, J. K. G., Stapleton, F. and Minassian, D. (1991b). *Lancet*, **338**, 1146–1147

30 De Jonkheere, J. and Van der Woorde, H. (1976). *Applied Environmental Microbiology*, **31**, 294–297

31 Devonshire, P., Munro, F. A., Abernethy, C. and Clark, B. J. (1993). *British Journal of Ophthalmology*, **77**, 41–45

32 DiGaetano, M., Stern, G. A. and Zam, Z. S. (1986). *Cornea*, **5**, 155–158

33 Donzis, P. B., Mondino, B. J., Weissman, B. A. and Bruckner, D. A. (1987). *American Journal of Ophthalmology*, **104**, 325–333

34 Donzis, P. B., Mondino, B. J., Weissman, B. A. and Bruckner, D. A. (1989). *American Journal of Ophthalmology*, **108**, 53–56

35 Driebe, W. T. (1989) *Survey of Ophthalmology*, **34**, 44–46

36 Duran, J. A., Refojo, M. F., Gipson, I. K. and Kenyon, K. R. (1987). *Archives of Ophthalmology*, **105**, 106–109

37 Efron, N., Wohl, A., Toma, N. G., Jones, L. W. J. and Lowe, R. (1991). *International Contact Lens Clinic*, **18**, 46–51

38 Evans, D. J., Allison, D. G., Brown, M. R. and Gilbert, P. (1991). *Journal of Antimicrobial Chemotherapy*, **27**, 177–184

39 Evans, D. J., Brown, M. R., Allison, D. G. and Gilbert, P. (1990). *Journal of Antimicrobiol Chemotherapy*, **25**, 585–591

40 Farb, M. D., Weissman, B. and Mondino, B. J. (1985). *Investigative Ophthalmology and Visual Science*, **26**, (suppl.) 275

41 Ficker, L., Hunter, P., Seal, D. and Wright, P. (1989). *American Journal of Ophthalmology*, **108**, 453

42 Galentine, P. G., Cohen, E. J., Laibson, P. R., Adams, C. P., Michaud, R. and Arentsen, J. J. (1984). *Archives of Ophthalmology*, **102**, 891–894.

43 Glastonbury, J. and Crompton, J. L. (1989). *Australia and New Zealand Journal of Ophthalmology*, **17**, 451

44 Grant, T., Kotow, M. and Holden, B. A. (1987). *Contax*, May, 5–8

45 Grant, T., Terry, R. and Holden, B. (1990). *Problems in Optometry*, **2**, 599–621

46 Gristina, A. G., Hobgood, C. D., Webb, L. X. and Myrvik, Q. N. (1987). *Biomaterials*, **8**, 423–429

47 Guillon, M., Guillon, J. P., Bansal, M., Maskell, R. and Rees, P. (1994). *Journal of the British Contact Lens Association*, **17**, 69–76

48 Hassman, C. and Sugar, J. (1983). *Archives of Ophthalmology*, **101**, 1549–1550
49 He, Y. G., McCulley, J. P., Alizadeh, H., Pidherney, M., Mellon, J., Ubelbaker, J. E. *et al.* (1992). *Investigative Ophthalmology and Visual Science*, **33**, 126–132
50 Holden, B. A., Sweeney, D. F., Vannas, A., Nilsson, K. T. and Efron, N. (1985). *Investigative Ophthalmology and Visual Science*, **26**, 1489–1501
51 Holland, E. J., Alul, I. H., Meisler, D. M., Epstein, R. J., Rotkis, W. M., Nathenson, A. L. *et al.* (1991). *American Journal of Ophthalmology*, **112**, 414–418
52 Holland, S., Ruseska, I., Alfonso, E., Lam, K., Miller, D., Costerton, J. W. *et al.* (1988). *Investigative Ophthalmology and Visual Science*, **29**, (suppl.) 279
53 Hovding, G. (1981). *Acta Ophthalmologica*, **59**, 387–401
54 Hyndiuk, R. A., Skorah, D. N., Burn, E. M. in Tabbara, K. F., and Hyndiuk, R. A. (eds) (1988). *Infection of the Eye*, Boston: Little, Brown & Co, 321–323.
55 John, T. (1991). *American Journal of Ophthalmology*, **111**, 766–768
56 John, T., Desai, D. and Sahm, D. (1989). *American Journal of Ophthalmology*, **108**, 658–664
57 Josephson, J. E. and Caffery, B. E. (1979). *International Contact Lens Clinic*, **6**, 223–241
58 Kersley, H. J. (1993). *Eye*, **7**, 718
59 Killingsworth, D. W. and Stern, G. A. (1989). *Archives of Ophthalmology*, **107**, 795–796
60 Kilvington, S. (1993). *Eye*, **7**, 535–538
61 Kilvington, S., Anthony, Y., Davies, D. J. G. and Meakin, B. J. (1991). *Review of Infectious Diseases*, **13**, (suppl. 5) S414–415
62 Klotz, S. A., Butrus, S. I., Misra, R. P. and Osato, M. S. (1989). *Current Eye Research*, **8**, 195–202
63 Koenig, S. B., Solomon, J. M., Hyndiuk, R. A., Sucher, R. A. and Gradus, M. S. (1987). *American Journal of Ophthalmology*, **103**, 832
64 Lancet (1988). Editorial. Disposable of Contact Lenses, **i**, 1437
65 Larkin, D. F. P., Kilvington, S. and Easty, D. L. (1990). *British Journal of Ophthalmology*, **74**, 133–135
66 Lawin-Brussel, C. A., Refojo, M. F., Leong, F. L., Hanninen, L. and Kenyon, K. R. (1990). *Archives of Ophthalmology*, **108**, 1012–1019
67 Lawin-Brussel, C. A., Refojo, M. F., Leong, F. L. and Kenyon, K. R. (1991). *Investigative Ophthalmology and Visual Science*, **32**, 657–662
68 Lindquist, T. D., Doughman, D. J., Rubenstein, J. B., Moore, J. W. and Campbell, R. C. (1988). *Cornea*, **7**, 300–303
69 Lindquist, T. D., Sher, N. A. and Doughman, D. J. (1988). *Archives of Ophthalmology*, **106**, 1202–1206
70 Ludwig, I. H., Meisler, D. M., Rutherford, I., Bican, F. E., Langston, R. H. S. and Visvesvara, G. S. (1986). *Investigative Ophthalmology and Visual Science*, **27**, 626–628
71 McBride, M. E. (1979). *Applied Environmental Microbiology*, **37**, 233–236
72 MacRae, S., Herman, C., Stulting, R. D., Lippman, R., Whipple, D., Cohen, E. *et al.* (1991). *American Journal of Ophthalmology*, **111**, 457–465
73 Marshall, K. C., Stout, R. and Mitchell, R. (1971). *Journal of General Microbiology*, **68**, 337–348
74 Matthews, T. D., Frazer, D. G., Minassian, D. C., Radford, C. F. and Dart, J. K. G. (1992). *Archives of Ophthalmology*, **110**, 1559–1562
75 Mayo, M. S., Cook, W. L., Schlitzer, R. L., Ward, M. A., Wilson, L. A. and Ahearn, D. G. (1986). *Journal of Clinical Microbiology*, **24**, 372–376
76 Mertz, G. W. and Holden, B. A. (1981). *Canadian Journal of Optometry*, **4**, (suppl. 4) 203–205
77 Miller, M. J. and Ahearn, D. G. (1987). *Journal of Clinical Microbiology*, **25**, 1392–1397
78 Miller, M. J., Wilson, L. A. and Ahearn, D. G. (1988). *Journal of Clinical Microbiology*, **26**, 513–517
79 Mondino, B. J. and Groden, I. R. (1980). *Archives of Ophthalmology*, **98**, 1767–1770
80 Mondino, B. J. and Kowalski, R. P. (1982). *Archives of Ophthalmology*, **100**, 1968–1971
81 Mondino, B. J., Kowalski, R., Ratajczak, H. V., Peters J., Culter, S. B. and Brown, S. I. (1981). *Archives of Ophthalmology*, **99**, 891–895
82 Mondino, B. J., Weissman, B. A., Farb, M. D. and Petit, T. H. (1986). *American Journal of Ophthalmology*, **102**, 58–65
83 Moore, M. B., McCulley, J. P., Luckenbach, M., Gelender, H., Newton, C., McDonald, M. B. *et al.* (1985). *American Journal of Ophthalmology*, **100**, 396–403

84 Moore, M. B., McCulley, J. P., Kaufman, H. E. and Robin, J. B. (1986). *Ophthalmology*, **93**, 1310–1315
85 Morgan, J. F. (1979). *Ophthalmology*, **86**, 1107–1119
86 Nickel, J. C., Ruseska, I., Wright, J. B. and Costerton, J. W. (1985). *Antimicrobial Agents and Chemotherapy*, **27**, 619–624
87 Nickel, J. C., Ruseska, I., Whitfield, C., Marrie, T. J. and Costerton, J. W. (1985). *European Journal of Clinical Microbiology*, **4**, 213–218
88 Niederkorn, J. Y., Ubelbaker, J. E., McCulley, J. P., Stewart, G. L., Meyer, D. R., Melton, J. A. *et al.* (1992). *Investigative Ophthalmology and Visual Science*, **33**, 104–112
89 Nilsson, S. E. and Montan, P. (1994). *Contact Lens Association of Ophthalmologists Journal*, **20**, 97–101
90 Ormerod, D. L. and Smith, R. E. (1986). *Archives of Ophthalmology*, **104**, 79–83
91 Osato, M., Pyron, M., Elizondo, M., Brown, E., Wilhelmus, K. and Jones, D. (1990). *Investigative Ophthalmology and Visual Science (suppl)*, **31**, 420
92 Panjwani, N., Zhao, Z., Baum, J., Pereira, M. and Zaidi, T. (1992). *Infection and Immunity*, **60**, 3460–3463.
93 Parker, W. T. and Wong, S. K. (1989). *American Journal of Ophthalmology*, **107**, 195
94 Penley, C. A., Willis, S. W. and Sickler, S. G. (1989). *Contact Lens Association of Ophthalmologists Journal*, **15**, 257–260
95 Pepose, J. S. (1988). *Contact Lens Association of Ophthalmologists Journal*, **14**, 165–168
96 Phillips, A. J., Badenoch, P. R., Grutzmacher, R. and Roussel, T. J. (1986). *International Eyecare*, **2**, 469–475
97 Poggio, E. C. and Abelson, M. (1993). *Contact Lens Association of Ophthalmologists Journal*, **19**, 31–39
98 Poggio, E. C., Glynn, R. J., Schein, O. D., Seddon, J. M., Shannon, M. J., Scardino, V. A. *et al.* (1989). *New England Journal of Medicine*, **321**, 779–783
99 Prosser, B. T., Taylor, D., Dix, B. A. and Cleeland, R. (1987). *Antimicrobial Agents and Chemotherapy*, **31**, 1502
100 Rabinowitz, S. K., Pflugfelder, S. C. and Goldberg, M. (1989). *Archives of Ophthalmology*, **107**, 1121
101 Rauschl, R. T. and Rodgers, J. J. (1978). *International Contact Lens Clinic*, **5**, 56–62
102 Ruseska, I., Robbins, J., Lashen, E. S. and Costerton, J. W. (1982). *Oil and Gas Journal*, 253–264
103 Schein, O. D., Buehler, P. O., Stamler, J. F., Verdier, D. D. and Katz, J. (1994). *Archives of Ophthalmology*, **112**, 186–190
104 Schein, O. D., Glynn, R. J., Poggio, E. C., Seddon, J. H. and Kenyon, K. R. (1989). *New England Journal of Medicine*, **321**, 773–778
105 Schnider, C. M., Zabkiewicz, K. and Holden, B. A. (1988). *International Contact Lens Clinic*, **15**, 124–129
106 Seal, D. V. and Hay, J. (1992). *Pharmacology Journal*, **248**, 717–719
107 Seal, D., Stapleton, F. and Dart, J. (1992). *British Journal of Ophthalmology*, **76**, 424–427
108 Silvany, S. E., Dougherty, J. M., McCulley, J. P.,Wood, T. S., Bowman, R. W. and Moore, M. B. (1990). *Ophthalmology*, **97**, 286–290
109 Slusher, M. M., Myrvik, Q. N., Lewis, J. C. and Gristina, A. G. (1987). *Archives of Ophthalmology*, **105**, 110–115
110 Smolin, G. (1979). *American Journal of Ophthalmology*, **88**, 543–547
111 Stapleton, F., Dart, J. K. G., Matheson, M. and Woodward, E. G. (1993). *Journal of the British Contact Lens Association*, **16**, 113–117
112 Stapleton, F., Dart, J. and Minassian, D. (1992). *Archives of Ophthalmology*, 110, 1601–1608
113 Stapleton, F., Dart, J. K. G. and Minassian, D. (1993). *Contact Lens Association of Ophthalmologists Journal*, **19**, 204–210
114 Stapleton, F., Davies, S. and Dart, J. K. G. (1991). *Investigative Ophthalmology and Visual Science*, **32**, (suppl.) 739
115 Stehr-Green, J. K., Bailey, T. M., Brandt, F. H., Carr, J. H., Bond, W. W. and Visvesvara, G. S. (1987). *Journal of the American Medical Association*, **258**, 57–60
116 Stehr-Green, J. K., Bailey, T. M. and Visvesvara, G. S. (1989). *American Journal of Ophthalmology*, **101**, 331–336

117 Stein, R. M., Clinch, T. E., Cohen, E. J., Genvert, G. I., Arentsen, J. J. and Laibon, P. R. (1988). *American Journal of Ophthalmology*, **105**, 632–636
118 Stern, G. A. and Zam, Z. S. (1986). *Journal of Clinical Microbiology*, **5**, 41–45
119 Theodore, F. H., Jacobiec, F. A., Juechter, K. B., MA, P., Troutman, R. C., Pang, P. M. and Iwamoto, T. (1985). *Ophthalmology*, **92**, 1471–1479
120 Thygeson, P. (1946). *Transactions of the American Academy of Ophthalmology and Otolaryngology*, **51**, 198–207
121 Tragakis, M. P., Brown, S. I. and Pearce, D. B. (1973). *American Journal of Ophthalmology*, **79**, 496–499
122 Vaughan, D. G. and Tabbara, K. F. (1986). Prevention of ocular infections. In: *Infections of the Eye*, edited by K. F. Tabbara and R. A. Hyndiuk. Boston: Little, Brown and Co. pp. 18–19
123 Visvesvara, G. S. and Stehr-Green, J. K. (1990). *Journal of Protozoology*, **37**, 25S–33S
124 Wilhelmus, K. R. (1987). *Contact Lens Association of Ophthalmologists Journal*, **13**, 211–214
125 Wilhelmus, K. R., Robinson, N. M., Font, R. A., Hamill, M. B. and Jones, D. B. (1988). *American Journal of Ophthalmology*, **106**, 708–714
126 Wilson, L. A. and Ahearn, D. G. (1986). *American Journal of Ophthalmology*, **101**, 434–436
127 Wilson, L. A., Schlitzer, R. L. and Ahearn, D. G. (1981). *American Journal of Ophthalmology*, **92**, 546–554
128 Wilson, L. A., Sawant, A. D. and Simmons, R. B. *et al.* (1990). *American Journal of Ophthalmology*, **110**, 193–198
129 Wilson-Holt, N. and Dart, J. K. G. (1989). *Eye*, **3**, 581–587
130 Zantos, S. G. (1984). *International Contact Lens Clinic*, **11**, 604–612

Index